MCQs and SBAs in Intensive Care Medicine

MCQs and SBAs in Intensive Care Medicine

Edited by

Lorna Eyre

Andrew Bodenham

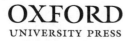

OXFORD
UNIVERSITY PRESS

OXFORD
UNIVERSITY PRESS

Great Clarendon Street, Oxford, OX2 6DP,
United Kingdom

Oxford University Press is a department of the University of Oxford.
It furthers the University's objective of excellence in research, scholarship,
and education by publishing worldwide. Oxford is a registered trade mark of
Oxford University Press in the UK and in certain other countries

© Oxford University Press 2021

The moral rights of the authors have been asserted

First Edition published in 2021

Published in the United States of America by Oxford University Press
198 Madison Avenue, New York, NY 10016, United States of America

British Library Cataloguing in Publication Data

Data available

Library of Congress Control Number: 2021940637

ISBN 978–0–19–875305–6

DOI: 10.1093/oso/9780198753056.001.0001

Printed and bound by
CPI Group (UK) Ltd, Croydon, CR0 4YY

DEDICATION

To my fabulous pack J, L, W, K, G, and R: love and creativity and inspiration and for all the eye rolling at the very mention of this book

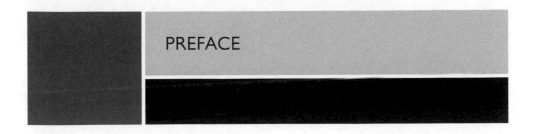

PREFACE

I started writing this book having gained enthusiasm (and possibly some knowledge) post the Diploma in Intensive Care exam. This now defunct qualification belays the evolution of the Faculty of Intensive Care over the last few years, and budding intensivists will now recognize a robust standalone curriculum, an e-portfolio spanning many domains and the now mandatory exam.

Regardless of the era, intensive care medicine needs eager, exuberant individuals with a wide breadth of knowledge who can bring the best care to patients, and so I hope this book goes someway in at least provoking some thought and reading around common themes found in the intensive care unit.

These last 12 months have probably been some of the most challenging times experienced by Critical Care staff up and down the country. Trainees have undoubtedly supported the resilience of intensive care units in the face of the Covid-19 pandemic. I am excited that this book therefore may play a role in helping to expand our community so that we can continue our robust efforts in understanding and managing critically ill patients.

CONTENTS

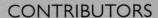
CONTRIBUTORS

James Beck Intensive Care Unit, St James's University Hospital, Leeds, UK

Richard Briscoe Intensive Care Unit, Bradford Royal Infirmary, Bradford, UK

Lorna Eyre Intensive Care Unit, St James's University Hospital, Leeds, UK

Simon Flood Intensive Care Unit, St James's University Hospital, Leeds, UK

Tom Lawton Intensive Care Unit, Bradford Royal Infirmary, Bradford, UK

Anand Padmakumar Intensive Care Unit, St James's University Hospital, Leeds, UK

Max Ridley The Leeds Teaching Hospitals Trust, Leeds, UK

Alex Scott Intensive Care Unit, St James's University Hospital, Leeds, UK

Brendan Sloan Intensive Care Unit, St James's University Hospital, Leeds, UK

Andrew Taylor The Leeds Teaching Hospitals Trust, Leeds, UK

Claire Tordoff Intensive Care Unit, St James's University Hospital, Leeds, UK

Laura Walton Intensive Care Unit, St James's University Hospital, Leeds, UK

1. **Regarding the Resuscitation Council (UK) adult advanced life-support algorithm, the following are true:**
   A. Adrenaline 1 mg is given after the second shock in VT/VF arrest
   B. Atropine is no longer recommended for asystole or pulseless electrical activity arrest
   C. In an out-of-hospital cardiac arrest (OOHA), evidence suggests that paramedics should perform 2 minutes of cardiopulmonary resuscitation (CPR) prior to defibrillation
   D. Use of adrenaline improves neurologically intact survival following cardiorespiratory arrest
   E. Waveform capnography can be used to assess the quality of chest compressions during CPR

2. **The following are true for electrocardiogram (ECG) interpretation:**
   A. A normal QRS is 70–100ms
   B. Partial right bundle branch block and ST elevation in V1 and V2 are findings of Brugada syndrome
   C. Prominent U waves occur most commonly during bradycardia
   D. The normal axis is −30° to +90°
   E. The speed is 25mm/s

3. **Regarding biomarkers for infection and inflammation, the following are true:**
   A. Procalcitonin is produced from the C cells of the thyroid gland and is a precursor to calcitonin
   B. Procalcitonin levels increase significantly in the presence of bacterial, fungal, and viral infections
   C. Procalcitonin has been shown to reduce antibiotic use
   D. Procalcitonin guided therapy improves outcomes in bacterial sepsis
   E. Procalcitonin discriminates between systemic inflammation with or without infection

4. **Echocardiography is frequently used in critical care, and the following are correct:**
   A. At higher frequencies, tissue penetration increases
   B. Echocardiographic machines use frequencies of 2–10MHz
   C. Sound velocity travels through a given material at variable speed
   D. Shorter wavelengths are associated with improved image resolution
   E. The tricuspid annular plane systolic excursion (TAPSE) can be used to assess right ventricular function

MCQs and SBAs in Intensive Care Medicine. Lorna Eyre and Andrew Bodenham, Oxford University Press. © Oxford University Press 2021.
DOI: 10.1093/oso/9780198753056.003.0001

5. **In relation to infective endocarditis (IE), the following statements are true:**
    A. Aortic lesions are the commonest type
    B. According to the Duke Classification, diagnosis can be confirmed with positive blood culture growth with a typical IE microorganism and fever >38°C
    C. According to the Duke Classification, diagnosis can be confirmed clinically by the presence of one major and three minor criteria
    D. Streptococcal infections are associated with the highest mortality
    E. The majority are caused by staphylococcal infections

6. **The following are typical findings in acute tubular necrosis:**
    A. Decreased urinary osmolarity
    B. Decreased urinary sodium
    C. Decreased N-acetylglucosaminidase (NAG)
    D. Raised cystatin C
    E. Tubular cells in the urine

7. **A young woman presents to A&E with progressive fatigable weakness, slurred speech, difficulty swallowing, and dyspnoea on lying flat. On examination she has marked ptosis and is tachypnoeic. The following are true:**
    A. Anti–muscle-specific receptor kinase antibodies are diagnostic in the majority of cases
    B. Computed tomography (CT) of the chest is recommended as part of the work up
    C. During a crisis, immunosuppression with a steroid remains the first-line management
    D. Electromyography (EMG) demonstrates normal baseline compound action potential with subsequent decrement following repetitive stimulation
    E. If intubation is required for respiratory failure, pyridostigmine should be given intravenously

8. **With regards to paracetamol overdose, the following are true:**
    A. Initial pH < 7.25 is one of the criteria for listing on the super-urgent liver transplantation list
    B. Lactate >3.5mmol/l on admission is one of the criteria for listing on the super-urgent transplant list
    C. N-acetylcysteine should not be given >24 hours after overdose of paracetamol
    D. Patients are asymptomatic in the first 24 hours following paracetamol overdose
    E. Paracetamol remains the leading cause of acute liver failure in the UK

9. **With regards to pancreatitis, the following are true:**
   A. Amylase rise is a good indicator of severity in pancreatitis in the first 48 hours
   B. Contrast-enhanced CT is investigation of choice
   C. Operative necrosectomy should be done immediately following diagnosis of necrotic pancreatitis
   D. Prophylactic antibacterial and antifungal agents are not recommended in patients with necrotizing pancreatitis
   E. Ranson score for pancreatitis includes amylase level

10. **You are called to assess a 28-year-old African man who has presented with severe abdominal pain and anaemia. The following are true:**
   A. A blood transfusion may be required to achieve Hb concentration > 10g/dl
   B. In sickle cell disease, the red cells can sickle at oxygen saturations of 85%
   C. Risk of infection with Klebsiella, Salmonella, and Group B Strep is much higher
   D. The 'sickledex' test diagnoses sickle cell disease
   E. There are no treatments available to reduce vaso-occlusive episodes and transfusion requirement other than good pain control

11. **Regarding diabetic ketoacidosis (DKA), the following are correct:**
   A. All DKA patients require aggressive fluid management
   B. Diagnosis includes capillary blood glucose >11 mmol/l; capillary ketones >4 mmol/l or urine ketones +++; and venous pH <7.35
   C. Low potassium results from a shift from the intracellular space and subsequent diuresis
   D. Mortality from DKA is <5%
   E. Patients are often hypernatraemic on initial presentation because of dehydration

12. **A patient is found to have a low plasma sodium of 120mmol/l. Clinically they are not dehydrated, and there are no signs of peripheral oedema or raised jugular venous pressure (JVP). They have no prior significant medical history or drug history, but do report a smoking history and recent weight loss of over 1 stone in the last 5 months. The following are correct:**
   A. An adrenocorticotropic hormone (ACTH) stimulation test should be considered
   B. Given the history, expected findings might include low plasma osmolality, high urine osmolality, and high urinary sodium
   C. Hypertonic saline is a first-line management
   D. Low plasma sodium is associated with muscle cramps and hyper-reflexia
   E. The above findings are most likely related to nephrotic syndrome

13. Fungal disease is increasing in the ICU. The following are true:

A. Candida and Cryptococcus are the fungi most commonly associated with infections in the critically ill
B. Early ophthalmic review is essential in candidaemia
C. Incidence of non-albicans species is increasing
D. Mortality may be up to 40% with candidaemia
E. Risk factors include haematological malignancy and faecal peritonitis

14. Regarding noninvasive positive pressure ventilation (NIPPV), the following are true:

A. NIPPV should only be instituted for an exacerbation of chronic obstructive pulmonary disease (COPD) if pH is >7.25
B. NIPPV is contra-indicated in the presence of a fixed upper airway obstruction
C. NIPPV when used following extubation in high-risk patients, reduces reintubation rates
D. NIPPV is not commonly associated with adverse haemodynamic effects
E. NIPPV is contra-indicated in asthma

15. The following statements are regarded as true regarding sepsis:

A. Organ dysfunction can be identified as a change in Sequential Organ Failure score (SOFA) ≥3 consequent to the infection
B. Sepsis is defined as infection and the coexistence of at least two or more systemic inflammatory response criteria
C. Specific infections may result in local organ dysfunction without generating a systemic host response
D. Sepsis is defined specifically as life-threatening organ dysfunction caused by a dysregulated host response
E. Sepsis-related hospital mortality is in excess of 40% when hypotension persists, and vasopressors are required to maintain a MAP ≥65mmHg and serum lactate is >2mmol/l despite adequate fluid volume resuscitation

16. Regarding fluid resuscitation, the following are true:

A. A large, blinded, randomized controlled trial (RCT) demonstrated that 4% albumin was superior to saline regarding rate of death or new organ failure
B. Fluid management should be considered in four distinct phases relating to rescue, optimization, stabilization, and de-escalation
C. In the Crystalloid versus Hydroxyethyl Starch Trial (CHEST) study involving 7000 adults in the ICU, the use of 6% hydroxyethyl starch (HES) 130/0.4, as compared with saline was associated with increased 90-day mortality
D. The early use of hypertonic saline in patients with traumatic brain injury has been shown to improve short- and long-term outcomes
E. The recommended dose of hydroxyethyl starch is 33–55ml per kilogram of body weight per day

17. In a patient undergoing right lower lobectomy and with one lung ventilation in the left lateral decubitus position, the following are true:

A. Clamping the right pulmonary artery will worsen any hypoxia

B. Positive end expiratory pressure (PEEP) applied to the left lung worsens any ventilation and perfusion mismatch

C. Reduced compliance of the dependent lung will result in increased shunt

D. The dependent left lung receives the greatest blood flow but because of ventilation and perfusion mismatch, causes an increase in dead space

E. The nondependent right lung compared to the dependent left lung receives the greatest blood flow, causing significant shunt

18. The following statements regarding the Sengstaken-Blakemore tube are true:

A. A Sengstaken-Blakemore tube will provide definitive control of bleeding from oesophago-gastric varices in up to 90% of patients

B. Bleeding from vessels through which gastric ulcers in the fundus of the stomach have eroded respond better to balloon tamponade with a Sengstaken-Blakemore tube than do lesions in the pyloric region of the stomach

C. Insertion of Sengstaken-Blakemore tubes require general anaesthesia and tracheal intubation to prevent aspiration of gastric contents

D. The tube consists of four major components: a gastric balloon, an oesophageal balloon, a gastric suction port, and an oesophageal suction port

E. The tube can be inserted via either the nostril or the mouth

19. Concerning the diagnosis of death, the following are true:

A. Best practice in the diagnosis of death requires confirmation of irreversible damage to vital centres in the brainstem

B. *Death* is defined by the Academy of Royal Colleges as 'the irreversible loss of the capacity for consciousness, combined with the irreversible loss of the capacity to breathe'

C. Patients in a vegetative state have retained the capacity for wakefulness and awareness

D. *Prolonged vegetative state* describes disordered consciousness for more than 6 months

E. There is no statutory definition of *death* within the UK

20. Regarding the diagnosis of brainstem death, the following are correct:

A. Is only valid if the patient's underlying condition is known to be irreversible

B. Should only be sought in patients wishing to donate organs after death

C. Requires an isoelectric electroencephalogram (EEG) confirming the absence of all electrical activity in the brain

D. Requires the involvement of two doctors, one of whom must be an intensive care consultant

E. Requires two sets of brainstem tests, a minimum of 4 hours apart

21. **A patient has been intubated and ventilated on the ICU for 8 days and is now in the process of weaning from mechanical ventilation. They become extremely agitated and demonstrate new-onset altered mental status. The following are true:**
    A. Avoiding constipation may prevent this situation
    B. Agitated, hyperactive delirium has a worse mortality outcome compared to the hypoactive form
    C. Agitated delirium is the commonest form on the ICU
    D. There is an association with decreased long-term cognitive function
    E. Their mortality will be expected to increase

22. **Epiglottitis rates have reduced dramatically over the years. The following remain true:**
    A. Commonest cause is Haemophilus influenzae
    B. Epiglottitis is associated with crack cocaine use
    C. Stridor is more common in children
    D. The incidence of epiglottitis remains the same in children but is increasing in adults
    E. The 'thumb sign' is diagnostic

23. **APACHE II is an ICU scoring system used to elucidate severity of illness. The following are true:**
    A. A maximum score of 71 can be calculated
    B. It is undertaken within the first 24 hours of hospital admission
    C. Points are given according to the patient's age
    D. Systolic blood pressure is a physiological variable
    E. There are 16 physiological variables

24. **Regarding the anatomy of the spinal cord includes, the following are true:**
    A. Blood supply to the spinal cord consists of one anterior spinal artery and two posterior spinal arteries
    B. Occlusion of the anterior spinal artery leads to flaccid paralysis and loss of pain and temperature sensation
    C. Radicular arteries supply the nerve roots, and many contribute to the spinal arteries
    D. The dural sac ends at approximately at the level of L2
    E. The epidural space is bound posteriorly by the posterior longitudinal ligament

25. **Regarding lactate, the following are true:**
    A. Generation is via pyruvate to lactic acid and then lactate + H^+
    B. It is only generated under anaerobic conditions
    C. Metformin can be implicated with higher levels of lactate, due to inhibition of glycolysis
    D. Type B is related to tissue hypoxia
    E. When there is an increase in glycolysis, the malate-aspartate shuttle is overwhelmed, and there is an increase in dihydronicotinamide adenine dinucleotide (NADH)

26. Regarding neuromuscular blockade, the following are true:
A. Atracurium consists of a mixture of 10 stereoisomers
B. Atracurium is associated with hypotension
C. Early neuromuscular blockade should be avoided in patients with acute respiratory distress syndrome (ARDS)
D. Immobilization of the critically ill patient results in an increased number of acetylcholine receptors
E. The action of suxamethonium is prolonged in liver disease and renal failure

27. The following are true regarding humidity:
A. *Absolute humidity* is defined as the mass of water vapour that a volume of gas contains at its critical temperature
B. As the temperature in a closed system increases, the relative humidity will increase
C. Fully saturated air at body temperature (37°C) contains 44g/m^3
D. Fully saturated air at room temperature (20°C) contains 25g/m^3
E. Relative humidity is the ratio of the water vapour pressure to the saturated water vapour pressure expressed as a percentage

28. In alcoholic hepatitis, the following are correct:
A. All the transaminases are grossly elevated (>1000U/l)
B. Alanine transaminase (ALT) is raised more than aspartate transaminase (AST)
C. Prednisolone should be given to patients with severe alcoholic hepatitis
D. Pentoxifylline shows no survival benefit in alcoholic hepatitis
E. The model for end-stage liver disease (MELD) score can be used to predict the need for steroids

29. Concerning refeeding syndrome, the following are true:
A. Feeding should be introduced at 50% energy requirements in at-risk patients
B. National Institute for Health Care Excellence (NICE) guidelines recommend electrolyte and fluid correction before feeding
C. Patients with a BMI below 19 kg/m^2 are at especially high risk
D. Patients starved for <10 days are not at high risk
E. Parenteral feeding is much higher risk than enteral nutrition

30. Lung ultrasound is increasingly used on the intensive care unit; the following are correct:
A. A lines are diagnostic for pneumothorax
B. B lines are generated by the juxtaposition of alveolar air and septal thickening (from fluid or fibrosis)
C. Lung Ultrasound has a higher diagnostic accuracy than physical examination and chest radiography combined
D. Two or more B lines between adjacent rib spaces are pathological
E. The lung point is a diagnostic finding for pneumothorax

Question 1 F T F F T

While there is greater emphasis on CPR throughout the algorithm, in OOHA there is no recommendation for CPR prior to defibrillation in unwitnessed arrest. A recent study, looking at over 9000 patients, demonstrated no difference in outcome with two minutes of CPR or immediate defibrillation. Previous studies have suggested that there might be a survival advantage with CPR, if time to defibrillation is more than 5 minutes.

Adrenaline is given after the third shock, although there is no evidence that it improves neurologically intact survival. A recent trial, PARAMEDIC2, suggested that the adrenaline arm had higher rates of return of spontaneous circulation, however the proportion of alive patients with severe neurological impairments was also higher.

Atropine is no longer recommended as arrest is not usually caused by excessive vagal tone.

In those patients with inadequate spontaneous respiration, intubation or ventilation via other airway devices (e.g. laryngeal mask airways) will be required. Wave form capnography can be used to monitor the quality of chest compressions during CPR. End-tidal CO_2 values are associated with compression depth and ventilation rate and a greater depth of chest compression will increase the value.

Stiell I, et al. Early versus later rhythm analysis in patients with out-of-hospital cardiac arrest. *New England Journal of Medicine* 2011;365:787–97.

Wik L, et al. Delaying defibrillation to give basic cardiopulmonary resuscitation to patients with out-of-hospital ventricular fibrillation: a randomized trial. *Journal of the American Medical Association* 2003;289:1389–95.

Resuscitation Council (UK). *Adult advanced life support*. www.resus.org.uk [accessed 30 July 2021].

Perkins GD, et al. on behalf of the PARAMEDIC2 Collaborators. A randomized trial of epinephrine in out-of-hospital cardiac arrest. *New England Journal of Medicine* 2018;379:711–21.

Question 2 T T T T T

All of the options are true.

The U wave is a small (0.5mm) deflection immediately following the T wave. It is best seen in leads V2 and V3. The exact cause of U waves remains uncertain, and a normal U wave can be seen when the heart rate falls to less than 65 beats per minute. The most common cause of prominent U waves (i.e. >1–2mm) is bradycardia, but this can also be seen in severe hypokalaemia.

Brugada syndrome is a sodium channelopathy, leading to sudden death in younger adults (mean age 41 years). There is a right bundle branch block with ST elevation (concave or convex) in V1-3. Urgent implantable cardioverter-defibrillator is often needed.

Hampton J. *The ECG made easy*. London: Churchill Livingstone, 2008.

Webster G, Beryl Cl. An update on channelopathies. *Circulation* 2013;127:126–40.

Question 3 T F T F F

Procalcitonin is the propeptide of calcitonin and is produced in the thyroid gland during normal health. Synthesis from extrathyroid tissue (mostly neuroendocrine cells in the lung and intestine) is triggered by bacterial endotoxin and inflammatory cytokines. There has been interest in its use as a biomarker for infection and serial measurement can guide antibiotic therapy; however, evidence has been conflicting. Several studies demonstrate its favourable use in guiding antibiotic duration but overall mortality has not shown to be improved with procalcitonin guided antibiotic use in sepsis.

Procalcitonin levels elevate primarily in bacterial sepsis and will recover with antibiotic therapy. Viral and fungal infections produce variable results, and procalcitonin levels may not rise at all. Procalcitonin may also be elevated post surgery and in patients with burns and trauma. Usually in these situations, the levels begin to fall within 24–48 hours. If levels remain elevated, this may indicate the advent of infection.

Bouadma L, et al; PRORATA trial group. Use of procalcitonin to reduce patients' exposure to antibiotics in intensive care units (PRORATA trial): a multicentre randomised controlled trial. *Lancet* Feb 2010;375(9713):463–74.

Becker K, Snider R, Nylen E. Procalcitonin assay in systemic inflammation, infection, and sepsis: clinical utility and limitations. *Critical Care Medicine* 2008;36:941–52.

Question 4 F T F T T

Echocardiography is increasingly being used to aid the clinical assessment of patients on the ICU. Echo machines use sound waves emitted at frequencies 2–10MHz. Shorter wavelengths produce better resolution but at higher frequencies, tissue depth is reduced. The velocity of sound through a given medium remains constant. However velocity varies with different mediums (e.g. sound velocity through blood is 1570m/s while the velocity through air is 330m/s).

TAPSE does represent the distance of systolic function of the right ventricular annular plane towards the apex, and it is measured in the M-mode.

Kaddoura S. *Echo made easy*, 2nd edition. London: Churchill Livingstone Elsevier, 2009.

Question 5 T F T F F

Staphylococcal infections account for approximately 25% of cases of endocarditis, although in the intravenous drug–using community, this can rise to approximately 60%. Most cases of endocarditis are actually caused by Streptococcal infections (50%–70%), with *Strep viridans* accounting for roughly half of these. IE caused by Staphylococcal infections or fungi have a high associated mortality compared with Streptococci or Enterococci.

Most lesions affect the left side of the heart, with right-sided lesions occurring most commonly in patients who inject drugs. The aortic valve is the most commonly affected valve.

The Duke Classification is divided into major and minor criteria. IE is demonstrated with either two major, one major and three minor, or five minor criteria.

Major blood culture criteria for IE include the following:

- Two blood cultures positive for organisms typically found in patients with IE
- Blood cultures persistently positive for one of these organisms, from cultures drawn more than 12 hours apart
- Three or more separate blood cultures drawn at least 1 hour apart

Major echocardiographic criteria include the following:

- An oscillating intracardiac mass on a valve or on supporting structures, in the path of regurgitant jets, or on implanted material, in the absence of an alternative anatomic explanation

- Myocardial abscess
- Development of partial dehiscence of a prosthetic valve
- New-onset valvular regurgitation

Minor criteria for IE include the following:

- Predisposing heart condition or intravenous drug use
- Fever of 38°C (100.4°F) or higher
- Vascular phenomenon, including major arterial emboli, septic pulmonary infarcts, mycotic aneurysm, intracranial haemorrhage, conjunctival haemorrhage, or Janeway lesions
- Immunologic phenomenon such as glomerulonephritis, Osler nodes, Roth spots, and rheumatoid factor
- Positive blood culture results not meeting major criteria or serologic evidence of active infection with an organism consistent with IE
- Echocardiogram results consistent with IE but not meeting major echocardiographic criteria

Beynon RP, Bahl VK, Prendergast BD. Infective endocarditis. *British Medical Journal* 2006;333:334–9.

Question 6 T F F T T

Acute tubular necrosis results in an inability to reabsorb sodium in the renal tubules. While the urinary sodium is raised, osmolarity is decreased as the disruption of the counter-current mechanism prevents urinary concentration.

Cystatin C is a more sensitive marker of reduced glomerular filtration rate (GFR) than creatinine. As tubular cells die, they are found in the urine, as opposed to the red cell casts of glomerulonephritis. NAG is a protein found in the renal epithelium released from damaged tubular cells.

Waldmann C, Soni N, Rhodes A (eds). *Oxford desk reference: critical care,* 1st edition. Oxford: Oxford University Press, 2008.

Kumar P, Clark M. *Clinical medicine,* 8th edition. London: Saunders, Elsevier, 2012.

Question 7 F T F T F

Myasthenia gravis is characterized by fatigable weakness, with proximal involvement more common. The majority of patients present with ocular symptoms, although bulbar weakness and respiratory muscle weakness may also occur.

Most patients with myasthenia gravis have antibodies directed against the post synaptic skeletal muscle acetylcholine receptors, and anti-AChR antibodies are diagnostic. Anti–muscle-specific receptor kinase antibodies are frequently found in the proportion of patients who are anti-AChR antibody negative (seronegative).

Thymoma is present in 20% cases, with 70% patients having thymic hyperplasia, so CT chest is necessary.

EMG demonstrates decremental reduction in compound action potential with repetitive stimulation.

A myasthenic crisis (i.e. weakness sufficient to require intubation) may be precipitated by infection, trauma, or surgery, or for no identifiable reason. Once the patient is intubated, pyridostigmine is not usually required. The mainstay of treatment for a crisis is either plasma exchange or intravenous immunoglobulin, both of which are equally effective. Long-term immunosuppression with corticosteroids or azathioprine is often required.

Waldmann C, Soni N, Rhodes A (eds). *Oxford desk reference: critical care,* 1st edition. Oxford: Oxford University Press, 2008.

Kumar P, Clark M. *Clinical medicine,* 8th edition. London: Saunders, Elsevier, 2012.

Question 8 F T F F T

The aetiology of acute liver failure remains unidentified in 20% cases, but paracetamol overdose remains the leading cause in the UK.

N-acetylcysteine (NAC) can be given at any time after overdose, but it provides optimal results when given within 10 hours. An adult patient should receive a total dose of 300mg/kg body weight over a period of 21 hours, and as NAC is relatively harmless (hypersensitivity has been reported), it is reasonable to start an infusion regardless of timing of overdose, especially if there has been concern of a staggered overdose.

Nausea and vomiting are fairly common in the first 24 hours, and as liver damage increases, right upper quadrant pain may occur.

The most commonly used criteria for liver transplantation was developed at King's College Hospital and includes pH <7.25 after adequate fluid resuscitation. A serum lactate >3.5mmol/l on admission or a lactate >3mmol/l after 24 hours of the overdose, and after fluid resuscitation, are also UK criteria for listing.

Bernal W, Wendon J. Acute liver failure. *New England Journal of Medicine* 2013;369:2525–34.

Question 9 F T F T F

Both a rise in serum amylase, and clinical assessment, are poor indicators of severity in the first 48 hours. Contrast-enhanced CT will confirm diagnosis and the presence of gallstones, and detect early abscess formation and necrosis of the pancreas. This should be done at initial presentation if the diagnosis is uncertain. However, if looking for local complications, this should be delayed 48–72 hours as necrosis may not be visualized early.

Ranson score is performed on admission and 48 hours later. Amylase is not included.

There is lack of evidence for routine prophylactic antibiotics; however, if there is evidence of an infected abscess or sepsis elsewhere, antimicrobials should be commenced.

If clinically appropriate surgery should be delayed 2–3 weeks to allow for demarcation of the necrotic pancreas. Delayed surgery is associated with increased survival.

Nathens Avery B, et al. Management of the critically ill patient with severe acute pancreatitis. *Critical Care Medicine* 2004;32:2524–36.

Question 10 F T T F F

Sickle cell disease is an inherited haemoglobinopathy, resulting in an amino acid substitution on the β-globin subunit. This gives rise to HbS, rather than the normal HbA variant. Patients may have sickle cell trait (approx. 30%–40% HbS) or sickle cell disease (approx. 100%HbS), with the latter sickling at oxygen saturations in the order of 85% (i.e. venous blood oxygen levels).

The disease principally consists of haemolytic anaemia and vaso-occlusive events, which can affect any organ (e.g. causing transient ischaemic attacks (TIAs) splenic infarcts, pulmonary infarcts, or aplastic crises). It is essential to avoid precipitants of sickling such as dehydration, infection, hypoxaemia, and cold.

Hydroxyurea increases the amount of fetal haemoglobin and has been shown to reduce frequency and severity of symptoms as well as need for transfusion.

Those with auto-infarction of the spleen need to be protected against encapsulated bacteria such as Neisseria meningitides, Haemophilus, and *Strep pneumonia*. Klebsiella, Salmonella, and Group B Strep are also encapsulated pathogens to which sickle cell patients are more susceptible.

In sickle cell disease, increased blood viscosity can cause complications when the haemoglobin exceeds 10g/dL even if this is due to simple transfusion. Red cell exchange can provide needed oxygen carrying capacity while reducing the overall viscosity of blood. Acute red cell exchange is useful in acute infarctive stroke, in acute chest and the multiorgan failure syndromes, the right upper quadrant syndrome, and possibly priapism.

Waldmann C, Soni N, Rhodes A (eds). *Oxford desk reference: critical care*, 1st edition. Oxford: Oxford University Press, 2008.

Kumar P, Clark M. *Clinical medicine*, 8th edition. London: Saunders, Elsevier, 2012.

Question 11 F F T T F

Diagnosis of DKA includes all of the following:

- Capillary blood glucose >11mmol/l
- Capillary ketones >3mmol/l or urine ketones > ++
- Venous pH <7.3 and/or bicarbonate <15mmol/l

There is a shift of intracellular potassium to the extracellular space as a consequence of hydrogen ion exchange, and much of the potassium is then lost via diuresis. There is a danger of further hypokalaemia as potassium then re-enters cells with glucose/insulin treatment.

As plasma osmolality is high in DKA, water moves from the intracellular to extracellular space and causes a dilutional hyponatraemia. Therapy with insulin lowers plasma osmolality, and water moves back into the cells causing hypernatraemia.

Excessive fluid management in *all* patients risks cerebral oedema, and guidelines are used to minimize this risk, although fluid management should be tailored to the individual's needs. Mortality is <5%.

Joint British Diabetes Societies Inpatient Care Group. *The management of diabetic ketoacidosis in adults*. https://www.diabetes.org.uk/professionals/position-statements-reports/specialist-care-for-children-and-adults-and-complications/the-management-of-diabetic-ketoacidosis-in-adults [accessed 30 July 2021].

Waldmann C, Soni N, Rhodes A (eds). *Oxford desk reference: critical care*, 1st edition. Oxford: Oxford University Press, 2008.

Question 12 T T F F F

Low plasma sodium (<135 mmol/l) can present with muscle cramps, lethargy, headache, nausea, and vomiting. Patients tend to demonstrate hyporeflexia, while other findings may include seizures, coma, and death.

On examining a patient, it is necessary to decide whether the patient is hypervolaemic (e.g. nephrotic syndrome), euvolaemic, or hypovolaemic as this will help differentiate between the many different causes. In this case, the patient appears to be euvolaemic and associated causes of low sodium include syndrome of inappropriate antidiuretic hormone (SIADH), hypothyroidism, and Addison's disease (hence, an ACTH stimulation test is appropriate).

The patient has a smoking history and weight loss, which may be relevant as small cell carcinoma of the lung is classically associated with SIADH (low plasma osmolality, higher urine osmolality with high urinary sodium). In the case of SIADH, fluid restriction is appropriate initially, but if the patient cannot tolerate this, judicious use of hypertonic saline may be considered, as may demeclocycline.

Sterns RH. Disorders of plasma sodium: causes, consequences, and correction. *New England Journal of Medicine* 2015;372:55–65.

Question 13 F T T T T

The incidence of fungal disease is increasing, with Candida and Aspergillus being the commonest causative organisms. Candida is a yeast, and the albicans species remains the most common cause of fungal disease, although non-albicans varieties are on the increase. Candida infections are mostly superficial, but once it enters the blood stream, it can spread to the liver, spleen, brain, eyes (hence ophthalmic review), and heart (echo should be considered) may occur, with mortality approaching up to 40%.

Beed M, Sherman R, Holden S. Fungal infections and critically ill adults. *Continuing Education in Anaesthesia, Critical Care & Pain* 2014;14:262–7.

Question 14 F T T T F

A pH of less than 7.25 is not a contraindication to NIPPV as long as appropriate monitoring is undertaken and recourse to intubation is timely if needed. Fixed upper airway obstruction is considered a contraindication.

Reintubation in patients at high risk of extubation failure is reduced if NIPPV is used early. Adverse haemodynamic effects are not frequently seen; cardiac output may even be improved.

There are some small trials showing possible benefits for NIPPV in acute severe asthma; compelling evidence to support its use is, however, lacking.

Ferrer M, et al. Early noninvasive ventilation averts extubation failure in patients at risk. *American Journal of Respiratory and Critical Care Medicine* 2006;173:164–70.

Lim, Mohammed A, et al. I. Non-invasive positive pressure ventilation for treatment of respiratory failure due to severe acute exacerbations of asthma. *Cochrane Database of Systematic Reviews* 2012;12:CD004360.

Question 15 F F T T T

A new definition for *sepsis* was released in 2016, which states that sepsis is life-threatening organ dysfunction caused by a dysregulated host response to infection.

Organ dysfunction can be identified as an acute change in total SOFA score ≥2 points consequent to the infection.

Patients with septic shock can be identified with a clinical construct of sepsis with persisting hypotension requiring vasopressors to maintain MAP ≥65mmHg and having a serum lactate level >2mmol/l despite adequate volume resuscitation. With these criteria, hospital mortality is in excess of 40%.

Sepsis is a syndrome shaped by pathogen factors and host factors (e.g. sex, race, and other genetic determinants; age; comorbidities; and environment) with characteristics that evolve over time. Infection alone is not associated with an aberrant or dysregulated host response and the presence of organ dysfunction.

SIRS criteria were largely excluded as their presence does not necessarily represent a dysregulated host response. SIRS criteria are present in many hospitalized patients who do not have an infection and indeed may be absent in those patients on ICU who have infection and new organ failure.

To help identify patients with sepsis, the Surviving Sepsis Campaign recommend the quick SOFA score (respiratory rate ≥22/min, altered mentation, systolic blood pressure ≤100mmHg).

Singer M, et al. The third international consensus definition for sepsis and septic shock. *Journal of the American Medical Association* 2016;15:801–10.

Question 16 F T F F T

In 2004, a large double-blind RCT involving almost 7000 adults was undertaken comparing saline with albumin (SAFE). The study showed no significant difference between albumin and saline with respect to the rate of death at 28 days (relative risk, 0.99; 95%CI, 0.91 to 1.09; P = 0.87) or the development of new organ failure. However, further analysis demonstrated a significant increase in the rate of death at 2 years among patients with traumatic brain injury with albumin resuscitation.

Hydroxyethyl starch has been shown to increase mortality (although this was not demonstrated in the CHEST study) and significantly increase the rate of renal replacement therapy, and it has somewhat fallen out of favour in recent times. Due to its accumulation in tissues, the recommended daily dose is 33–55ml per kilogram of body weight per day.

Concern about sodium and water overload associated with saline resuscitation has resulted in the concept of 'small volume' crystalloid resuscitation with the use of hypertonic saline (3%, 5%, and 7.5%) solutions. However, the early use of hypertonic saline for resuscitation, particularly in patients with traumatic brain injury, has not improved either short-term or long-term outcome.

Fluid therapy is complex and requires consideration of the goal of what is trying to be achieved. More recently a working group considered four distinct phases of resuscitation: rescue, optimization, stabilization, and de-escalation.

SAFE Study Investigators, The. A comparison of albumin and saline for fluid resuscitation in the intensive care unit. *New England Journal of Medicine* 2004;350:2247–56.

Finfer S, et al. Hydroxyethyl starch or saline for fluid resuscitation in intensive care. *New England Journal of Medicine* 2012;367:1901–11.

Cooper DJ, et al. Prehospital hypertonic saline resuscitation of patients with hypotension and severe traumatic brain injury: a randomized controlled trial. *Journal of the American Medical Association* 2004;291:1350–7.

ADQI XII Investigators Group, The. Four phases of intravenous fluid therapy: a conceptual model. *British Journal of Anaesthesia* 2014;113:740–7.

Question 17 F F T F F

When lying in the left lateral decubitus position, the left dependent lung receives greater pulmonary blood flow due to the effects of gravity. The right nondependent lung will have preferential ventilation due to improved compliance.

When the right lung is collapsed to facilitate surgery it will receive pulmonary flow resulting in a large shunt. However compared to the left dependent lung, that blood flow is less and is further reduced by hypoxic pulmonary vasoconstriction.

The left lung receives greater blood supply, but has less compliance due to the weight of the mediastinum and displacement of diaphragm and abdominal organs cephalad. Again this resultant compliance reduction leads to atelectasis and further shunt.

The reduced compliance of the left lung and reduced ventilatory surface area results in hypoxic pulmonary vasoconstriction and increased resistance of blood flow in the left pulmonary artery, with diversion of blood flow to the nondependent right lung and worsening shunt fraction.

Managing hypoxia during one lung ventilation requires a systematic approach ensuring equipment is connected with no blockages or malposition of airway apparatus. Double lumen tubes can easily be displaced, and confirmation of correct positioning is essential.

Fractional inspired oxygen can be increased, and continuous positive airway pressure can be applied to the nondependent lung.

In cases of persistent hypoxia, the surgeon should be made aware and may clamp the nondependent pulmonary artery to reduce the shunt. Alternatively two-lung ventilation may have to be resumed.

PEEP applied to the dependent lung, in theory, may impede flow to the ventilated lung and worsen the shunt, but in reality it is often used. Caution should be taken not to over ventilate the dependent lung.

Eastwood J, Mahajan R. One-lung anaesthesia. *Continuing Education in Anaesthesia, Critical Care & Pain* 2002;2:83–7.

Question 18 F F F F T

The control of torrential bleeding from oesophago-gastric varices makes use of balloon tamponade techniques including the use of Sengstaken-Blakemore, Minnesota, and Linton-Nachlas tubes.

A Sengstaken-Blakemore tube has three major components: gastric and oesophageal balloons and a gastric suction port. A later adoption to the Sengstaken-Blakemore tube incorporated an oesophageal suction port with an aim to reduce the possibility of aspiration of oesophageal content—this is known as a Minnesota tube. In contrast, the Linton-Nachlas tube has only a single gastric balloon.

Although haemorrhage form peptic ulcer disease represents the majority of upper gastrointestinal haemorrhage in the UK, the use of Sengstaken-Blakemore tubes plays no role in their management.

Although many patients receive general anaesthesia and tracheal intubation for the placement and maintenance of balloon tamponade tubes, it is not a prerequisite to placement, and many patients tolerate the procedure awake with or without sedation.

The Sengstaken-Blakemore tube should be lubricated and inserted via the mouth or nose, the latter providing a greater degree of patient comfort in the awake patient. In the awake patient, topicalization of the oropharynx with local anaesthetic facilitates tube passage and oesophageal intubation.

The balloon is passed until the 55cm mark aligns with the incisors, as this indicates positioning well below the gastro-oesophageal junction. Inflation of the gastric balloon with water or air reduces the chance of accidental displacement, followed by gentle traction and inflation of the oesophageal balloon to deliver the required tamponade effect. The position of the tube should then be confirmed with chest radiograph.

It should be noted that commonly the oesophageal balloon does not require insufflation in order to gain haemorrhage control, and if it does, then pressure should be limited to <40cmH$_2$O, and it should be deflated for 15 minutes every 4 hours to reduce the incidence of oesophageal necrosis. Bleeding will be controlled in up to 90% of cases—however, this should not be considered definitive therapy, as, following balloon deflation, rebleeding occurs in approximately 50% of patients.

Moore KL, Dalley AF. *Clinically oriented anatomy,* 5th edition. London: Lippincott Williams & Wilkins, 2006.

Waldmann C, Soni N, Rhodes A (eds). *Oxford desk reference: critical care,* 1st edition. Oxford: Oxford University Press, 2008.

Question 19 T T F F T

There is no statutory definition of *death* within UK law. *Death* is defined in the Academy of Medical Royal Colleges' Code of Practice for the Diagnosis and Confirmation of Death as the irreversible loss of the capacity for consciousness, combined with irreversible loss of the capacity to breathe.

The vegetative state is wakefulness without awareness. Vegetative state is considered prolonged if it has lasted more than 4 weeks. It is considered permanent when it has persisted for more than 1 year after traumatic brain injury and more than 6 months after other brain injuries.

The diagnosis of death always requires confirmation that there has been irreversible damage to vital centres in the brainstem. In the case of death following cardiac arrest, this reflects the length of time in which the circulation to the brain has been absent.

Academy of Medical Royal Colleges. *A code of practice for the diagnosis and confirmation of death.* 2008. http://www.aomrc.org.uk/doc_view/42-a-code-of-practice-for-the-diagnosis-and-confirmation-of-death [accessed 12 June 2014].

Royal College of Physicians. *Prolonged disorders of consciousness.* 2013. https://www.rcplondon.ac.uk/guidelines-policy/prolonged-disorders-consciousness-national-clinical-guidelines [accessed 12 June 2014].

Question 20 T F F F F

A diagnosis of brainstem death in the UK does not require cessation of all brain electrical activity. The diagnosis is based on a set of bedside clinical tests and does not routinely require an EEG.

The diagnosis of brainstem death requires at least two doctors to perform brainstem tests on at least two occasions. Both doctors must have been professionally registered for more than 5 years and be competent in the conduct of brainstem testing. At least one of the doctors must be a consultant. Those carrying out the tests must not have, or be perceived to have, any clinical conflict of interest with regard to the results of the testing process. Neither doctor should be a member of the transplant team.

A complete set of tests should be performed by the two doctors working together, and on two separate occasions. Doctor A may perform the tests while Doctor B observes; this would constitute the first set. Roles may be reversed for the second set. The tests, in particular the apnoea test, are therefore performed only twice in total.

Several specialties have experience in conducting brainstem tests, including critical care, emergency medicine, neurosurgery, and neurology. There is no recommended minimum period between sets of tests.

Arguably, death is an important diagnosis to make in any patient. Confirmatory brainstem death testing provides a patient's family and other clinical staff with the certainty of a diagnosis rather than merely a prognosis. One of the prerequisites to conducting brainstem death tests is that the patient's underlying pathology is known to be irreversible.

Academy of Medical Royal Colleges. *A code of practice for the diagnosis and confirmation of death.* 2008. http://www.aomrc.org.uk/doc_view/42-a-code-of-practice-for-the-diagnosis-and-confirmation-of-death [accessed 12 June 2014].

Question 21 T F F T T

Delirium is a clinical syndrome, and it consists of acute change in mental state, inattention, and disorganized thinking which is fluctuant in nature. Incidence of delirium on the ICU is highly variable in studies, but a diagnosis is associated with an increase in mortality (estimated as a 10% increase in the relative risk of death for each day of delirium) and decreased long-term cognitive function. The hypoactive form is characterized by inattention, disordered thinking, and a decreased level of consciousness without agitation. Pure agitated delirium affects less than 2% of patients with delirium in the ICU. Patients with hypoactive delirium are the least likely to survive. Avoiding risk factors, including constipation, can help prevent delirium.

Reade M, Finfer S. Sedation and delirium in the intensive care unit. *New England Journal of Medicine* 2014;370:444.

Question 22 T T T F T

The commonest cause of epiglottitis in adults remains *Haemophilus influenzae* type b. This historically had also been the commonest cause of epiglottitis in children, but following the Hib vaccine, non-type b *H influenzae* has been implicated as a leading infectious cause. Non infectious causes include thermal damage (smoking crack cocaine and marijuana), caustic ingestion, and chemotherapy.

As a result of the Hib vaccine, incidence of epiglottitis has decreased in children but has remained relatively constant in adults. Stridor, drooling, and high temperature are all classic features in children, whereas in adults, sore throat, muffled voice, and odynophagia are more common features.

Enlarged epiglottis (thumb sign) on radiographs is associated with airway obstruction. Lateral neck radiographs should be reserved for the stable patient and are increasingly being replaced by direct nasopharyngoscopy.

Waldmann C, Soni N, Rhodes A (eds). *Oxford desk reference: critical care,* 1st edition. Oxford: Oxford University Press, 2008.

Guldfred LA, Lyhne D, Becker BC. Acute epiglottitis: epidemiology, clinical presentation, management and outcome. *Journal of Laryngology & Otology* Aug 2008;122(8):818–23.

Question 23 T F T F F

The APACHE II is a routinely used severity of disease scoring system. It is calculated within the first 24 hours of ICU admission, and an integer score of 0–71 can be achieved. Higher scores correlate with greater disease severity and higher risk of death. The score is calculated from the patient's age, and 12 physiological variables, including mean arterial pressure.

Bouch C, Thompson J. Severity scoring systems in the critically ill. *Continuing Education in Anaesthesia, Critical Care & Pain* 2008;8:181–5.

Question 24 T T T F F

The epidural space is bound posteriorly by the ligamentum flavum and laminae. The spinal cord ends at L1/L2, but the dural sac ends at S2. The dural sac contains the spinal cord and cauda equina. The blood supply consists of an anterior spinal artery, arising from the vertebral arteries, and two posterior vertebral arteries, arising from the inferior cerebellar arteries. Radicular branches supply the nerve roots and may contribute to the spinal arteries. One of the largest radicular branches, artery of Adamkiewicz, makes a major contribution to the blood supply of the lower two thirds of the spinal cord, and compromise of this artery can lead to paraplegia. Occlusion of the anterior spinal cord causes ischaemia of the anterior central part of the cord.

Yentis S, Hirsh N, Smith G. *Anaesthesia and intensive care A to Z: an encyclopaedia of principles and practice.* London: Butterworth Heineman, 2003.

Question 25 T F F F T

Lactate is generated via pyruvate → lactic acid (catalysed by lactate dehydrogenase) and then → lactate + H^+ (the H^+ can be used to generate ATP with oxidative phosphorylation, but if there is a reduction in these pathways e.g. critical illness, H^+ increases). Pyruvate to lactate also utilizes:

NADH → NAD^+. The supply of NADH controls pyruvate → lactate.

To keep NADH levels low, the "ox-phos" shuttle (including malate-aspartate and glycerol-phosphate shuttles) converts NADH → NAD^+. Under conditions where there is increased glycolysis (hypoxaemia, anaemia, shock, vasopressors, inotropes, and exercise), the "ox-phos" shuttle is overwhelmed, and there is an increase in NADH levels, and hence lactate.

Increases in lactate occur due to increased production (anaerobic metabolism, excessive glycolysis, reduced oxidative phosphorylation, and increased substrate) or reduced clearance. Lactate is metabolized mainly in the liver, mostly by gluconeogenesis (which can be inhibited by biguanides and alcohol). Renal clearance accounts for <5% excretion.

Classically type A is tissue hypoxia, and type B reflects drugs, underlying conditions, and inborn errors of metabolism.

Phypers B, Pierce JMT. Lactate physiology in health and disease. *Continuing Education in Anaesthesia, Critical Care & Pain* 2006;6:128–32.

Question 26   T T F F T

Atracurium is a benzylisoquinolinium compound consisting of 10 stereoisomers. It may precipitate release of histamine, which can result in hypotension and bronchospasm.

Immobilization and burns can result in an increased number of postsynaptic nicotinic receptors. Structurally, these receptors differ from normal acetylcholine receptors, being of the fetal–type with a gamma subunit rather than the adult type with an epsilon subunit. They occur extrajunctionally. While suxamethonium is metabolized rapidly by plasma cholinesterase, activity may be reduced by liver disease and renal failure, leading to a prolonged block. The ACURSYS trial suggests early neuromuscular blockade in patients with severe ARDS may confer a mortality benefit.

Appiah-Ankam J, Hunter JM. Pharmacology of neuromuscular blocking drugs. *Continuing Education in Anaesthesia, Critical Care & Pain* 2004;4:2–7.

Papazian L, et al. Neuromuscular blockers in early acute respiratory distress syndrome. *New England Journal of Medicine* 2010;363:1107–16.

Tripathi S, Hunter J. Neuromuscular blocking drugs in the critically ill. *Critical Care Medicine* 2006;6:119–23.

Question 27   F F T F T

Absolute humidity is defined as the mass of water vapour per unit volume of gas, measured in grams per cubic metre. Absolute humidity bears no relationship to critical temperature.

Relative humidity is the ratio of the actual mass of water vapour in a volume of gas to the mass of water vapour required to saturate that volume of gas. It is expressed as a percentage. Relative humidity can be calculated as the water vapour pressure over the saturated water vapour pressure expressed as a percentage. As the temperature in a closed system increases, the relative humidity decreases.

Maximal water content varies with temperature so warmer gases can contain greater amounts of water vapour. If a gas is heated, the actual amount of water vapour remains the same (i.e. absolute humidity remains constant, but the amount of water vapour for full saturation will increase, thus reducing the relative humidity). Fully saturated air at room temperature (20°C) contains 17g/m^3 water while fully saturated air at body temperature (37°C) contains 44g/m^3 water.

Middleton B, Philips J, Thomas R. *Physics in anaesthesia*. Banbury: Scion Publishing, 2012.

Question 28   F F T F F

Characteristically the transaminases are only mildly elevated (200–300U/l) and AST is usually higher than the ALT. This elevation of AST above ALT is quite sensitive for alcoholic hepatitis but can also occur in autoimmune or ischaemic hepatitis.

Following meta-analyses of use of steroids in alcoholic hepatitis (as the process is driven by inflammation), prednisolone 40mg daily is recommended for at least 7 days, with continuation to 1 month if there is improvement in liver function tests.

Pentoxyifylline is a nonselective phosphodiesterase inhibitor which blocks tumour necrosis factor (TNF) synthesis and has been shown in an initial RCT to demonstrate a survival advantage; however, more trials are required.

The modified (or Maddrey) discriminant function score is used to predict the need for steroids.

Jackson P, Gleeson D. Alcoholic liver disease. *Continuing Education in Anaesthesia, Critical Care & Pain* 2010;10(3):66–71.

Mathurin P, et al. Early change in bilirubin levels is an important prognostic factor in severe alcoholic hepatitis treated with prednisolone. *Hepatology* 2003;38:1363–9.

Madhotra R, Gilmore IT. Recent developments in the treatment of alcoholic hepatitis. *Quarterly Journal of Medicine* 2003;96:391–400.

Question 29 T F F F

Patients at very high risk of refeeding are those with: a BMI <16kg/m^2, starvation periods of more than 10 days, weight loss of >15% over 3 months, or pre-existing electrolyte derangement.

Patients starved for >5 days are at increased risk, and feed should be started at 50% calculated energy requirements after starvation for 5 or more days to reduce the risk of refeeding.

The NICE guidelines recommend concurrent correction of electrolytes to avoid prolongation of malnourishment. There is no significant difference in risk between enteral and parenteral routes.

National Institute for Health and Clinical Excellence. *Nutrition support in adults clinical guideline CG32.* 2006. https://www.nice.org.uk/guidance/CG32 [accessed 30 July 2021].

Question 30 F T T F T

Lung ultrasound (LUS) can be performed quickly, obviates the need for risky transfers, and has higher diagnostic accuracy than physical examination and chest radiography combined. Any of the ultrasound (USS) probes (curvilinear, cardiac, or linear) can be used. When USS is transmitted across mediums with differing impedances, some waves of the sound waves are transmitted across the boundary, whereas some are reflected as an echo. Soft tissue and air reflect 99.9%, rendering this interface virtually impenetrable to USS. A lines are horizontal lines generated between the USS waves bouncing back and forth between the pleura and the transducer. Because they demonstrate the presence of air below the pleura, they are present both in normal lungs and in pneumothorax. As the parietal and visceral pleura are tightly opposed with a small layer of fluid between them, the lung appears to slide with normal respiration. M-mode depicts this sliding as the 'seashore' sign. Lung sliding will be absent in any condition in which the pleura are not directly opposed (e.g. pneumothorax, effusion). M-mode in a pneumothorax is the horizontal straight lines 'barcode/ stratosphere' sign.

B lines are vertical hyperechoic 'comet tails' which move with lung sliding. They are generated by the juxtaposition of alveolar air and septal thickening (from fluid or fibrosis). Three or more between rib spaces (or close together in a transverse image) are pathological. When oedema becomes more severe (ground-glass appearance on CT), B lines become more numerous and closely spaced.

USS findings that suggest pneumothorax include: absence of lung sliding, absence of B lines, and a lung point. The lung point, as you move the probe from anterior to a more lateral position, is where the parietal and visceral pleura become opposed again, with the reappearance of lung sliding. Absent lung pulse (cardiac pulsation when the two pleural layers are opposed) also suggests pneumothorax.

Miller A. Practical approach to lung ultrasound. *British Journal of Anaesthesia Education* 2016;16:39–45.

paper
2

MCQ QUESTIONS

1. **Regarding trauma patients, the following statements are correct:**
   A. Acute traumatic coagulopathy (ATC) is an endogenous coagulation dysfunction which starts within minutes of major trauma and is solely due to a consumptive process
   B. Damage control resuscitation includes permissive hypotension, haemostatic resuscitation, and damage control surgery
   C. Fluid boluses should continue for as long as the patient is fluid responsive
   D. Permissive hypotension is appropriate for all trauma patients
   E. There is a significant increase in odds of survival for trauma victims being managed at a Major Trauma Centre

2. **A patient is brought into the Emergency Department (ED) having been found collapsed for an unknown amount of time. He has sustained an acute kidney injury, and the creatinine kinase (CK) result is awaited. The following are true of rhabdomyolysis:**
   A. Diagnosis of rhabdomyolysis relies on a CK >2000 units/l
   B. Early complications relate to muscle necrosis and include hyperkalaemia and hypercalcaemia
   C. Ecstasy ingestion has been implicated as a cause
   D. Myoglobin binds to Tamm–Horsfall proteins, which can obstruct renal tubules, and this is attenuated by an acid urine
   E. The pathophysiology relates to the destruction and disintegration of smooth muscle

3. **Most patients in the intensive care unit (ICU) will have invasive arterial blood pressure monitoring, and the following are true:**
   A. During mechanical ventilation, there is a reduction in venous return during inspiration to the right side of the heart
   B. Elderly patients tend to have a lower diastolic blood pressure
   C. Regular calibration is not necessary when pulse contour analysis is used to obtain cardiac output
   D. Systolic pressure is determined by stroke volume and systemic vascular resistance
   E. The dicrotic notch will shift upwards in a patient with severe sepsis

MCQs and SBAs in Intensive Care Medicine. Lorna Eyre and Andrew Bodenham, Oxford University Press. © Oxford University Press 2021.
DOI: 10.1093/oso/9780198753056.003.0002

4. **Measurement of cardiac output using an oesophageal Doppler probe is based on the following assumptions:**
    A. All red blood cells (RBC) are travelling at the same velocity
    B. Blood flow through the descending aorta is about 70% of total cardiac output
    C. Flow calculations are independent of aortic cross-sectional area
    D. The angle between incident ultrasound beam and aortic blood flow is 90°
    E. There is minimal flow during diastole

5. **You are referred, for consideration of a critical care admission, a 72-year-old lifelong smoker, who has recently been admitted with an infective exacerbation of chronic obstructive pulmonary disease (COPD). The following are true:**
    A. COPD is characterized by fully reversible airflow obstruction
    B. COPD patients have pulmonary function tests in keeping with $FEV_1/FVC >0.7$
    C. FEV_1 <50% predicts an increased risk of dying with respiratory failure within 1 year
    D. Noninvasive ventilation is contraindicated in a patient who has depressed level of consciousness and with a type II respiratory failure pattern
    E. Poor outcome at ICU referral can be predicted by the presence of new-onset atrial fibrillation

6. **A postoperative cardiac patient on the ICU suddenly goes into an abnormal heart rhythm. The pulse is irregularly irregular, and the electrocardiogram (ECG) reveals a normal QRS but absent p waves. The blood pressure is significantly compromised, and the heart rate is >150 beats per minute. The following are correct:**
    A. Control of the rate, rather than the rhythm, remains the initial priority
    B. Digoxin may be considered in patients undergoing cardiothoracic surgery, to reduce postoperative atrial fibrillation
    C. Preferentially, rhythm control should be achieved chemically in this critically ill patient
    D. Synchronized DC cardioversion occurs during the refractory portion of the cardiac cycle
    E. When pharmacological cardioversion is attempted, either flecainide or amiodarone are suitable in the presence of known structural heart disease

7. **Regarding tuberculosis (TB), the following are true:**
    A. Efficacy of antituberculosis treatment regimens is good in critically ill patients when using the enteral route
    B. In patients with active TB requiring mechanical ventilation for respiratory failure, the prognosis is similar to that of acute respiratory distress syndrome (ARDS) due to any cause
    C. The standard treatment for non–multidrug resistant TB involves combination therapy of three or more drugs
    D. Tuberculosis leads to an increase in HIV replication and accelerates progression of HIV infection
    E. The Bacillus Calmette–Guerin (BCG) vaccine is approximately 90% effective for the prevention of tuberculosis

8. Concerning contrast-induced nephropathy (CIN), the following are true:

A. There is a very high incidence of CIN in ICU patients undergoing contrast-enhanced scans

B. The volume of contrast is not related to the risk of nephropathy

C. There is good evidence for N-acetylcysteine (NAC) prophylaxis

D. There is good evidence for prophylactic hydration

E. There is good evidence for mannitol prophylaxis

9. Regarding aortic stenosis (AS), the following are true:

A. AS becomes haemodynamically significant with a valve area of approximately 2cm²

B. AS causes diastolic dysfunction

C. AS reduces myocardial oxygen supply

D. Maintenance of preload is important

E. Signs of AS include a 'water hammer' pulse

10. Regarding severe acute pancreatitis, the following are true:

A. An amylase rise is the most sensitive and specific biomarker for acute pancreatitis

B. Alcohol-related pancreatitis is the commonest cause of severe acute pancreatitis in case series

C. Early computed tomogram (CT) of the abdomen on admission with contrast is helpful in determining associated complications

D. *Severe acute pancreatitis* is defined by local complications and organ failure extending beyond 72 hours

E. USS confirmed gallstone-related pancreatitis and acute cholangitis mandates early endoscopic retrograde cholangiopancreatography (ERCP)

11. The following statements are correct regarding tetanus:

A. A wound is always apparent once symptoms occur

B. It is a toxin-mediated disease caused by the bacterium Clostridium tetani

C. It can cause autonomic instability

D. It causes a flaccid paralysis

E. The toxin prevents the synaptic release of neurotransmitter from the presynaptic GABA-ergic inhibitory interneurons

12. Relating to Central Venous Catheterization, the following are true:

A. Before central venous catheter (CVC) insertion, platelets should be given to correct patient's thrombocytopaenia when the platelet level is 45 × 10⁹/l

B. CXR is necessary to confirm the tip position, when a central line is inserted in a vessel other than the femoral veins

C. Differential time to positivity aids diagnosis of catheter-related blood stream infection (CRBSI) when blood from the CVC demonstrates microbial growth at the same time as that detected in blood collected simultaneously from a peripheral vein

D. The normal central venous waveform is comprised of three upstrokes ('a', 'c', and 'v' waves) and two descents ('x' and 'y' descents)

E. Thoracic duct injury is more commonly associated with a left subclavian approach to central venous access than a left internal jugular approach

13. **A 38-year-old patient with severe pancreatitis develops type 1 respiratory failure for which he is intubated and ventilated, with pressure support of 18cm H_2O and a positive end expiratory pressure of 5cm H_2O. A chest radiograph shows diffuse bilateral infiltrates. A transthoracic echo is normal. His PaO_2 is 8.1kPa with an FiO_2 of 0.8. The following are true:**

A. Diuretics should be considered if the patient does not have signs of intravascular depletion

B. Peak pressures should be less than 30cm H_2O

C. This patient has acute respiratory distress syndrome (ARDS)

D. There is evidence to support the use of high-frequency oscillation ventilation (HFOV) in this patient

E. Ventilation with a tidal volume of 6ml/kg actual body weight would be in keeping with ARDSnet recommendations

14. **Inhaled nitric oxide (NO) can be used as a therapy for ARDS, and the following statements are correct:**

A. Concentration is kept normally at 80 parts per million (ppm)

B. It improves survival

C. It improves oxygenation significantly in ARDS

D. It can cause pulmonary oedema and methemoglobinemia in high concentrations

E. Use of NO has been associated with renal impairment

15. **When adrenaline is infused intravenously, the following occur:**

A. A type A lactataemia results

B. Coronary artery constriction can cause ischaemia

C. Histamine release from mast cell degranulation is reduced

D. Serum glucose rises as a result of insulin resistance

E. There is an antithrombotic effect during endotoxaemia

16. **The following features are necessary for the underwater seal component of an intercostal chest drain (ICD):**

A. A three-bottle system can be used in which the first bottle acts as an underwater seal; the second as a fluid trap; and the third allows application of suction

B. The volume of tubing extending from the drain to the chest drain bottle should exceed the patient's maximal inspiratory volume to prevent aspiration of water into the chest during inspiration

C. The volume of water above the end of the patient tube within the chest drain bottle must exceed half of the patient's maximal inspiratory volume

D. The chest drain tubing submerged in the chest drain bottle must be at least 10cm below the surface of the water to prevent air entrainment during vital capacity breaths

E. Suction applied to the chest drain should be approximately 10 to 20cm H_2O

17. **When conducting brainstem death tests, the following statements are correct:**

    A. Alternative causes of apnoea should be excluded
    B. Plasma levels of sedative drugs should be routinely measured
    C. The oculo-vestibular reflex is tested by injecting 50ml of ice cold water into each external auditory meatus over 1 minute with the patient at a 30° head-up tilt
    D. The patient's temperature should be greater than 34°C
    E. The pupillary light reflex tests cranial nerves I and II

18. **A 3 year-old child presents to the ED lethargic, with a high temperature, and nonblanching rash. The child is cool to touch peripherally, with a very weak and thready pulse and unrecordable blood pressure. Correct further management includes:**

    A. Albumin is contraindicated
    B. Give intravenous ceftriaxone initially 1g
    C. Give a fluid bolus of 20ml/kg 0.9% NaCl
    D. Perform a lumbar puncture immediately as meningitis is likely
    E. Start dexamethasone 0.15mg/kg

19. **Fires rarely occur within the critical care setting; however, the sequelae may be devastating. The following statements are true:**

    A. Foam extinguishers can be used for electrical fires
    B. In evacuation, the sickest patients should be removed first
    C. Medical gas supplies cannot be turned off locally
    D. Oxygen cylinders should be safely placed on patient's beds during transfer
    E. The fire triad comprises an oxidizer, an ignition source and fuel

20. **Peripherally Inserted Central Venous Catheters (PICC lines) are increasingly used on the ICU. The following statements are true:**

    A. The basilic vein is often chosen for the site of insertion as it lies superficially along the lateral side of the arm
    B. The cephalic vein can also be used but is likely to result in greater placement failure
    C. The brachial veins are closely related to the ulnar nerve
    D. The axillary vein is formed by the basilic and cephalic vein
    E. The complications may include thrombosis, tip migration, and pneumothorax

21. **The described abnormalities of coagulation tests may be seen under the following circumstances:**

    A. Disseminated intravascular coagulation: a prolonged prothrombin time (PT), prolonged activated partial thromboplastin time (APTT), and increased fibrinogen
    B. Haemophilia A: a prolonged PT and normal APTT
    C. Subtherapeutic warfarin: a prolonged PT and normal APTT
    D. Supra-therapeutic Fondaparinux: a slight prolongation of PT and prolonged APTT
    E. Von Willebrand disease: a normal PT and prolonged APTT

22. **Regarding the cardiac action potential, the following are true:**

    A. Cardiac muscle action potential lasts approximately 100ms

    B. Diastolic relaxation is an active process

    C. It is similar to the action potential seen in nerves

    D. Much of the calcium influx seen in the plateau phase is due to opening of the L-type calcium channels

    E. Pacemaker cells exhibit a stable resting membrane potential

23. **Pre surgery, a patient is being given intravenous unfractionated heparin. The following are correct:**

    A. Heparin naturally occurs in mast cell granules

    B. Heparin enhances the rate of formation of the antithrombin III-thrombin complex 100-fold

    C. Heparin inhibits factor Xa

    D. Heparin can be reversed by protamine

    E. Thrombocytopaenia associated with heparin is always immune-mediated

24. **Regarding pharmacology, the following are true:**

    A. At a pH below their pK_a weak acids will be mostly unionized

    B. High lipid solubility of a drug results in a rapid onset of action

    C. In a severely burnt patient, the effect of a given dose of a drug may have a significantly exaggerated effect

    D. More potent drugs have a faster onset of action

    E. Only unionized drug can cross a cell membrane

25. **The following are true of defibrillators:**

    A. Biphasic defibrillators improve defibrillation rates by delivering a higher peak current than monophasic defibrillators

    B. In a simple defibrillator, an inductor is used to increase the shock duration

    C. The shock energy is stored temporarily in a capacitor

    D. Shock duration is typically 100ms

    E. Transthoracic impedance is typically 50–150 Ohm

26. **Regarding pulse oximetry, the following are true:**

    A. Light-emitting diodes (LED) emit radiation at red and ultraviolet wavelengths

    B. Each LED is alternatively switched on and off to allow for the pulsatility of arterial blood flow

    C. In the presence of carboxyhaemoglobin, oxygen saturation is falsely high

    D. Fetal haemoglobin falsely increases oxygen-saturation reading

    E. Using pulse oximetry, oxygen saturation tends towards 85% in the presence of increasing methaemoglobin

27. **Following a road traffic accident, a 67-year-old woman, who was a passenger in the car, is found to be profoundly hypotensive, with a blood pressure of 60/35mmHg; hypoxic; and a raised jugular venous pressure. While an echo is being organized, the following are true:**
    A. An exaggerated fall in systemic arterial blood pressure during the inspiratory phase of spontaneous breathing is in keeping with cardiac tamponade
    B. Clinical signs and symptoms of tamponade occur when at least 750ml of fluid has accumulated
    C. Echocardiographic signs of left-sided diastolic chamber collapse and ventricular interdependence are highly suggestive of cardiac tamponade
    D. Electrical alternans on the ECG is a highly specific finding to cardiac tamponade
    E. These clinical findings could be attributable to a type B aortic dissection

28. **The following statements are true regarding the physiological response to significant blood loss:**
    A. Decrease in cardiac output and subsequent chemoreceptor activation
    B. Increase in baroreceptor discharge as blood pressure falls
    C. Renin release from juxtaglomerular apparatus
    D. Secretion of atrial natriuretic peptide increases
    E. Systemic vascular resistance to pre haemorrhage values via compensatory mechanisms

29. **With regard to dexmedetomidine and the use of sedation on the ICU, the following are correct:**
    A. Daily sedation holds are essential in reducing duration of mechanical ventilation and length of ICU stay
    B. Dexmedetomidine is an α2 antagonist
    C. Dexmedetomidine is far superior to midazolam when length of ICU stay is compared
    D. Protocolized sedation may limit mechanical ventilation and length of stay
    E. There is no reversal to overcome dexmedetomidine

30. **In patients who have sustained a traumatic brain injury, the following statements are true:**
    A. A 1 g bolus of tranexamic acid should be given to patients with a Glasgow coma scale (GCS) 8-13 and presenting within 3 hours of injury
    B. Dexamethasone reduces surrounding oedema
    C. Intracranial pressure (ICP) monitoring results in better outcomes
    D. In ventilated patients, a target $PaCO_2$ of 3.2kPa improves cerebral blood flow
    E. Measures should be taken to prevent deep vein thrombosis (DVT), including the use of prophylactic low molecular weight heparin on admission

Question 1 F T F F T

The delivery of trauma care has changed in the UK in recent years and is managed by major trauma centres (MTC), who manage trauma victims with injury severity scores >15. There is a significant increase in the odds of survival of trauma victims since the implementation of the MTC, and this may be multifactorial relying on higher volumes of patients, greater consultant input, alteration of major haemorrhage protocols, and the use of rapid imaging and tranexamic acid.

Changes in initial management have centred on damage control resuscitation, which included permissive hypotension, haemostatic resuscitation and damage control surgery.

- Permissive hypotension: restricted fluid resuscitation and permitting a lower than normal perfusion pressure until haemorrhage is controlled.
- Haemostatic resuscitation: the use of blood and blood products as first line resuscitation fluid after severe injury.
- Damage control surgery: initial surgery aimed at control of haemorrhage and contamination, while definitive repair is delayed until the patient is stable.

European guidelines suggest systolic pressures of 80–100mmHg are sufficient unless there is traumatic brain injury (systolic must be >90mmHg). ATC can occur within minutes of trauma, and it appears to be modulated by tissue damage, inflammatory mediator release, hypotension, and disruption of the equilibrium between platelets, vascular endothelium, and pro- or anticoagulant factors, not just consumption of coagulation factors and platelets.

Spahn D, et al. Management of bleeding and coagulopathy following major trauma: an updated European guideline. *Critical Care* 2013;17:R76.

Moran C, et al. Changing the system: major trauma patients and their outcomes in the NHS (England) 2008–2017. *Lancet Clinical Medicine* 2018;2:13–21.

Question 2 F F T F F

Rhabdomyolysis describes the disintegration and necrosis of striated muscle. Cell damage leads to the accumulation of cytoplasmic calcium and hence initial plasma hypocalcaemia. Cell death leads to hyperkalaemia.

Causes of rhabdomyolysis can be divided into traumatic (e.g. crush syndromes, acute compartment syndromes, ischaemic limbs, and extreme exercise, for example seen in military recruits undertaking training), and in nontraumatic causes, including drugs (e.g. statins, ecstasy overdose), infectious causes (e.g. legionella, salmonella), autoimmune causes (e.g. polymyositis), metabolic and or endocrine causes (e.g. hyperosmolar conditions), and genetic enzyme deficiencies.

Clinically, muscle pain, weakness, and dark urine may also be accompanied by fever, malaise, confusion, and oligo-anuria.

Within the renal tubules, myoglobin interacts with the protein Tamm–Horsfall to form brown granular casts, and this results in tubular obstruction. This process is favoured when the urine is acidic. Creatine kinase >5000 units/l is diagnostic, but ultimately significant rises denote muscle damage, and trends in levels may be important.

Petejova N, Martinek A. Acute kidney injury due to rhabdomyolysis and renal replacement therapy: a critical review. *Critical Care* 2014;18:224.

Question 3   T T F T F

Systolic blood pressure is primarily influenced by stroke volume and vascular capacitance. Diastolic pressure depends on the ability of the proximal arteries to recoil and continue to squeeze the blood forwards against the resistance offered by the peripheral vascular beds. Elderly patients tend to have a stiff noncompliant vascular system, resulting in a lower diastolic pressure.

The dicrotic notch represents closure of the aortic valve (aortic pressure >pressure in left ventricle). In marked vasodilation, such pressure gradients occur later in the cardiac cycle, and there is a downward shift of the dicrotic notch.

During mechanical ventilation there is a transient increase in venous return to the left atrium during inspiration. However on the right side of the heart, an increase in intra-thoracic pressure during the inspiratory phase will be associated with an immediate reduction in venous return, and, therefore, the left ventricular stroke volume will decrease after the initial increase. This interaction is exaggerated in hypovolaemia and is seen as a 'swing' on the arterial pressure waveform trace.

The size of the pulsatile component of the arterial waveform is linked to the stroke volume, vascular capacitance, and systemic vascular resistance. Under stable conditions, stroke volume becomes the major determinant of pulse pressure and area under the systolic portion of the waveform, and this can be used to measure cardiac output using pulse contour analysis. If there is a change in the mathematical relationships (i.e. from a change in vascular capacitance due to new sepsis), the estimates of cardiac output become inaccurate.

Lamia B, et al. Clinical review: interpretation of arterial pressure wave in shock states. *Critical Care* 2005;9(6):601–6.

Question 4   T T F F T

The Doppler principle has been used to measure cardiac output by using the formula:

$$\Delta F = 2.F_0.v.\cos\theta/c$$

(ΔF = observed frequency; F_0 = emitted frequency; v = velocity of flow; θ = angle of incident ultrasound beam to long axis of blood flow; and c = velocity of ultrasound in that medium).

Spectral analysis of the Doppler shift is used to generate velocity-time curves. However, employment of this technique involves a number of assumptions, including all red blood cells (RBC) travel at the same velocity (a Doppler shift in frequency occurs when the ultrasound wave is reflected back from moving RBCs, with the shift in frequency proportional to the velocity of the blood flow), and blood flow through the descending aorta is approximately 70% of total cardiac output. Measurement is combined with the cross-sectional area of the descending aorta (using a nomogram based on age, weight, and height). Minimal or no blood flow in the descending aorta will be detected by the oesophageal Doppler probe during diastole.

The cosine of 90° is 0, and hence the angle of incident ultrasound should be 45°–60°, as the oesophagus is normally parallel to the aorta. Small changes in angulation can result in errors of up to 30%.

Berton C, Cholley B. Equipment review: new techniques for cardiac output measurement – oesophageal Doppler, Fick principle using carbon monoxide, and pulse contour analysis. *Critical Care* 2002;6(3):216–21.

Question 5 F F F F T

COPD is characterized by airflow obstruction that is not fully reversible. The airflow obstruction is usually progressive and is predominately caused by smoking. As there is an obstructive pattern, the FEV_1/FVC is <0.7.

Noninvasive ventilation (NIV) often has a role in acute hypercapneic respiratory failure. Reduced level of consciousness is a relative contraindication to the use of NIV, but may help stave of intubation in this situation. A low GCS and the use of NIV in Type 2 respiratory failure should prompt the need for closer monitoring in an appropriate environment and early appraisal as to whether there is clinical improvement or need for intubation and ventilation. In addition NIV may not only improve gas exchange, but in cases of palliation, also improve symptoms of breathlessness and facilitate timeliness of family discussions.

Prognostic features at referral include failure to improve during current admission, ongoing acidosis, and physiological disturbance including new arrhythmias. An FEV_1 <30% predicts an increased risk of death with respiratory failure within 1 year.

Chronic obstructive pulmonary disease. Management of chronic obstructive pulmonary disease in adults in primary and secondary care (partial update). June 2010. http://www.nice.org.uk/guidance/cg101/resources/guidance-chronic-obstructive-pulmonary-disease-pdf [accessed 14 June 2014].

Davidson A, et al. BTS/ICS guideline for the ventilatory management of acute hypercapnic respiratory failure in adults. *Thorax* 2016;71(Suppl 2).

Question 6 F F F F F

Atrial fibrillation (AF) is characterized by absent p waves and an irregularly irregular ventricular response. New-onset AF occurs frequently on the ICU and is often a reversible manifestation of the critical illness. The aetiology tends to differ from that of AF in the community, and many of the risk factors are potentially reversible (e.g. sepsis). AF may occur in 5%–15% septic patients and has a greater incidence in postsurgical patients, especially cardiac.

Immediate management should take into account haemodynamic instability. If there is haemodynamic compromise, management should correct reversible causes and proceed to synchronized DC cardioversion (synchronized with the R wave and not the T wave) for rhythm control.

Flecainide is not suitable in the presence of structural heart disease. If there is no haemodynamic compromise, aim to correct any reversible causes and opt for rate control with a standard beta blocker (unless contraindicated) or calcium channel blocker.

In patients undergoing cardiothoracic surgery, the risk of postoperative AF can be reduced with a beta blocker, rate limiting calcium antagonist, or amiodarone. Digoxin should not be offered.

Atrial fibrillation: the management of atrial fibrillation. https://www.nice.org.uk/guidance/cg180/resources/atrial-fibrillation-management-35109805981381 [accessed 19/07/2021].

Question 7 F F T T F

There is a significantly higher in-hospital mortality for patients requiring mechanical ventilation for TB in comparison to ARDS of any cause.

Critically ill patients on the ICU potentially will have unreliable enteral absorption. Enterally administered antituberculous drugs are likely to be subtherapeutic, causing a slow clinical response or treatment failure. Where possible, drugs should be converted to parenteral and therapeutic levels measured. In the individual host the two pathogens, *M. tuberculosis* and HIV, potentiate one another, accelerating the deterioration of immunological functions and resulting in premature death if untreated. Some 14 million individuals worldwide are estimated to be co-infected.

The BCG vaccine has an overall efficacy of approximately 50%.

Hagan G, Nathani N. Clinical review: tuberculosis on the intensive care unit. *Critical Care* 2013;17:240–4.

Getahun H, Gunneberg C, Granich R, Nunn P. HIV infection-associated tuberculosis: the epidemiology and the response. *Clinical Infectious Diseases* 2010;50(Suppl 3):S201–S207.

Question 8 F F F T F

CIN is associated with larger volumes of iodinated contrast. Studies of critically ill patients have demonstrated a CIN rate of up to 14% following contrast-enhanced scans. Hydration has been shown to reduce incidence of CIN. Despite initially promising reports, recent large, randomized controlled trials (RCTs) and meta-analysis have refuted the role of NAC. Mannitol provides no benefit in CIN.

Lakhal K, et al. Acute Kidney Injury Network definition of contrast-induced nephropathy in the critically ill: incidence and outcome. *Journal of Critical Care* 2011;26:593–9.

ACT Investigators. Acetylcysteine for prevention of renal outcomes in patients undergoing coronary and peripheral vascular angiography: main results from the randomized Acetylcysteine for Contrast-Induced Nephropathy Trial (ACT). *Circulation* 2011;124:1250–9.

Question 9 F T T T F

The normal aortic valve area is 2.6–3.5cm^2, and haemodynamic significance is seen at around 1cm^2. Compensatory left ventricular hypertrophy develops causing diastolic dysfunction—consequently preload and atrial contractility is important to maintain.

A slow-rising pulse is a sign of stenosis, whilst a 'water hammer', or collapsing, pulse is associated with aortic regurgitation.

Myocardial oxygen demand is increased due to the left ventricular hypertrophy. Simultaneously, oxygen supply is reduced due to the decreased gradient between aortic and left ventricular diastolic pressures.

Brown J, Morgan-Hughes N. Aortic stenosis and non-cardiac surgery. *CEACCP* 2005;5(1):1–4.

Question 10 F F T F T

Serum amylase peaks a few hours after the onset of symptoms and falls back to normal levels within 3 to 5 days; therefore, levels may be normal on admission in up to 20% of patients. Serum lipase is more specific and remains elevated for longer.

Acute pancreatitis secondary to gallstones is the commonest form in most case series, with alcohol accounting for 20%–25% of cases, and 20% of cases remaining idiopathic. There is therefore a recommendation that transabdominal ultrasound is undertaken for all patients with acute pancreatitis, as it may identify a biliary cause or acute cholangitis (which warrants early ERCP). Early contrast CT may not be that helpful, unless exact aetiology is unclear, but where doubt of cause exists, contrast CT provides good evidence of presence or absence of pancreatitis. The strength of contrast CT performed later allows identification of interstitial oedematous pancreatitis from necrotizing pancreatitis, and, of course, it will also help identify associated complications including peri-pancreatic collections and pseudocysts, all of which are defined with time.

Severe acute pancreatitis is defined as organ failure lasting >48 hours, with or without local complications. Mortality from acute severe pancreatitis is in the order of 30% but may increase in the presence of infected necrosis.

Johnson CD, Besselink MG, Carter R. Acute pancreatitis. *BMJ* 2014;349:1–8.

Question 11 F T T F T

Tetanus is indeed caused by C. tetani, an anaerobic Gram-positive bacterium that produces an extremely potent toxin. The bacterial spores are present primarily in soil and in human or animal faeces, and infection tends to spread by the contamination of a wound with the spores.

The toxin prevents the release of neurotransmitters from the presynaptic GABA-ergic inhibitory neurons, which leads to uncontrolled skeletal muscle activity as well as disinhibited autonomic nervous system activity. As a result, patients tend to present with skeletal muscle rigidity and spasm as well as autonomic dysfunction.

In many cases, the original wound is never found.

Cook TM, Protheroe RT, Handel JM. Tetanus: a review of the literature. *BJA* 2001;87:477–87.

Question 12 F F F T T

Thrombocytopaenia is common amongst the population who frequently require central venous access. Current practice in many countries is to correct thrombocytopaenia with platelet transfusions prior to CVC insertion, in order to mitigate the risk of serious peri- or postprocedural bleeding. The platelet count threshold recommended prior to CVC insertion varies significantly from country to country. In the UK, the current threshold is $50 \times 10^9/l$ (BCSH 2003), whereas in Germany and the United States, they will accept levels of $10 \times 10^9/l$ and $20 \times 10^9/l$, respectively. In isolation, and if there are no obvious additional bleeding risks, a level of $45 \times 10^9/l$ is probably sufficient for a straightforward CVC line insertion (thus mitigating risks of platelet transfusion and cost).

CXR is not always necessary to confirm tip position. For example PICC insertion is amenable to ECG-guided confirmation of tip placement.

CRBSI is suggested when blood from the CVC demonstrates microbial growth at least 2 hours earlier than growth is detected in blood collected simultaneously from a peripheral vein.

The components of the venous waveform include:

- A wave—due to atrial contraction. Absent in AF. Enlarged in tricuspid stenosis, pulmonary stenosis, and pulmonary hypertension.
- C wave—due to bulging of tricuspid valve into the right atrium or possibly transmitted pulsations from the carotid artery.
- X descent—due to atrial relaxation.
- V wave—due to the rise in atrial pressure before the tricuspid valve opens. Enlarged in tricuspid regurgitation.
- Y descent—due to atrial emptying as blood enters the ventricle.

The thoracic duct passes laterally to the left boarder of the oesophagus and arches laterally in the root of the neck, posterior to the carotid sheath, anterior to the sympathetic trunk and vertebral arteries, finally entering the left brachiocephalic vein at the junction of the subclavian and internal jugular vessels.

Estcourt L, et al. Comparison of different platelet transfusion thresholds prior to insertion of central lines in patients with thrombocytopaenia. *Cochrane Database of Systematic Reviews* 2015;12:CD011771.

Gahlot G, et al. Catheter related bloodstream infections. *International Journal of Critical Illness and Injury Science* 2014;4:162–7.

Moore KI, Dalley AF. *Clinically oriented anatomy,* 5th edition. London: Lippincott Williams & Wilkins, 2006.

Question 13 T F T F F

The clinical scenario fits a diagnosis of ARDS (see Table 2.1). ARDS is an acute diffuse, inflammatory lung injury, leading to increased pulmonary vascular permeability, increased lung weight, and loss of aerated lung tissue and thus subsequent hypoxemia and bilateral radiographic opacities. The Berlin definition of ARDS includes:

* Acute, meaning onset 1 week or less
* Bilateral opacities consistent with pulmonary oedema must be present and may be detected on CT or chest radiograph
* PF ratio <300mmHg with a minimum of 5cm H_2O PEEP (or CPAP)
* Must not be fully explained by cardiac failure or fluid overload, in the physician's best estimation using available information—an 'objective assessment' (e.g. echocardiogram) should be performed in most cases if there is no clear cause such as trauma or sepsis.

Table 2.1 Definition of ARDS

ARDS Severity	Pa/FIO$_2$ ratio (Peep 5 cm)	Observed Mortality
Mild	200-300	27%
Moderate	100-200	32%
Severe	<100	45%

ARDSnet recommendations are 6ml/kg *ideal* body weight. Plateau pressure target is less than 30cm H_2O as per ARDSnet.

No mortality benefit has been shown for a restrictive fluid regime, but a reduction in days ventilated and days on ICU has been shown.

Two recent randomized control trials have shown either no benefit or increased mortality when HFOV is used in ARDS.

The Acute Respiratory Distress Syndrome Network. Ventilation with lower tidal volumes as compared with traditional tidal volumes for acute lung injury and the acute respiratory distress syndrome. *New England Journal of Medicine* 2000;342:1301–8.

Wiedmann HP, et al. Comparison of two fluid-management strategies in acute lung injury. *New England Journal of Medicine* 2006;354:2564–75.

Ferguson ND, et al. High-frequency oscillation in early acute respiratory distress syndrome. *New England Journal of Medicine* 2013;368:795–805.

Question 14 F F T T T

Nitric oxide is a component of smog that can be measured in urban area air at 10 to 100 parts per billion (ppb). It is naturally produced endogenously by NO synthase and has numerous physiological functions. It has a major role as a messenger molecule in most human organ systems. In the kidney, as well as in other solid organs, physiologic concentrations of NO function as a tonic vasodilator. However, higher concentrations can be toxic, damaging cellular constituents (such as DNA).

Inhaling very high levels of NO can be lethal, causing pulmonary oedema and methaemoglobinaemia. However, there is little evidence of such toxicity when the concentration is kept in the normal concentration range (1 to 80ppm).

Starting doses of inhaled nitric oxide (iNO) are usually 5ppm, titrating up to 10 ppm and then 20ppm gradually every 30 minutes. There is negligible risk of methaemoglobinaemia in adults using concentrations of 40ppm.

Two large, randomized control trials using iNO as a treatment for ARDS have been performed. Unfortunately, neither demonstrated improved survival, although iNO does improve oxygenation for a short period. In addition the risk of renal dysfunction associated with iNO therapy was first reported in an RCT of patients with ARDS, in which iNO was found to double the risk of the need for renal replacement therapy compared with controls.

Role of NO in management of ARDS. *Annals of Thoracic Medicine* 2008 Jul–Sep;3(3):100–3.

Rossaint R, Falke K, Lopez F, Slama K, Pison U, Zapol WM. Inhaled nitric oxide for the adult respiratory distress syndrome *New England Journal of Medicine* 1993;328:399–405.

Dellinger R, et al. Effects of inhaled nitric oxide in patients with acute respiratory distress syndrome: results of a randomized phase II trial. *Critical Care Medicine* 1998;26:15–23.

Lundin S, Mang H, Smithies M, Stenqvist O, Frostell C. Inhalation of nitric oxide in acute lung injury: results of a European multicentre study. The European study group of inhaled nitric oxide. *Intensive Care Medicine* 1999;25:911–19.

Question 15 F F T F T

Adrenaline administration causes a type B lactataemia, by increasing aerobic glycolysis, not by inducing tissue hypoxia (the basis of a type A lactataemia). Serum glucose rises as a result of glycolysis, inhibition of insulin secretion, stimulation of glucagon secretion, and an increase in ACTH release. Insulin sensitivity is enhanced.

Ischaemia results as a consequence of increased myocardial oxygen demand, and adrenaline may cause coronary vasodilation. Adrenaline may have a beneficial effect by reducing microvascular thrombosis in endotoxaemia.

Adrenaline infusion is recommended in the treatment of anaphylactic shock since it inhibits mast cell degranulation and histamine release.

Levy B. Bench-to-bedside review: is there a place for epinephrine in septic shock? *Critical Care* 2005;9:561–5.

McLean-Tooke AP, Bethune CA, Fay AC, Spickett GP. Adrenaline in the treatment of anaphylaxis: what is the evidence? *British Medical Journal* 2003;327:1332–5.

Question 16 F F T F T

ICDs are most commonly connected to an underwater seal device, which allows unidirectional flow of air from the pleural cavity. The underwater seal should have a number of features:

- The tube connecting the ICD to the underwater seal bottle must be wide to reduce resistance, and its volumetric capacity must exceed half of the patient's maximal inspiratory volume. This prevents water being aspirated into the chest during inspiration.
- The end of the tube, within the underwater seal bottle, should have a volume of water above it that exceeds half the patient's maximal inspiratory volume. This prevents air being drawn into the interpleural cavity during inspiration.
- The end of the tube, within the underwater seal bottle, should not be more than 5cm below the surface of water, as air will not be sufficiently drained.
- The drain should be at least 45cm below the patient.
- Suction may be applied, no more than 10–20cm H_2O. Portable suction drains are often used post thoracic surgery, which allow application of suction and measurement of air leak.

- A three-bottle system may be used, although far less common. The first bottle acts as a fluid trap. The second bottle provides the underwater seal, while the third bottle can be used for suction.

Miller KS, Sahn SA, Review. Chest tubes, indications, technique, management and complications. *Chest* 1987;91:258–64.

Laws D, Neville E, Duffy J, on behalf of the British Thoracic Society Pleural Disease Group, a Sub-Group of the British Thoracic Society Standards of Care Committee. BTS guidelines for the insertion of a chest drain. *Thorax* 2003;58(Suppl II):ii53–ii59.

Yentis S, Hirsh N, Smith G. *Anaesthesia and intensive care A to Z: an encyclopaedia of principles and practice.* London: Butterworth Heineman, 2003.

Question 17 T F T T F

A central temperature of less than 34°C can lead to an impaired level of consciousness. Brainstem reflexes are often lost below 28°C. Core temperature should therefore be greater than 34°C at the time of brainstem death testing.

The persistence of neuromuscular blocking drugs is one reversible cause of immobility, unresponsiveness and lack of spontaneous respiration. Their presence should be excluded by testing deep-tendon reflexes and by the demonstration of adequate neuromuscular conduction with a conventional nerve stimulator.

In a similar fashion, hypnotics and narcotics must be excluded as a cause of apparent coma, although plasma levels of sedative drugs are not routinely required. Clinicians should be confident after considering the dose and duration of sedatives, temperature, age, and renal/hepatic function that the patient's unconscious state is not a result of residual drug effects. Occasionally plasma levels of thiopentone or midazolam may assist in this assessment.

The pupillary light reflex tests the integrity of the second and third cranial nerves. Testing of the oculo-vestibular reflex should be preceded by direct otoscopy to ensure direct access to an undamaged tympanic membrane bilaterally. In a brainstem dead patient, no eye movements are seen during or following the slow injection of at least 50mls of ice cold water over 1 minute into each external auditory meatus in turn. The head should be at 30 degrees to the horizontal plane unless an unstable spinal injury is suspected.

Academy of Medical Royal Colleges. *A code of practice for the diagnosis and confirmation of death.* 2008. http://www.aomrc.org.uk/doc_view/42-a-code-of-practice-for-the-diagnosis-and-confirmation-of-death [accessed 12 June 2014].

Question 18 F T T F T

The concern with the clinical scenario is that this child may be suffering from meningococcal disease. Meningococcal disease presents as meningitis (15% cases), septicaemia (25% cases) or a combination of both (60% cases). Meningococcal disease is the leading infectious cause of death in early childhood.

Intravenous ceftriaxone should be immediately given in the presence of a petechial rash that is spreading or becoming purpuric, or where bacterial meningitis or meningococcal septicaemia is suspected. Antibiotics should not be delayed to facilitate lumbar puncture.

Where meningococcal septicaemia is suspected, 0.9% NaCl fluid boluses in 20ml/kg aliquots should be given. Human albumin 4.5% may be given as an alternative, and once the third bolus has been administered, it is prudent to start vasoactive agents. In cases of bacterial meningitis, dexamethasone 0.15mg/kg four times daily for 4 days should be started within 4 hours of antibiotics; however, in the case of meningococcal septicaemia, do not treat with high-dose corticosteroids, although low-dose corticosteroids (hydrocortisone) may be used for shock refractory to vasoactive agents.

Visintin C, et al. Management of bacterial meningitis and meningococcal septicaemia in children and young people: summary of NICE guidance. *British Medical Journal* 2010;340:c3209.

Question 19 F F F F T

Fires require an oxygen supply, an ignition source, and a fuel source that is capable of participating in combustion. Thankfully, fire is relatively rare, but it is essential that those working within the ICU are aware of fire exits, extinguishers, gas shut-off valves (located within the unit and ideally visibly located), fire sheets, and the evacuation policy.

Foam extinguishers are not suitable for electrical fires, and their use may corrode nearby equipment. Carbon dioxide extinguishers are preferable. An ICU should have three fire escape routes and separate fire-safe areas that provide protection for up to 30 minutes.

In general the triage of patients during evacuation means the least unwell go first, and the sickest last, but clearly it will take into account those at most direct danger from the fire and the practical aspects of discontinuing many of the specific critical care therapies.

Following a fire caused by an oxygen cylinder, a number of recommendations on the safe use of oxygen cylinders have been put in place, which include opening valves slowly, setting the cylinder up for use before placing it close to the patient, and not placing cylinders on beds.

Kelly FE, et al. Managing the aftermath of a fire on intensive care caused by an oxygen cylinder. *Journal of the Intensive Care Society* 2014;15:283–7.

Question 20 F T F F F

Insertion of a PICC has benefits compared to catheters accessed by more central routes—including the avoidance of pneumothorax, haemothorax, and major arterial bleeding, since local haemostasis is easier to achieve. There may also be less risk of CRBSI.

Despite the ease and general safe use of PICCs, there are well-recognized complications, including venous thrombosis, phlebitis, CRBSI, malposition, and tip migration.

The basilic vein is often chosen for PICC insertion. Distally it runs superficially within the subcutaneous fat on the medial side of the upper arm. At the junction of the middle and inferior thirds of the upper arm, the basilic vein penetrates the brachial deep fascia and then ascends to join the brachial veins to become the axillary vein. The brachial veins are related to the median nerve, which also lies within the brachial sheath.

The cephalic vein may also be used for PICC insertion. While superficial and free of surrounding nerves, it is often a tortuous course as it penetrates the fascial layers in the deltopectoral groove, and enters the axillary vein at an acute angle, making PICC placement more difficult.

Hudman L, Bodenham A. Practical aspects of long-term venous access. *Continuing Education in Anaesthesia, Critical Care & Pain* 2013;13:6–11.

Question 21 F F T T T

Disseminated intravascular coagulation is characterized by activation of the coagulation cascade and therefore results in marked deposition of fibrin and microvascular thrombosis, as well as consumption of platelets and coagulation proteins, leading to severe bleeding. Fibrinogen is therefore low.

Haemophilia A (deficiency in factor VIII) prolongs APTT not PT. Subtherapeutic warfarin may prolong the PT. Fondaparinux, a synthetic pentasaccharide factor Xa inhibitor, can cause the described abnormalities. Anti Xa activity is, however, normally used to monitor its effect. Von

Willebrand disease is a genetic disorder caused by missing/defective von Willebrand factor, which under normal circumstances binds factor VIII. Therefore the APTT may be mildly prolonged (low levels of VIII) while the PT is in reference range.

Smogorzewska A, et al. Effect of fondaparinux on coagulation assays: results of College of American Pathologists proficiency testing. *Archives of Pathology & Laboratory Medicine* 2006;130(11):1605–11.

Bersten AD, Soni N. *Oh's intensive care manual*, 6th edition. London: Butterworth Heinemann, 2009.

Question 22 **F T F T F**

The cardiac action potential, of non-pacemaker cells in the myocardium, is quite different from that of nerves. There are a number of phases, and the process takes in the order of 300ms:

- Phase 0 is depolarization and results from opening of fast sodium channels. Phase 1 is partial repolarization from decrease in sodium permeability.
- Phase 2 is the plateau phase resulting from the opening of L-type calcium channels. This maintains depolarization and lengthens the action potential.
- Phase 3 is repolarization as an inward potassium current that replaces the now inactivated calcium movement.
- The resting potential in phase 4 results from the sodium-potassium ATPase pump, which creates a negative intracellular potential.

Pacemaker cells have no phase 1 or 2 and do not have a stable resting potential. Diastolic relaxation is an active process.

Smith T, et al. (eds). *Fundamentals of anaesthesia*, 3rd edition. Cambridge: Cambridge University Press, 2009.

Question 23 **T F T T F**

Heparin occurs naturally in liver and mast cell granules. The inactive anti-thrombin III-thrombin complex, which inhibits clot formation, is enhanced by heparin 1000-fold. Heparin at lower concentration will also inhibit factor X_a.

Low platelets seen with heparin may be due to immune-mediated mechanisms (i.e. heparin-induced thrombocytopaenia, HIT) or may be due to non-immune mechanisms, which tend to be seen earlier and have a more indolent course.

Protamine (positively charged) indeed reverses the effects of heparin (negatively charged) by forming an inactive complex, which is then cleared by the reticulo-endothelial system.

Hill S, Peck T, Williams M. *Pharmacology for anaesthesia and intensive acre*, 2nd edition. London: Greenwich Medical Media, 2003.

Question 24 **T F T F T**

The lipophilic nature of the cell membrane means that only the unionized portion of a drug can cross the cell membrane. pK_a is the pH at which 50% of the drug molecules are ionized. At a pH below their pK_a, weak acids will be mostly unionized.

High lipid solubility does not guarantee fast onset. Alfentanil, despite being less lipid-soluble than fentanyl, has a more rapid onset partly because of a smaller volume of distribution but also because it is less potent (relatively more has to be given and a greater concentration gradient exists), and more is unionized at physiological pH.

In burns patients, lower plasma albumin will result in less drug-protein binding, and therefore the proportion of unbound drug at the same dose may be greater.

Hill S, Peck T, Williams M. *Pharmacology for anaesthesia and intensive acre*, 2nd edition. London: Greenwich Medical Media, 2003.

Question 25 F T T F T

A capacitor is used rather than directly powering from the battery or mains due to the high discharge rate required. In a classic monophasic defibrillator, this is combined with an inductor to increase the shock duration, which is typically under 10ms. Biphasic defibrillators use a lower peak current which can theoretically reduce complications.

Weisz MT. Physical principles of defibrillators. *Anaesthesia & Intensive Care Medicine* 2009 Aug;10(8):367–9.

Question 26 F F T F T

LEDs within the probe of a pulse oximeter use monochromatic light at red (660nm) and infrared (940nm) wavelengths. Each LED is switched on and off alternatively as the detecting photodiode is unable to differentiate between the wavelengths. Carboxyhaemoglobin will give a false high oxygen-saturation reading. Fetal haemoglobin has no effect, while methaemoglobin with lead to readings of 85%.

Smith T, et al. (eds). *Fundamentals of anaesthesia,* 3rd edition. Cambridge: Cambridge University Press, 2009.

Question 27 T F F T T

Cardiac tamponade is a potentially life-threatening pathology. It results from accumulation of fluid within the potential cardiac space, and when this accumulation is faster than the pericardium's ability to stretch, then increased pressure on the right ventricle results in less filling of the left ventricle and reduced cardiac output.

Beck triad (falling blood pressure, rising jugular venous pressure, and muffled heart sounds) may be present, as may electrical alternans on the ECG (height of normally conducted QRS alters with each beat). A volume of 100ml may be sufficient to cause tamponade in acute circumstances (trauma, myocardial rupture, and aortic dissection), whereas volumes of 1500ml may accumulate in chronic causes (malignancy, uraemia, pericarditis, and radiation).

Malignancy is a cause of subacute tamponade and is often secondary to lung cancer, although it may also be caused by breast cancer and lymphoma. Pericardial window may be necessary for recurrent pericardial effusions.

Potentially a type B aortic dissection could propagate proximally towards the ascending aorta and cause bleeding into the pericardial sac. Most blunt aortic injuries occur in the proximal thoracic aorta, although any portion of the aorta is at risk.

The proximal descending aorta, where the relatively mobile aortic arch can move against the fixed descending aorta (ligamentum arteriosum), is at greatest risk from the shearing forces of sudden deceleration.

Spodick D. Acute cardiac tamponade. *New England Journal of Medicine* 2003;349:684–90.

Question 28 T F T F F

Following significant blood loss, there is an immediate reduction in venous return and a decrease in discharge rates of baroreceptors in the carotid sinus and aortic arch. Decreased cardiac output causes activation of chemoreceptors. Both reflexes result in reduced parasympathetic activity (increase in heart rate from reduced vagal tone) and increased sympathetic tone. Sympathetic activation results in; increase in peripheral vascular resistance, redistribution of blood away from cutaneous and splanchnic circulations, stimulation of adrenal catecholamines, increase in vasopressin and renin release. Reduced renal blood flow results in an increase in renin release (and subsequent angiotensin and aldosterone). Venous hypotension decreases atrial natriuretic peptide (so renal blood flow and sodium and water excretion are also reduced). Stroke volume is restored via compensatory mechanisms but not back to pre haemorrhage values, while the reflex response will heighten the systemic vascular resistance to values higher, than before onset of blood loss.

Bricker S. *Short answers in anaesthesia.* Cambridge: Cambridge University Press, 2005.

Question 29 F F F T F

Dexmedetomidine is an α_2 agonist, resulting in sedation, anxiolysis, analgesia, and attenuation of the stress response. Several studies have demonstrated its strengths; however, no firm conclusions can be made regarding 'vast' superiority to other forms of sedation.

There is good evidence to support protocolized sedation in reducing mechanical ventilation and length of ICU stay; however, daily sedation holds are not essential in achieving this outcome.

Atipamezole is a selective α_2 antagonist that can reverse sedation and analgesia associated with clonidine and dexmedetomidine.

Adams R, Brown GT, Davidson M. Efficacy of dexmedetomidine compared with midazolam for sedation in adult intensive care patients: a systematic review. *British Journal of Anaesthesia* 2013;111:703–10.

Kress JP, et al. Daily interruption of sedative infusions in critically ill patients undergoing mechanical ventilation. *New England Journal of Medicine* 2000; 342:1471–7.

Mehta S, et al; SLEAP Investigators; Canadian Critical Care Trials Group. Daily sedation interruption in mechanically ventilated critically ill patients cared for with a sedation protocol: a randomized controlled trial. *Journal of the American Medical Association* 2012;308:1985–92.

Question 30 T F T F F

Traumatic brain injury (TBI) can be divided into primary (the initial insult) and secondary brain injury, whereby inflammation and neurotoxic processes result in vasogenic fluid accumulation, raised ICP, decreases cerebral perfusion, and subsequent ischaemia. Initial priorities in management are to prevent hypoxia and hypotension. In the setting of TBI, an elevated d-dimer has been associated with progressive haemorrhagic brain injury and possible worse outcome. Analysis of the CRASH-3 data supports recommendation of tranexamic acid within 3 hours of injury in patients with moderate TBI.

The Brain Trauma Foundation guidelines suggest that collecting ICP data facilitates outcome prediction, targeted management of cerebral perfusion pressure, avoidance of over aggressive ICP treatment (and the consequent side effects), and allowing rapid detection of clinical deterioration. Protocols using ICP data lead to improved results and high-volume trauma centres, which regularly utilize ICP data and generate superior outcomes. Prevention of additional complications, such as DVT, is also essential, and for that reason, graduated compression stockings should be placed on admission (unless there are contraindications).

Evidence supports the use of prophylactic low molecular weight heparin (LMWH); however, timing of initiation is less clear. It is probably safe to introduce LMWH 48–72 hours post TBI in the stable patient.

Prophylactic hyperventilation to produce $PaCO_2$ of 3.2kPa is not recommended. While hyperventilation reduces elevated ICP, it does so by reducing cerebral blood flow and therefore increases the risk of iatrogenic cerebral ischaemia. Prolonged periods of hyperventilation should be avoided. Conversely hypercapnia should also be avoided.

In the 1960s steroids were introduced as a treatment for brain oedema, and were seen to have a positive effect in patients with tumours. However the 2004 CRASH trial (a large RCT randomizing methylprednisolone in patients with TBI) was stopped early because mortality was increased in the steroid group compared to controls.

Brain Trauma Foundation. *Guidelines for the management of severe traumatic brain injury.* https://braintrauma.org/guidelines/guidelines-for-the-management-of-severe-tbi-4th-ed#/ 2016 [as accessed 30th July 2021]

CRASH Collaborators. Effects of intravenous corticosteroids on death within 14 days in 10,008 adults with clinically significant head injury. *Lancet* 2004;364:1321–8.

Dinsmore J. Traumatic brain injury: an evidence-based review of management. *Continuing Education in Anaesthesia, Critical Care & Pain* 2013;13:189–95.

CRASH Collaborators. Effects of tranexamic acid on death, disability, vascular occlusive events and other morbidities in patients with acute traumatic brain injury (CRASH-3): a randomised, placebo-controlled trial. *Lancet* 2019;394:1713–23.

1. **In cases of near-drowning, the following are true:**
   A. Cardiac arrhythmia can occur and is not uncommon when core body temperature is 32°C or below
   B. Death may occur as a result of acute respiratory distress syndrome (ARDS)
   C. Immersion into water <25°C increases minute ventilation and reduces cardiac output
   D. Patients hypothermic and in cardiac arrest on scene can be declared dead when CPR has been unsuccessful for some time
   E. The diving reflex, which may be protective, is mediated by the ophthalmic nerve

2. **With respect to pulmonary embolism (PE), the following are true:**
   A. Echocardiogram is the investigation of choice
   B. Shunt is primarily responsible for the cardio-respiratory decline seen in massive PE
   C. The vast majority of patients present with haemoptysis, chest pain, and dyspnoea
   D. The severity of PE depends on its size and location
   E. The pulmonary embolism severity index (PESI) score is used to predict the clinical probability of having a PE

3. **Regarding the monitoring of intracranial pressure (ICP), the following are true:**
   A. Monitoring of intracranial pressure reduces mortality after traumatic brain injury
   B. Microtransducer ICP monitors must be regularly recalibrated due to the zero drift of the sensor
   C. Lundberg 'A' waves are seen when there is reduced cerebral perfusion
   D. Pressure monitoring in the brain parenchyma is associated with reduced infection rates, compared with ventricular monitoring
   E. The reference point for pressure measurement is the Foramen of Munroe

4. **You are asked to review the electrocardiogram (ECG) of an unwell patient. You note a QT interval of 490ms. The following are true:**
   A. Hyperkalaemia is a cause of long QT
   B. QT <350ms is regarded as normal
   C. QT lengthens with faster heart rates
   D. This patient has a higher risk of ventricular arrhythmia
   E. This represents prolonged ventricular depolarization

MCQs and SBAs in Intensive Care Medicine. Lorna Eyre and Andrew Bodenham, Oxford University Press. © Oxford University Press 2021.
DOI: 10.1093/oso/9780198753056.003.0003

5. **Regarding Guillain-Barre Syndrome (GBS), the following are true:**
   A. GBS is more common in females
   B. GBS is frequently preceded by an infectious precipitant (e.g. gastroenteritis)
   C. GBS is characterized by a symmetrical proximal polyneuropathy
   D. GBS may include autonomic instability
   E. GBS requires prompt treatment with corticosteroids

6. **A 30-year-old obese woman, with an uncomplicated pregnancy, presents at term with abdominal pain, diarrhoea, and possible spontaneous rupture of membranes. She is found to be tachycardic, hypotensive with BP 80/42 and has a mild temperature of 37.9°C. The following are true:**
   A. As labour is not established, she ought to return home until contractions are regular
   B. Co-amoxiclav should be prescribed as an initial broad-spectrum antibiotic
   C. Differential diagnosis includes thromboembolism, which remains the leading cause of maternal death to date
   D. Intravenous immunoglobulin should be considered
   E. Sepsis in pregnancy is most often caused by α-haemolytic Strep

7. **A patient with known cirrhosis presents with haematemesis. With regards to the management of variceal bleeding, the following are true:**
   A. Antibiotic prophylaxis should be instituted when patients are admitted with acute variceal bleeding
   B. Endoscopy should be delayed until the patient is stable
   C. Isosorbide mononitrate can be used if beta-blockers are contra-indicated, to decrease the risk of variceal bleeding in patients with medium and large oesophageal varices
   D. Prophylactic band ligation is useful in preventing variceal bleeding in patients with medium and large oesophageal varices
   E. Vasoactive treatment (vasopressin, somatostatin, and their analogues) should be maintained for 24 hours in patients with oesophageal variceal bleeding

8. **A critically ill female patient undergoes intubation (using fentanyl, propofol, and cisatracurium) for deteriorating type I respiratory failure. Following successful intubation, the patient's blood pressure is no longer recordable, she is difficult to ventilate and develops widespread flushing of her torso, arms, and face. The following are true:**
   A. A normal tryptase level excludes anaphylaxis
   B. Allergic anaphylaxis is mediated by IgE, IgG, or complement associated immune reactions
   C. Allergic anaphylaxis is more common in females
   D. A history of prior drug exposure is essential for allergic anaphylaxis to occur
   E. This is most likely to be allergic anaphylaxis rather than the nonallergic type

9. **A 42-year-old female presents to the Emergency Department experiencing her 'worst headache ever'. She complains of neck stiffness and photophobia. On examination, she has a Glasgow Coma Scale of 14 and appears to be a little confused, with some dysphasia. Her blood pressure is 170/94mmHg. The following are true:**

    A. Most subarachnoid haemorrhages are due to trauma
    B. Subarachnoid haemorrhage accounts for 25% of strokes
    C. She has a World Federation of Neurosurgical Societies (WFNS) severity of subarachnoid haemorrhage grade of five
    D. To ensure adequate cerebral perfusion, her blood pressure should not be lowered
    E. The preferred management is endovascular coiling (if an aneurysm is seen on imaging), as studies demonstrate superior outcomes in term of death and dependence, as well as rebleed risk and need for further treatment

10. **The following are risk factors for acute kidney injury associated with acute illness:**

    A. Age >65 years
    B. Cognitive impairment
    C. Heart failure
    D. Liver disease
    E. Magnetic resonance imaging (MRI) associated use of gadolinium-contrast

11. **The following biochemical abnormalities are found in refeeding syndrome:**

    A. Hypophosphataemia
    B. Hypomagnesaemia
    C. Hyponatraemia
    D. Hypokalaemia
    E. Uraemia

12. **Concerning blood products, the following are true:**

    A. Cryoprecipitate contains significant amounts of factor X
    B. FFP can be stored for a maximum of 180 days
    C. Platelets are stored at 4°C
    D. Red cells can be stored for up to 35 days
    E. The volume of a unit of red cells is around 280mls

13. **Regarding meningitis, the following are true:**

    A. Bacterial infection is the commonest cause
    B. Dexamethasone should be given in cases of bacterial meningitis
    C. In viral meningitis, cerebrospinal fluid (CSF) analysis typically shows an increased lymphocyte count, a raised protein count, and a low glucose
    D. If suspected, initial treatment is with cefotaxime 2g intravenously
    E. Listeria monocytogenes is a commoner cause of meningitis in children, compared to adults

14. **A provisional diagnosis of disseminated intravascular coagulation (DIC) is made in a patient on the intensive care unit (ICU). The following would be true:**
    A. A low platelet count correlates with markers of thrombin generation
    B. A normal plasma fibrinogen may be seen
    C. Antifibrinolytic treatments may be appropriate if the patient is overtly bleeding
    D. DIC may occur in isolation without a predisposing clinical condition
    E. The International Society for Thrombosis and Haemostasis (ISTH) DIC scoring system correlates with mortality

15. **Antibiotic resistance is an increasingly recognized problem in the critically ill patient. The following are true:**
    A. A mechanism by which bacteria acquire resistance, is enzyme production
    B. Cell wall permeability may change in bacteria that have become resistant to a class of antibiotic
    C. First-line management for extended spectrum β-lactamase-producing (ESBL) organisms would include a cephalosporin
    D. Patient mortality increases with infection with vancomycin-resistant enterococci
    E. Transfer of bacterial resistance occurs through mechanisms such as transformation, transduction, and plasmid formation

16. **With regards to pressure control ventilation (PCV), the following are true:**
    A. PCV delivers a constant pressure during the inspiratory phase
    B. PCV allows an assessment of elastic and resistive properties of the lung from observation of pressure trace
    C. PCV is always time cycled
    D. PCV has level one evidence to show superiority to volume control ventilation in patients with ARDS
    e) PCV can be delivered to the patient despite ventilator settings configured in terms of tidal volume

17. **The following are true regarding the Berlin Criteria for ARDS:**
    A. Does not require exclusion of cardiac failure
    B. Requires onset within 10 days of a physiological insult
    C. Requires bilateral opacities consistent with pulmonary oedema on chest radiograph
    D. Requires PaO_2/FiO_2 <300mmHg
    E. The ability to predict mortality using the Berlin definition of ARDS is superior to the previous American-European Consensus Conference definition of *ARDS*

18. **With regards to prone positioning in ARDS, the following are true:**
    A. Alveolar recruitment is a time-dependent phenomenon
    B. A recent trial demonstrated that early application of prolonged prone positioning resulted in a significant reduction of all-cause 28-day and 90-day mortality in ARDS patients
    C. Postpyloric feeding is recommended in prone positioning
    D. Prone positioning improves ventilation via its effect on pleural pressure and lung compression
    E. Spinal instability is a relative contraindication to prone positioning

19. **In critical illness, the delivery and uptake of oxygen by tissues is often abnormal, and for this reason, supplemental oxygen therapy is often required. With regards to oxygen therapy, the following are true:**
    A. At pressures of three atmospheres and FiO_2 1.0, dissolved oxygen is approximately 60ml/ l plasma
    B. Humidification is an essential component of high- and low-flow devices
    C. Hyperbaric oxygen is provided in a sealed chamber at pressures of pressures of 5 atmospheres
    D. Low-flow systems such as the Venturi-type masks provide a constant FiO_2 by delivering gas flows that exceed the patients' peak inspiratory flow rate
    E. The nonrebreather mask is a variable performance high-flow system delivering fractional inspired oxygen concentrations (FiO_2) of up to nearly 1.0

20. **The following antimicrobials are used in selective decontamination of the digestive tract (SDD):**
    A. Cefotaxime to treat overgrowth of 'normal' bacteria such as *Staphylococcal aureus*
    B. Fluconazole to treat gut overgrowth of yeasts
    C. Metronidazole to treat C.difficile
    D. Polymyxin E with tobramycin to treat anaerobes
    E. Vancomycin to treat MRSA

21. **Regarding ventricular assist device (VAD) therapy, the following are true:**
    A. Cardiopulmonary resuscitation may cause VAD catheter displacement
    B. Continuous-flow devices are preferred to pulsatile systems
    C. Insertion requires sternotomy
    D. Left VAD therapy is associated with gastrointestinal haemorrhage
    E. Presence of a VAD is associated with higher incidence of fungal infection

22. **The following are correct regarding cardiovascular criteria for the diagnosis of death:**
    A. Confirmation of the absence of pupillary light reflexes
    B. Invasive arterial pressure monitoring if the patient wishes to be an organ donor
    C. The presence of two doctors at the time of diagnosis
    D. The absence of residual sedative medication
    E. Three minutes of asystole

23. According to UK advanced life support resuscitation guidelines, the following should occur during a paediatric cardiac arrest:

A. Adrenaline should be given 1ml/kg of 1:10000 solution

B. Cardiopulmonary resuscitation should commence with 5 initial breaths and then at a rate of 15:2

C. For an infant, defibrillator pad size should be 4.5cm and applied just below the right clavicle and midaxillary line

D. If using an automated external defibrillator (AED), an adult shock energy can be selected for a child older than 6 years old

E. Nonshockable rhythms are more common findings in paediatric arrest

24. Care bundles are frequently used within the intensive care unit. The following are true:

A. A key principle for success is high levels of adherence

B. Audit of care bundles routinely measure how well interventions are performed

C. Care bundles comprise three to five evidence-based interventions, which, when used together, have a better outcome than when used individually

D. Care bundles provide a means of assessing quality of care

E. Components of a care bundle must be supported by high grades of evidence

25. A 65-year-old patient is receiving intravenous heparin on intensive care 6 days after a laparotomy and bowel resection for ischaemic small bowel. Their platelet count falls from 230 to 50. The following are true:

A. Alternative anticoagulation is necessary

B. Fondaparinux would be a reasonable alternative anticoagulant

C. Heparin-induced thrombocytopaenia (HIT) is likely

D. Heparin should be continued until discussion with the consultant surgeon

E. If a diagnosis of HIT is confirmed then, after 3 days, warfarin should be considered

26. Which of the following statements regarding levosimendan are true:

A. It is an inodilator

B. It is instigated with a bolus dose followed by a continuous infusion

C. It is metabolized by the liver to inactive metabolites

D. It has no effect on diastolic dysfunction

E. It has little effect on myocardial oxygen demand

27. In Wolff-Parkinson-White (WPW) syndrome, the following are correct:

A. PR interval is prolonged

B. QRS complex is widened

C. T wave inversion may be seen

D. The most common arrhythmia is atrial fibrillation (AF)

E. Theta waves are pathognomonic ECG findings

28. In alcoholic liver disease (ALD), the following are true:

A. Alcoholic hepatitis presents with jaundice, tender hepatomegaly, and fever
B. Male patients with ALD have a worse outcome
C. There are three histological subtypes
D. The risk of ALD depends on the type of alcohol consumed
E. The majority of heavy drinkers develop cirrhosis

29. A 37-year-old pregnant female presents with a type 1 respiratory failure. She has a 4 day history of feeling feverish, with myalgia, cough, and headache. The following are true:

A. Influenza infection has been associated with paralysis
B. Influenza B causes similar morbidity and mortality as influenza A
C. Risks for complicated influenza include diabetes, pregnancy, and morbid obesity (BMI >40 kg/m^2)
D. Therapy should include oseltamivir 75mg bd, once viral PCR results confirm influenza
E. Zanamivir can be administered via nebulizer or intravenously

30. It is correct that the following are all recognized causes of low sodium:

A. Congestive cardiac failure
B. Cerebral salt wasting syndrome
C. Lithium
D. Multiple myeloma
E. Syndrome of inappropriate antidiuretic hormone (SIADH)

Question 1 F T F F F

Near-drowning is defined as initial survival following immersion in liquid. Subsequent death may follow the consequences of aspiration of water into the lungs, or subsequent to complication from hypothermia. Cold shock reflexes after immersion into cold water increase respiratory drive. Peripheral vasoconstriction and tachycardia increase cardiac output. As you submerge under water, the diving reflex can occur. This is mediated by the ophthalmic division of the trigeminal nerve and leads to apnoea, bradycardia, and peripheral vasoconstriction. When breath holding is overcome, involuntary gasping occurs, leading to aspiration and laryngospasm. Ventricular fibrillation occurs at temperatures <28°C, and bradycardia and asystole at temperatures <24–26°C. Temperatures between 32–34°C can be associated with an impaired level of consciousness and brain-stem reflexes tend to be lost if the temperature falls below 28°C. These deficits are potentially reversible. Core temperature should be greater than 34°C before death can be confirmed.

Academy of the Medical Royal Colleges. *A code of practice for the diagnosis and confirmation of death.* London, 2008. www. aomrc.org.uk/reports.aspx [accessed 26 July 2021].

Question 2 F F F F F

Venous thromboembolism resulting in 30%–50% occlusion of the pulmonary artery leads to an abrupt increase in pulmonary vascular resistance. In turn, this leads to a rapid increase in right ventricular afterload, and acute right ventricular failure, which results in hypotension and significant dead space. In patients with a patent foramen ovale (up to one third of the adult population), a right-to-left shunt will also be present.

The classic triad of haemoptysis, pleuritic chest pain, and shortness of breath occurs in a minority of patients, although symptoms can vary, and can include tachycardia, tachypnoea, fever, chest pain, or syncope.

The 'severity' of the PE is defined in terms of the risk of early (30 day) mortality. This is considered high (>15%) in patients with hypotension and shock; intermediate (3%–15%) in those with right ventricle dysfunction and, or myocardial injury, but without hypotension; and low (<3%) in those with no clinical features of shock and right ventricular dysfunction or myocardial injury. Clearly clinical presentation will alter with the burden of emboli and location; however, for example, mortality is not necessarily increased in patients with saddle embolus.

The Wells score is used to estimate the clinical probability of PE. The PESI is a clinical tool used to stratify risk of 30 day mortality once the diagnosis of PE has been made. It takes into account clinical severity of the acute event and the comorbidity of the patient, and the subsequent score puts the patient into one of five categories (classes III–V are high risk).

An echocardiogram is only the investigation of choice in PE associated with syncope and hypotension, where the patient is too unstable for a computer tomography pulmonary angiogram.

The Task Force for the Diagnosis and Management of Acute Pulmonary Embolism of the European Society of Cardiology (ESC). Guidelines on the diagnosis and management of acute pulmonary embolism. *European Heart Journal* 2008;29:2276–315.

Pathak R, Giri S, Aryal M. Comparison between saddle versus non-saddle pulmonary embolism: insights from nationwide inpatient sample. *Blood* 2014;124:3514.

Question 3 F F T T T

While ICP monitoring does not confer a direct mortality benefit, there are several advantages associated with using it (it may be the first indication of worsening pathology), and protocols incorporating ICP data tend towards improved patient outcomes. The Foramen of Munroe is the standard reference point, but for simplicity the external auditory meatus can be used.

Microtransducer monitors are subject to drift, but cannot be recalibrated once in situ. Lundberg 'A' waves are always pathological and represent early herniation.

Smith M. Monitoring intracranial pressure in traumatic brain injury. Anesthesia & Analgesia 2008 Jan;106(1):240–8.

Chesnut RM, et al. A trial of intracranial-pressure monitoring in traumatic brain injury. *New England Journal of Medicine.*2012 Dec 27;367(26):2471–81.

Question 4 F F F T F

The QT interval represents the time taken for ventricular depolarization *and* repolarization. It is normally <440ms, and the QT interval is inversely proportional to heart rate. The corrected QT interval (QT$_c$) estimates the QT interval at a heart rate of 60 beats per minute.

A QT <350ms is abnormally short and may also predispose to ventricular arrhythmia. QT$_c$ >440ms (men) and >460ms (women) is prolonged and increases risk of ventricular arrhythmia (increased risk with QT$_c$ >500ms). Hypokalaemia is associated with prolonged QT, as are a number of drugs. Similarly myocardial disease and genetic cardiac ion channel mutations can also increase QT duration.

Hampton J. *The ECG made easy*, 7th edition. London: Churchill Livingstone, 2008.

Question 5 F T F T F

GBS is an acute demyelinating peripheral polyneuropathy, with several subtypes, and is characterized by a progressive ascending symmetrical weakness evolving over a few days. It is associated with the formation of auto-antibodies (following an infectious agent), which produce characteristic demyelination. Often distal paraesthesia, pain, and numbness occur early, with progression to respiratory muscle and autonomic involvement. Reflexes are diminished or absent.

GBS may be preceded by a recognized flu-like illness or gastroenteritis (66% cases), although the causative agent may not always be identified. *Campylobacter jejuni*, *Mycoplasma pneumoniae*, CMV, EBV, and HIV have all been implicated.

GBS is more common in males and is managed with supportive care and immunotherapy in the form of either plasma exchange or intravenous immunoglobulin. Corticosteroids are ineffective.

Richards K, Cohen A. Guillain-Barre syndrome. *Continuing Education in Anaesthesia, Critical Care & Pain* 2003;3:46–9.

Question 6 F F T F F

The eighth report into the Confidential Enquiries into Maternal Deaths highlights the importance of early recognition of sepsis in pregnancy, which was the leading cause of direct deaths between 2006–2008. However the more recent surveillance 2015–2017 highlights thrombosis and thromboembolism as the leading cause of direct maternal death during and up to 6 weeks after the end of pregnancy.

Genital tract sepsis commonly arises from community-acquired β haemolytic streptococcus Lancefield Group A. Group A Strep (GAS) can be carried on the skin, or in the throat, and GAS should be considered in all mothers who report sore throat and or flu-like illness. The most common organisms identified in pregnant women dying from sepsis are Lancefield Group A beta-haemolytic streptococcus and *E.coli*.

Maternal sepsis often has an insidious course with nonspecific symptoms, and can present late, with a delay in appropriate antibiotics resulting in collapse and death. Persistent tachycardia, hypotension, abdominal pain, diarrhoea, and vomiting should all trigger a low threshold for observation (using Modified Early Obstetric Warning Scores). Other clinical features, including rash, PV discharge, cough, and urinary symptoms, need to be considered.

If sepsis is suspected, blood cultures, vaginal and throat swabs, and urine samples may all be taken to help identify the cause. Broad-spectrum antibiotics should be given within 1 hour of recognition of sepsis. Co-amoiclav does not cover MRSA or *Pseudomonas*, and there is concern about an increase in the risk of necrotizing enterocolitis in neonates exposed to co-amoxiclav in utero. Piperacillin with tazobactam provides good cover (except for MRSA). Intravenous immunoglobulin (IVIG) is recommended for severe invasive streptococcal or staphylococcal infection if other therapies have failed. IVIG has an immunomodulatory effect, and in staphylococcal and streptococcal sepsis, it also neutralizes the superantigen effect of exotoxins, and inhibits production of tumour necrosis factor and interleukins. The Department of Health has recommendations regarding the use of IVIG for invasive streptococcal and staphylococcal infection.

Royal College of Obstetricians and Gynaecologists. *Sepsis in pregnancy, bacterial (Green-top Guideline No. 64a)*. https://www.rcog.org.uk/en/guidelines-research-services/guidelines/gtg64a/ [accessed 26 July 2021].

MBRRACE-UK. Mothers and babies: reducing risk through audits and confidential enquiries across the UK. https://www.npeu.ox.ac.uk/assets/downloads/mbrrace-uk/reports/MBRRACE-UK%20 Maternal%20Report%202019%20-%20WEB%20VERSION.pdf [accessed 26 July 2021].

Question 7 T F F T F

Nonselective beta-blockers remain the drug of choice in prophylaxis against variceal bleeding. They reduce cardiac output and induce splanchnic vasoconstriction and thus reduce portal pressure. Isosorbide mononitrate used alone, or in combination with beta-blockers, does not seem to reduce bleeding, and may result in a greater number of side effects.

Endoscopic variceal ligation (EVL) is also effective, as prophylaxis against variceal bleeding. Although the frequency of adverse effects of EVL is small, their severity is greater. Choice between nonselective beta blockade and EVL therefore depends on patient characteristics, together with local resources.

Antibiotics should be instituted on admission to prevent bacterial infections and or spontaneous bacterial peritonitis. Infection occurs in 33%–66% patients with cirrhosis and gastrointestinal bleeds.

Endoscopy should be done as soon as possible after admission, ideally within 12 hours, and especially in patients with clinically significant bleeding, or patients with features suggesting cirrhosis. Vasoconstrictor treatment should be maintained for 3–5 days. Terlipressin has an improved side-effect profile and can be given as a bolus.

Tripathi D, Stanley AJ, Hayes PC UK guidelines on the management of variceal haemorrhage in cirrhotic patients. *Gut* 2015;64:1680–704.

Question 8 F T T F T

Allergic anaphylaxis describes an immunological reaction (IgG, IgE, or complement mediated), with antibody formation occurring on exposure to antigen. Antibody-mediated mast cell degranulation and release of mediators (histamine, tryptase, leukotrienes, and prostaglandins) subsequently occurs, producing the characteristic clinical features.

In contrast, in nonallergic anaphylaxis, mast cell and basophil activation are caused by direct drug action, with no immune trigger. Clinically, however, they are indistinguishable.

Allergic anaphylaxis has an incidence of between 1:5000–1:20,000, with a female preponderance and a mortality of between 3%–6%. Prior drug exposure is not necessary, but a prior history of atopy, asthma, and environmental exposure (with toiletries, detergents, and fruit all exhibiting cross-reactivity) may be helpful.

Approximately 60% of anaesthesia-related anaphylaxis is thought to be due to neuromuscular blocking drugs. Suxamethonium is most likely to be associated with allergic anaphylaxis. Atracurium and mivacurium are associated with nonallergic anaphylaxis. Cisatracurium, although sharing a benzylisoquinolinium structure, is not associated with nonallergic anaphylaxis, although several cases of allergic anaphylaxis have been reported.

Mast cell tryptase has a half-life of 2 hours, peaking at 1 hour after onset of reaction. Relative concentrations are often more helpful than absolute levels, and a normal level does not exclude anaphylaxis.

Ryder SA, Waldmann C. Anaphylaxis. *Continuing Education In Anaesthesia, Critical Care & Pain* 2004;4:111–13.

Mills A, Sice P, Ford S. Anaesthesia-related anaphylaxis :investigation and follow up. *Continuing Education In Anaesthesia, Critical Care & Pain* 2014;14:57–62.

AAGBI Safety Guideline. Suspected anaphylactic reactions associated with anaesthesia. *Anaesthesia* 2009;64:199–211.

Question 9 F F F F F

Subarachnoid haemorrhage (SAH) accounts for only 5% of strokes, but is a major cause of mortality and morbidity. SAH can be congenital or acquired, and intracranial aneurysms account for 85% of all SAH. Other causes include arterio-venous malformation and trauma. Hypertension, smoking, and cocaine all increase the risk.

There are a number of grading scales to help direct management and prognosis, and the WFNS grading system uses the Glasgow Coma Scale and presence or absence of focal neurological deficits to grade the severity of subarachnoid haemorrhage.

- Grade 1: GCS 15, no motor deficit
- Grade 2: GCS 13–14, without deficit
- Grade 3: GCS 13–14, with focal neurological deficit
- Grade 4: GCS 7–12, with or without deficit
- Grade 5: GCS <7, with or without deficit

While it is paramount to avoid hypotension, the risk of rebleeding in an unsecured aneurysm increases with higher BP; therefore, it is prudent to lower the systolic pressure to <160mmHg and ensure MAP <110mmHg.

Endovascular coiling is the preferred management, as death and disability outcomes have been shown to be superior. However there is a longer term risk of rebleeding, and the need for delayed retreatment is higher.

Molyneux AJ, et al; for the ISAT collaborators. Risk of recurrent subarachnoid haemorrhage, death or dependence, and standardised mortality ratios after clipping or coiling of an intracranial aneurysm in the International Subarachnoid Aneurysm Trial: long-term follow up. *Lancet Neurology* 2009;8:427–33.

Question 10 T T T T T

The National Institute for Health and Care Excellence (NICE) guideline on acute kidney injury identifies a number of risk factors, including chronic kidney disease, diabetes, heart failure, liver disease, and sepsis. Patient age is also an independent risk factor with those aged older than 65 years at higher risk. Patients with cognitive or neurological deficit may be at higher risk of dehydration due to reliance on assistance. Gadolinium is widely employed as a contrast agent for MRI and has generally been considered to be safe. However as with iodinated radiocontrast, concern for contrast-induced nephropathy does exist with gadolinium-contrast, as it possesses many similar qualities (e.g. it is hyperosmolar and undergoes renal excretion via glomerular filtration). It has also been implicated in a rare condition known as nephrogenic systemic fibrosis.

National Institute for Health and Care Excellence. *Acute kidney injury: prevention, detection and management of acute kidney injury up to the point of renal replacement therapy.* (Clinical guideline 169) 2013. https://pubmed.ncbi.nlm.nih.gov/25340231/ [accessed 4 July 2021].

Perazella M. Gadolinium-contrast toxicity in patients with kidney disease: nephrotoxicity and nephrogenic systemic fibrosis. *Current Drug Safety* 2008;3:67–75.

Question 11 TTFTF

A cardinal feature of refeeding syndrome is hypophosphataemia, thought to occur secondary to the re-establishment of ATP-dependent metabolic pathways with the subsequent demand for phosphate. Hypokalaemia and hypomagnesaemia are also seen, with the switch from fat to carbohydrate metabolism. Reintroduction of carbohydrate metabolism also results in retention of sodium, which can lead to fluid overload and pulmonary oedema, especially as a starved individual may have depleted cardiac muscle mass. In addition thiamine levels will fall dramatically as there will be uptake into the Krebs cycle. Uraemia does not typically occur.

National Institute for Health and Clinical Excellence. *Nutrition support in adults Clinical guideline* CG32. 2006 https://www.nice.org.uk/guidance/cg32/documents/nutrition-support-in-adults-clinical-guideline-first-consultation-nice-guideline2 [accessed 26 July 2021].

Question 12 F F F T T

Platelets are stored at room temperature (20–24°C), and so have a higher risk of bacterial contamination, with a shelf life of 5 days. Fresh frozen plasma is stored at −30°C, and can be kept for up to 2 years. Red cells are stored at 2–6°C, for up to 35 days. The volume of each unit varies, but averages 280mls. Cryoprecipitate contains mainly Factor VIII, von Willebrand factor, and fibrinogen.

Joint United Kingdom Blood Transfusion and Tissue Transplantation Services Professional Advisory Committee. *Transfusion handbook*, 5th edition. 2014. http://www.transfusionguidelines.org.uk/transfusion-handbook/3-providing-safe-blood/3-3-blood-products [accessed 26 July 2021].

Question 13 F T F T F

Viral meningitis is the most common form of infective meningitis, and CSF analysis typically shows increased lymphocytes, slightly raised protein, and a normal glucose. Listeria monocytogenes is more commonly seen in neonates and older patients (>55 years). Cefotaxime is used as a first-line medication, and ampicillin 2g should be added if at risk of listeria monocytogenes. Dexamethasone at a dose of 0.15mg/kg should be given with the first dose of antibiotics, and every 6 hours subsequently.

Meningitis (bacterial) and meningococcal septicaemia in under 16s: recognition, diagnosis, and management. Clinical Guideline 102. https://www.nice.org.uk/guidance/cg102/evidence [accessed 26 July 2021].

Question 14 T T F F T

DIC never occurs in isolation, and recognizing that a patient has a clinical disorder which may result in the development of DIC is the key to appropriate investigation and management. DIC may arise in patients with a wide spectrum of disorders including sepsis, malignancy, trauma, and complications relating to pregnancy.

DIC is characterized by activation of the coagulation cascade, leading to massive fibrin generation and clot production, which may in turn lead to organ failure through localized thrombosis. Concomitant consumption of platelets and coagulation factors may then lead to bleeding.

Fibrinogen levels will often fall. However as fibrinogen is an acute phase protein, levels may remain normal for some time after the DIC process has started.

Treatment should always be directed at the underlying mechanism. Platelets should be given if the patient is bleeding, and the platelet count is <50 × 10⁹/l. Treatment with products (e.g. fresh frozen plasma and cryoprecipitate) should be based on the clinical picture as well as laboratory test results. Fibrin deposition is a key factor in DIC, and, therefore, inhibition of fibrinolysis is not recommended.

The International Society for Thrombosis and Haemostasis (ISTH) DIC scoring system provides objective measurement of DIC. A strong correlation between an increasing DIC score and mortality has been demonstrated by several studies.

The International Society for Thrombosis and Haemostasis (ISTH) DIC scoring system

Risk assessment:

- Does the patient have an underlying disorder known to be associated with overt DIC?

If yes, proceed:

Order global coagulation tests (prothrombin time, platelet count, fibrinogen, fibrin related marker)

Score the test results:

- Platelet count (>100 × 10 ^{9}/l = 0, <100 × 10⁹/l = 1, <50 × 10⁹/l = 2)
- Elevated Fibrin marker (i.e. D-dimer (no increase = 0, moderate increase = 1, strong increase = 2))
- Prolonged PT (<3s = 0, 3-6s = 1, >6s = 2)
- Fibrinogen level (>1 g/l = 0, <1 g/l = 1)

Calculate score:

- ≥5 compatible with overt DIC, repeat score daily

Guidelines for the diagnosis and management of disseminated intravascular coagulation. *British Journal of Haematology* ;145:24–33.

Question 15 T T F F T

Mechanisms by which bacteria acquire resistance include enzyme production (e.g. extended spectrum β-Lactamase-producing (ESBL) organisms), target site modification, structural changes to cell walls, active expulsion of antibiotic molecules, and formation of alternative metabolic pathways (e.g. MRSA).

Resistance is reliant on mutation and intercell transfer, which can be undertaken by transformation (uptake of naked DNA by bacteria), transduction (viral infection of bacteria), and plasmid formation (circles of DNA within bacteria but distinct from their chromosomes).

Vancomycin-resistant enterococci have increased, and their effect is not thought to increase mortality directly (isolates are no more virulent but more difficult to eliminate). Carbapenems are the most active against ESBL bacteria.

Barley AJ, Williams H, Fletcher S. Antibiotics resistance in the intensive care unit. *Continuing Education In Anaesthesia, Critical Care & Pain* 2009;9:114–18.

Question 16 T F T F T

Pressure control ventilation does apply a constant pressure during inspiration, as such, the airway pressure trace does not allow assessment of airway resistance or pulmonary elastance. PCV is always time cycled. Whilst there is evidence to support low- (6ml/kg ideal body weight) volume ventilation and plateau pressure minimization (<30cm H_2O), there is no consensus on, or evidence for, superiority of different ventilation modes. Various manufactures provide the ability to set a tidal volume but deliver gas flow in a pressure control manner (terms vary with manufacturer but include VC + and Autoflow).

Gattinoni L, Caironi P. Refining ventilatory treatment for acute lung injury and acute respiratory distress syndrome. *Journal of the American Medical Association* 2008;299:691–3.

Question 17 T F F T F

Onset should be within 7 days of a defined insult. Bilateral opacities can be identified on chest x-ray or computed tomography scan. Cardiac failure no longer needs excluding; instead, respiratory failure needs to be 'not *fully* explained by cardiac failure or fluid overload'.

PaO_2/FiO_2 200–300mmHg (on 5cm H_2O PEEP) is mild ARDS, 100–200 is moderate and <100 is severe. The increased power of the new Berlin definition to predict mortality compared to the American-European Concensus Conference (AECC) definition, in truth, is still poor, with an area under the curve of only 0.577, compared to 0.536 for the old definition.

The ARDS Definition Task Force. Acute respiratory distress syndrome: the Berlin definition. *Journal of the American Medical Association* 2012;307(23):2526–33.

Question 18 T T T T F

ARDS is a complex condition affecting critically ill patients, resulting from direct or indirect lung injury. Prone positioning has been proposed as a potential option for treatment of acute lung injury and ARDS.

The main physiological aims of prone positioning are: i) to improve oxygenation; ii) to improve respiratory mechanics; iii) to homogenize the pleural pressure gradient, the alveolar inflation, and the ventilation distribution; iv) to increase lung volume and reduce the amount of atelectatic regions; v) to facilitate the drainage of secretions; and vi) to reduce ventilator-associated lung injury.

In 2013, the Proning Severe ARDS Patients (PROSEVA) trial randomly assigned 466 patients with severe ARDS in European ICUs to early (<36 hours after intubation), lengthy (goal 16 hours daily), or intermittent prone positioning, or to a standard supine position. *Severe ARDS* was defined as a P:F ratio of <150mmHg with FiO_2 >60% and PEEP ≥5cm H_2O. At 28 days, the prone group had a 51% relative and 17% absolute reduction in all-cause mortality when compared to the supine group (16.0% vs 32.8%; NNT 6). Importantly, PROSEVA incorporated low-tidal ventilation and therapeutic paralysis, suggesting that prone positioning confers a survival benefit beyond that seen with the standard of care.

Spinal instability is considered as an absolute contraindication. Enteral feeding is possible and preferred with prone positioning. To avoid complications associated with enteral feeding, postpyloric feedings, or promotility agents are recommended to prevent aspiration.

Guérin C, et al. Prone positioning in severe acute respiratory distress syndrome. *New England Journal of Medicine* 2013;368(23):2159–68.

Question 19 T F F F F

Supplemental oxygen therapy can be divided into low-flow devices and high-flow devices. Low-flow devices can be further subdivided into variable performance devices (e.g. nasal cannulae, Hudson face masks, and nonrebreather masks) or fixed performance devices (e.g. Venturi-type masks). High-flow systems, which are generally not ubiquitous throughout hospital wards, provide a constant FiO_2 by delivering gas at flow rates that exceed the patient's peak inspiratory flow rate (and they entrain a fixed proportion of room air). High-flow systems require humidification, but low-flow systems are frequently used in the absence of humidification.

The hypoxic patient often has increased inspiratory flow and loss of the respiratory pause. Thus, with a low-flow device, the patient's inspiratory effort will exceed oxygen flow rate, draining the reservoir and entraining room air, which reduces the delivered oxygen concentration.

Hyperbaric oxygen is provided at 2–3 atmospheres, and at 3 atmospheres it has the ability to dissolve oxygen up to 60ml/l in plasma, which is almost sufficient to supply the resting total oxygen requirement. In contrast, at 1 atmosphere, dissolved plasma oxygen concentration is only 3ml/l plasma.

Leach RM, Rees P, Wilmshurst P. Hyperbaric oxygen therapy. *British Medical Journal* 2008;24:1140–3.

Question 20 T F F F T

Antimicrobials used in SDD are:

- Cefotaxime, to treat overgrowth of 'normal' flora (*S.pneumoniae, H.influenzae, E.coli, and S.aureus*)
- Amphotericin B, to treat overgrowth of yeasts (e.g. C.albicans)
- Polymixin E with tobramycin, to treat aerobic Gram-negative bacilli (Klebsiella, Enterobacter, Citrobacter, Proteus, Morganella, Serratia, Acinetobacter, and Pseudomonas)
- Vancomycin, to treat MRSA

Silvestri L, Cal MA de la, Saene HKF van. Selective decontamination of the digestive tract: the mechanism of action is control of gut overgrowth. *Intensive Care Medicine* 2012;38(11):1738–50.

Question 21 T T F T T

Continuous-flow devices have been demonstrated to be superior to pulsatile systems in freedom from stroke or reoperation and in survival. LVAD therapy is associated with gastrointestinal haemorrhage, both as a result of anticoagulant therapy and independent of such treatments.

Manufacturers recommend avoidance of CPR, if possible, as ventricular or aortic cannulae may be displaced.

Transcatheter percutaneous devices are appearing on the market, such as the Abiomed Impella® device.

Chronic immune activation can cause immunosuppression and sensitivity to fungal infection.

Pagani FD, et al. Extended mechanical circulatory support with a continuous-flow rotary left ventricular assist device. *Journal of the American College of Cardiology* 2009;54:312–21.

Suarez J, Patel CB, Felker GM, Becker R, Hernandez AF, Rogers JG. Mechanisms of bleeding and approach to patients with axial-flow left ventricular assist devices. *Circulation and Heart Failure* 2011 Nov;4(6):779–84.

Holman WL, et al. Infection in ventricular assist devices: prevention and treatment. *The Annals of Thoracic Surgery* 2003;75(6 Suppl):S48–S57.

Question 22 T F F F F

Cardiovascular criteria, for the diagnosis of death, are outlined by the Academy of Royal Colleges 'A code of practice for the diagnosis and confirmation of death'. Death may be diagnosed after a continuous 5 minute period of cardio-respiratory arrest in patient in whom resuscitation has failed or deemed not appropriate. The absence of mechanical cardiac function may be confirmed by the absence of a central pulse on palpation or the absence of heart sounds on auscultation. In hospital settings this is usually supplemented with asystole on a continuous ECG monitor, a lack of pulsatile flow on invasive arterial pressure monitoring or the absence of contractile activity on continuous echocardiography.

Any return of spontaneous cardiac or respiratory activity should prompt another period of observation from the next point of cardio-respiratory arrest. After 5 minutes of no cardiac or respiratory activity, the absence of a pupillary response to light, of corneal reflex, and of motor response to supra orbital pressure should be confirmed. Death can be diagnosed by a registered medical practitioner or other appropriately trained and qualified individual.

Academy of Medical Royal Colleges. *A code of practice for the diagnosis and confirmation of death.* 2008. http://www.aomrc.org.uk/doc_view/42-a-code-of-practice-for-the-diagnosis-and-confirmation-of-death [accessed 12 June 2014].

Question 23 F T T F T

According to the Resuscitation Council (UK) Guidelines 2015, secondary arrests caused by respiratory failure or circulatory failure are more common than primary arrests caused by arrhythmia, and non shockable rhythms predominate. Five initial breaths followed by cardiopulmonary resuscitation at a ratio of 15:2 and at a compression rate of 100–120 should be commenced while the defibrillator paddles are attached under the right clavicle and in the midaxillary line. Once the child is intubated, compressions can be continuous with a respiratory rate of 10–12 breaths per minute. Adrenaline is given 10mcg/kg (0.1ml/kg of 1:10000 solution) every 3–5 minutes. Using an AED, an adult shock can be selected for children over 8 years. In patients younger than 8 years old, use a paediatric attenuated shock or, if using a manual defibrillator, use energy 4J/kg.

Resuscitation Council (UK). *Paediatric advanced life support.* 2015. www.resus.org.uk/resuscitation-guidelines/paediatric-advanced-life-support (accessed 2nd September 2019).

Question 24 T F T T F

Care bundles were developed over 20 years ago and provide a means of assessing quality of care. The care bundle is a valuable tool for audit, but this assesses the delivery of interventions rather than how well these interventions are performed. Care bundles consist of three to five evidence-based interventions. Ideally the grade of evidence should be high for each specific intervention; however, frequently many components arise from lower levels of evidence and expert opinion. This means that bundles should constantly be reappraised and updated. Adherence to all interventions is mandatory for success.

Horner DL, Bellamy MC. Care bundles in intensive care. Continuing Education In Anaesthesia, Critical Care & Pain 2012;12(4):199–202.

Question 25 T T T F F

The 4T's HIT score estimates the probability of HIT, based on its characteristic features. Points are allocated as in Table 3.1. A score of 0–3 is unlikely to be HIT; 4–5 makes HIT likely; and 6–8 makes HIT highly likely.

The description given matches a patient with a 4T score of at least 4, as such heparin should be stopped immediately, and alternative anticoagulation started. Fondaparinux is a logical alternative, but controlled trials do not exist, however.

Warfarin should be considered, especially in patients with thrombosis, although not before 7 days, though, as a paradoxical worsening can occur. It is important to bear in mind the other myriad causes of thrombocytopaenia seen in critical care.

Table 3.1 The 4 Ts Clinical Scoring System for HIT

Category	2 Points	1 Point	0 Points
Thrombocytopaenia	Greater than 50% fall or nadir of 20–100×10^9/l	30%–50% fall or nadir 10–19×10^9/l	Less than 30% fall or nadir less than 10×10^9/l
Timing of platelet count fall	5–10 days or <1 day with recent (30 days) previous exposure	Beyond day 10 or <1 day if previous exposure in last 30–100 days	No recent heparin use
Thrombosis or other sequelae	Proven thrombosis after injection	Progressive or recurrent thrombosis	None
Other causes	None	Possible	Definite

Hall A, Thachil J, Martlew V. Heparin-induced thrombocytopaenia in the intensive care unit. *Journal of the Intensive Care Society* 2010;11(1):20–5.

Question 26 T T F F T

Levosimendan is a calcium channel sensitizer that has inodilator effects without increasing intracellular calcium concentrations and without increasing myocardial oxygen demand. It improves systolic and diastolic dysfunction. The half-life is approximately 1.3 hours with two active metabolites, both of which with much longer half-lives. Treatment is with a 10-minutes loading bolus followed by infusion.

Waldmann C, Soni N, Rhodes A (eds). *Oxford desk reference: critical care*, 1st edition. Oxford: Oxford University Press, 2008.

Question 27 F T T F F

In patients with WPW, pre-excitation occurs along accessory pathway causing shortening of PR interval, delta waves (slurred and broadened QRS complexes), and occasional abnormal repolarization (T wave changes). Arrhythmias tend to be atrioventricular tachycardias (AVRT)— orthodromic (most common) or antidromic (least common). Although AF occurs more commonly in patients with WPW syndrome than in normal individuals, it is less common than orthodromic AVRTs.

Stouffer GA. *Practical ECG interpretation: clues to heart disease in young adults.* Chichester: Wiley-Blackwell, 2009.

Question 28 T T T F F

Steatosis (accumulation of lipid within liver cells), alcoholic hepatitis (ethanol metabolism and generation of free oxygen radicals promoting inflammation), and cirrhosis (longstanding hepatocellular damage and collagen deposition with fibrosis) are the three histological subtypes.

Acute hepatitis may indeed present with jaundice, fever, and hepatomegaly. Chronic signs of increased alcohol intake may include palmar erythema, spider naevi, and in the presence of portal hypertension, ascites, splenomegaly, and caput medusae. The single biggest risk factor is the quantity of alcohol ingested, irrespective of what form it takes. Other risk factors include hepatitis C infection and obesity. For reasons not well-established, only 8%–20% of heavy drinkers will develop cirrhosis. Obesity and Hepatitis C are also risk factors for development of ALD. Alcohol-related deaths are twice as frequent in males; however, the incidence is increasing in both sexes.

Jackson P, Gleeson D. Alcoholic liver disease. *Continuing Education In Anaesthesia, Critical Care & Pain* 2010;10:66–71.

Question 29 T F T F T

Influenza A, B, and C are RNA viruses. The three types have many strains depending on antigenic differences. Type A is the cause of worldwide pandemics (e.g. H1N1 swine flu pandemic in 2009). Types B and C tend to produce milder disease. Influenza tends to present with nonspecific symptoms of fever, headache, cough, sore throat, arthralgia, and myalgia. Risks for complicated disease (hospital admission, lower respiratory tract or neurological involvement) include chronic disease, diabetes, immunosuppression, age >65 years, pregnancy, and morbid obesity. First-line treatment is oseltamivir, and this should be commenced if influenza is suspected before confirmation with test results. Zanamivir should be started in those patients with severe immunosuppression. It is normally inhaled but can be nebulized or given intravenously (unlicensed). Complications of influenza include secondary bacterial infection but also neurological complications such as encephalitis and GBS (leading to paralysis).

Johnston C, Hall A, Hart I. Common viral illnesses in intensive care: presentation, diagnosis, and management. *Continuing Education In Anaesthesia, Critical Care & Pain* 2014;14:213–19.

Question 30 T T F T T

All can lead to low sodium except for lithium. Multiple myeloma can lead to a pseudohyponatraemia as there are elevated levels of immunoglobulins. Lithium can result in nephrogenic diabetes insipidus, which results in hypernatraemia.

Rassam S, Counsell D. Perioperative electrolyte and fluid balance. *Continuing Education in Anaesthesia, Critical Care & Pain* 2005;5:157–60.

paper
4

MCQ QUESTIONS

1. **A 45-year-old man has sustained significant injuries following a road traffic accident. The following are true:**
   A. Fluid responders should be managed with urgent surgery, and this takes priority over invasive lines or completion of the secondary survey
   B. *Major trauma* is defined as an injury severity score >15
   C. There is evidence to use of recombinant Factor VII with continued bleeding
   D. Tranexamic acid should be given as early as possible
   E. Transfusion of fresh frozen plasma (FFP) should occur once the prothrombin time (PT) and activated partial thromboplastin time (APTT) >1.5 × normal

2. **Regarding cardiac output monitoring using a pulmonary artery catheter (PAC), the following are true:**
   A. A thermocouple is used to detect temperature changes
   B. Cardiac output can be directly measured
   C. PAC tip position in West Zone III can be confirmed by a lateral chest x-ray
   D. Systemic vascular resistance can be directly measured
   E. The Stewart-Hamilton equation is used to calculate cardiac output

3. **The following statements regarding β-haemolytic Group A streptococci are true:**
   A. It is a Gram-positive rod
   B. It may be found on asymptomatic carriers in the throat, or on the skin, in up to 30% of the population
   C. It may lead to scarlet fever, which is a notifiable disease
   D. It directly causes rheumatic fever, which is a notifiable disease
   E. It results in high levels of neonatal death

4. **With regards to fulminant acute liver failure, the following are true:**
   A. All patients should be given prophylactic antibiotics
   B. Arterial blood lactate measurement rapidly identifies patients who will die from paracetamol-induced acute liver failure
   C. If coagulopathy is present, FFP should be given
   D. Portal vein thrombosis is a cause of acute liver failure
   E. Subacute liver failure is diagnosed if the time from the onset of jaundice to encephalopathy is between 7 days and 4 weeks

MCQs and SBAs in Intensive Care Medicine. Lorna Eyre and Andrew Bodenham, Oxford University Press. © Oxford University Press 2021.
DOI: 10.1093/oso/9780198753056.003.0004

5.   A 55-year-old patient presents to A&E with a history of painful rash, fever, cough, and general malaise. On examination, the patient has a heart rate of 100 beats per minute, a blood pressure of 85/45mmHg and has a widespread erythematous rash, involving the mucus membranes and covering >50% of the body surface area. Areas of the rash have become blisters, and there is evidence of epidermal detachment. The following are true:

   A. Diagnosis is most likely Staphylococcal scalded skin syndrome
   B. Diagnosis is most likely Stevens-Johnson syndrome
   C. Most causes are idiopathic
   D. Mortality relates to a secondary septic insult
   E. Steroids can be used to manage the skin manifestation

6.   Complications following massive blood transfusion may include the following:

   A. Dilutional coagulopathy
   B. Hypoxaemia
   C. Hypothermia
   D. Hyperthermia
   E. Increase in ionized calcium levels

7.   In the assessment of community-acquired pneumonia, which of the following are true?

   A. Mortality risk increases in those older than 65 years old
   B. Mortality is 15% of a CURB65 pneumonia score 3
   C. The mini-mental test is used to assess severity of pneumonia
   D. The use of moxifloxacin increases the risk of MRSA
   E. Urine can be used to detect Legionella and Mycoplasma pneumonia

8.   An 18-year-old patient is admitted to the intensive care unit (ICU) with a life-threatening exacerbation of asthma. His PaCO2 is 8.1kPa with a pH of 7.29. He remains profoundly bronchospastic. The following are true:

   A. An I:E ratio of 1:3.5 is an appropriate initial setting
   B. Disconnection from the ventilator may be required if ventilation becomes more difficult
   C. PEEP is contraindicated
   D. Permissive hypercapnia should be employed
   E. The ventilator should be set at a rate of at least 15 to help normalize the pH

9.   Regarding dobutamine, the following are true:

   A. Acts on dopamine receptors to release noradrenaline
   B. Dobutamine is a pure β1-adrenergic agonist
   C. Infusion is indicated in treatment of acute heart failure with shock
   D. Infusion increases atrio-ventricular AV-nodal conduction
   E. Infusion may cause hypotension

10. Regarding speaking valves, the following are true:

A. The Passy-Muir valve is an open-position speaking valve

B. The Passy-Muir valve opens during patient inhalation and closes during expiration

C. The Passy-Muir valve closes at the end of the inspiratory cycle and requires patient expiratory effort

D. The Passy-Muir valve improves olfaction

E. The Montgomery speaking valve is a closed-position speaking valve

11. With regards to the apnoea test in brainstem death testing, the following are true:

A. All electrolytes must be in the normal range before testing proceeds

B. Arterial blood analysis should confirm that the initial (pretest) pCO_2 is at least 6.0kPa and the arterial blood pH is greater than 7.40

C. If maintenance of apnoeic oxygenation is problematic then CPAP may be utilized

D. It cannot be conducted reliably in patients with a chronically elevated pCO_2

E. The apnoea test should not be performed if any of the preceding brainstem tests confirm the presence of brainstem reflexes

12. Regarding the paediatric airway, the following are true:

A. Cuffed endotracheal tubes remain relatively contraindicated because of the risk of tracheal necrosis

B. In a child who is difficult to ventilate and intubate, surgical cricothyroidotomy is a reasonable next-line alternative

C. Risk of upper-airway obstruction occurs when the child is on a flat surface such as a spinal board

D. The glottic opening is the narrowest part of the upper airway

E. The oral cavity is relatively smaller and tongue relatively larger compared to the adult airway

13. When considering insertion of percutaneous tracheostomy on the ICU, it is true that the following are important landmarks to consider:

A. The cricoid cartilage lies at a level anterior to the fourth cervical vertebra

B. The recurrent laryngeal nerve lies in the groove between the trachea anteriorly and the oesophagus posteriorly

C. The cricothyroid membrane extends from the inferior boarder of the thyroid cartilage to the superior boarder of the cricoid cartilage

D. The cricoid cartilage comprises the most inferior boarder of the larynx

E. The isthmus of the thyroid overlies the second to fourth tracheal rings anteriorly

14. It is true that donated blood is routinely screened for the following:

A. cytomegalovirus (CMV)

B. Human T-lymphotropic virus (HTLV)

C. Hepatitis B

D. HIV

E. Syphilis

15. **A 65-year-old woman with a history of diabetes presents to A&E severely unwell, dehydrated, and with a capillary blood glucose 60mmol/l. Capillary ketones are 2.5mmol/l and pH is 7.32. The following are true:**

A. Hypotonic fluid resuscitation should be instituted

B. Insulin should be started at a fixed rate 0.1 units/kg/hr Actrapid

C. Management should follow the diabetic ketoacidosis protocol

D. Mortality is up to 20%

E. Osmolality can be estimated by $(2 \times Na) + urea + glucose$

16. **An obese, short-necked patient is being intubated on the ward for transfer to ICU. The patient is known COPD and requires mechanical ventilation for a community-acquired pneumonia. The ICU trainee, on first look with the laryngoscope, is unable to intubate the patient. The following are true:**

A. Cricoid pressure should be maintained at 10N throughout

B. In the absence of more senior help, the trainee should attempt intubation with the aid of a bougie or video laryngoscope up to five times

C. The patient should be repositioned so that there is extension of the lower cervical vertebrae and head

D. The trainee should attempt insertion of second generation supraglottic airway if intubation remains unsuccessful

E. There should be a maximum of three attempts of insertion of supraglottic airway device if the patient cannot be intubated

17. **Regarding haemoglobin, the following are true:**

A. A haem molecule consists of a protoporphyrin ring and a central iron ion in the ferric state Fe^{3+}

B. Binding oxygen to a haem molecule induces changes in adjacent globin chains

C. Haemoglobin contains four globin chains, each containing a haem molecule, which reversibly bind to oxygen

D. In health, the average amount of methaemoglobin is 5%

E. The Haldane effect describes the ability of oxyhaemoglobin to carry more oxygen than deoxyhaemoglobin

18. **Regarding antiarrythmics currently used, the following are true:**

A. Adenosine can be used to convert atrial fibrillation and flutter back into sinus rhythm

B. Digoxin inhibits Na^+/K^+ ATPase which leads to an increase in inotropy

C. Digoxin slows conduction by increasing acetylcholine at the muscarinic receptors

D. Digoxin cardiac toxicity is precipitated in the presence of hyperkalaemia

E. Dialysis should be used for digoxin toxicity

19. The following statements about vasopressin are true:

A. It is synthesized in the posterior pituitary

B. It is released in response to hypoxia

C. It can be used to treat diabetes Insipidus caused by lithium

D. Noradrenaline stimulates release

E. Vasopressin will also cause vasodilatation

20. Regarding gases used on ICU, the following are true:

A. Heliox (21% He, 79% O_2) reduces airway resistance in small airways in asthma by reduced gas density compared with air

B. Increasing the oxygen flow rate above the recommended value of Venturi mask will result in an inappropriately high concentration of oxygen being delivered to the patient

C. 'Laminar flow' describes the situation where all gas particles are moving at the same speed along a tube

D. Resistance to laminar flow in an endotracheal tube is proportional to the fourth power of the internal radius

E. Warming inspired gases from room temperature (approx. 20°C) to approx. 40°C halves gas density

21. It is true that the following have been shown to be of benefit:

A. Early enteral feeding in pancreatitis

B. Glutamine supplements in burns

C. High carbohydrate diet in acute respiratory distress syndrome (ARDS)

D. Immune enhancing nutrition in severe sepsis

E. Selenium supplementation in sepsis

22. When measuring a patient's blood pressure, the following are true:

A. Noninvasive intermittent automatic measurements utilize an oscillometer

B. Optimal damping of a system occurs when the damping factor is <0.7

C. The System International unit of pressure is used

D. When blood pressure is assessed by auscultation, the third Korotkoff sound represents diastolic pressure

E. With continuous invasive arterial blood pressure measurement, the natural frequency of the system should be the same as the fundamental frequency

23. Regarding drugs used to modulate coagulation, the following are correct:

A. A prolonged specimen transport time can cause supratherapeutic anti-Xa levels

B. Causes of subtherapeutic anti-Xa levels include renal failure

C. Fondaparinux has both antithrombin activity and activity against factor Xa

D. Low molecular weight heparin activity is reported in international units per ml

E. Rivaroxiban directly inhibits factor Xa

24. **When interpreting the thromboelastogram (TEG), the following are true:**
    A. The R-time (reaction time) is prolonged by severe hypofibrinogaemia
    B. The K-time represents clot formation time, and can be measured from the end of the R-time to a TEG amplitude of 10mm
    C. The alpha angle is decreased with thrombocytopaenia
    D. The maximum amplitude represents clot strength
    E. The LY30 (lysis after 30 minutes post maximum amplitude) is elevated with administration of t-PA

25. **When interpreting a chest radiograph, the following are true:**
    A. Pleural effusions of approximately 75ml can be detected on the erect chest x-ray
    B. The radiation dose is equivalent to 28 days of exposure to natural background radiation
    C. The diaphragm should be seen at the level of the eighth through tenth anterior ribs during full inspiration
    D. The right lung has two lobes, and the left lung has three lobes
    E. The deep sulcus sign is seen on the erect chest x-ray and is indicative of a pneumothorax

26. **A patient who has suffered severe postoperative complications and now has an open abdomen is being weaned from the ventilator with tracheostomy and no current sedation. There is a plan to take this patient back to theatre for surgical re-exploration. The following are true:**
    A. According to the Mental Capacity Act 2005, it is not necessary to assume capacity, and any action you take in the patient's best interest will protect you from liability
    B. It is safe to assume that this patient will not have the capacity to consent
    C. It is reasonable to make best-interest decisions based on age and condition
    D. If this patient is anaesthetized for surgery, there is an automatic deprivation of liberty
    E. This patient should be anaesthetized and taken to theatre as this is in the patient's best interest

27. **Regarding acid-base status, the following are correct:**
    A. Anion gap equates to $([Na^+] + [K^+]) - ([Cl^-] + [HCO_3])$ and is between 3 and 11mmol/l
    B. Anion gap is underestimated in hypoalbuminaemia
    C. Base excess reliably helps to identify the mechanism of acid-base disturbance
    D. Strong anions include Cl^-, HCO_3. and lactate
    E. When interpreting blood gas results $[H^+]$, pCO_2 and $[HCO_3-]$ are measured directly

28. **It is true that methillin-resistant *Stapylococcal aureus* (MRSA) on the ICU is associated with the following:**
    A. Linezolid is superior to vancomycin in treating MRSA pneumonia
    B. Nasal MRSA colonization is not a risk factor for MRSA infection
    C. The multidrug efflux genes qacA and qacB also confer resistance to chlorhexidine
    D. The use of quinolone antibiotics is a risk factor for subsequent MRSA isolation
    E. Universal decolonization with mupirocin and chlorhexidine is no more effective than screening and isolation of MRSA-positive patients in reducing ICU-attributable MRSA-positive clinical cultures on an ICU

29. **Regarding the use of high-flow nasal oxygen therapy (HFNOT), the following are true:**
    A. During respiratory distress, respiratory flow rates may be as high as 120l/min
    B. HFNOT provides warmed, humidified gases at flows of up to 60l/min
    C. HFNOT reduces dead space and work of breathing
    D. HFNOT produces a positive end expiratory pressure of at least 5cm H_2O
    E. HFNOT can reduce mortality and intubation rate in patients with noncardiogenic acute respiratory failure

30. **The following are true regarding severe aortic stenosis:**
    A. CPR is often ineffective
    B. Patients may be dependent on atrial kick to maintain cardiac output
    C. The valve area is less than $0.5cm^2$
    D. The peak gradient is 41–70mmHg
    E. Tachycardia is poorly tolerated

Question 1 T T F T F

The management of major trauma (defined as an injury severity score >15) has changed, and is now undertaken at high-volume major trauma centres, with clinical priority being aimed at damage control resuscitation (including permissive hypotension, haemostatic resuscitation, and damage control surgery). In-hospital management should be a continuation of prehospital care, and patients who remain fluid responders should be transferred to the operating theatre. The CRASH-2 study reported a reduction in mortality when tranexamic acid was administered early (there was an increase in mortality if administered 3 hours after the point of injury). Recombinant Factor VII is not licensed for trauma. It may promote thrombosis and has not been accepted in the use of haemostatic control. Haemostatic resuscitation is the use of whole blood components being used as initial fluid resuscitation, in an attempt to counteract the negative effects of ongoing bleeding and trauma-induced coagulopathy. There is some uncertainty regarding exact ratios of transfusion (i.e. FFP to packed red blood cells (PRBCs)), and the timing of platelets and cryoprecipitate, but there is acceptance that higher ratio FFP:PRBC and early platelets and cryoprecipitate are superior to the older methods of waiting for clotting results.

Shakur H, Roberts I; CRASH-2 Trial Collaborators. Effects of tranexamic acid on death, vascular occlusive events, and blood transfusion in trauma patients with significant haemorrhage (CRASH-2): a randomised, placebo-controlled trial. *Lancet* 2010;376:23–32.

Brasel K. Advanced trauma life support (ATLS®): the ninth edition. *Journal of Trauma and Acute Care Surgery* 2013;74(5):1363–6.

Question 2 F T F F T

PAC has been used for several decades as a gold standard for cardiac output monitoring. Due to the lack of evidence on improvement in clinical outcomes, and the risk of complications, newer, less-invasive, methods have evolved over time.

Directly measured PAC data include temperature, central venous pressure, pulmonary artery wedge pressure (surrogate marker of left atrial pressure), pulmonary artery pressure, cardiac output (thermodilution method using a PAC tip thermistor), and mixed venous saturations. Derived values include stroke volume, systemic vascular resistance, and pulmonary vascular resistance (and the indexed forms).

The Stewart-Hamilton equation uses the integral of blood temperature changes over time to calculate cardiac output. West Zones are functional models and dynamic in nature, changing with alterations in pulmonary venous and alveolar pressures (therefore they cannot be readily confirmed on x-ray).

Wigfull J, Cohen AT. Critical assessment of haemodynamic data. *Continuing Education in Anaesthesia, Critical Care & Pain* 2005;5(3):84–8.

Waldmann C, Soni N, Rhodes A (eds). *Oxford desk reference: critical care*, 1st edition. Oxford: Oxford University Press, 2008.

Question 3 F T T F F

Beta-haemolytic Group A streptococci are spherical Gram-positive bacteria. Asymptomatic carriage is common and may be up to 30% of the population.

Group A strep (GAS) infections can be noninvasive or invasive. Noninvasive infections such as pharyngitis and impetigo are common and not severe. Scarlet fever is a noninvasive infection caused by GAS and is a notifiable disease in the UK. Invasive GAS disease, such as toxic shock syndrome and necrotizing fasciitis, are also notifiable to Public Health England.

GAS does not directly cause rheumatic fever. The latter is a consequence of untreated GAS, where antibodies form leading to cross-reactivity and inflammatory disease. GAS is not specifically associated with high levels of neonatal death. Group B strep can cause neonatal pneumonia and meningitis.

Health Protection Agency. Interim UK guidelines for management of close community contacts of invasive group A streptococcal disease. Health Protection Agency, Group A Streptococcus Working Group. *Communicable Disease and Public Health* 2004;7:354–61.

Question 4 T T F F F

Acute liver failure can be subdivided depending on the time from the onset of jaundice to the development of encephalopathy:

- Hyperacute: under 7 days
- Acute: between 7 days and 4 weeks
- Subacute: longer than 4 weeks

There are multiple causes of acute liver failure:

- Paracetamol and idiosyncratic reactions (NSAIDS, halothane, antibiotics, antiepileptics, isoniazid, herbal, and ecstasy/cocaine)
- Viral causes (Hepatitis A, B, E, CMV, EBV, and HSV)
- Autoimmune
- Pregnancy (acute fatty liver of pregnancy)
- Toxins (Amanita phalloides)
- Vascular (hepatic vein thrombosis (Budd Chiari), ischaemic hepatitis, and hepatic veno-occlusive disorder)
- Metabolic (alpha 1 antitrypsin, Wilson disease)
- Other (malignant infiltration)

Infections should be treated aggressively and promptly with broad-spectrum antibiotics and antifungals. Sepsis is a common cause of clinical deterioration and death, and antimicrobials should be given prophylactically.

By correcting coagulopathy, PT cannot be used as a prognostic indicator and may influence decision to list for transplantation. In rare cases, FFP may be given to control active bleeding; however, this is best discussed with a regional liver unit, if transplantation is a likely consideration.

Lactate levels can be used to prognosticate mortality in patients with acute liver failure secondary to paracetamol overdose.

Bernal W, Wendon J. Acute liver failure. *New England Journal of Medicine* 2013; 369:2525–34.

Question 5 F F F T F

Staphylococcal scalded skin syndrome is caused by an exfoliative toxin produced by roughly 5% of *Staphylococcus aureus*. These toxins act at a remote site leading to a red rash and separation of the epidermis beneath the granular cell layer. Bullae form and diffuse sheetlike desquamation occurs. It occurs very rarely in adults.

Stevens-Johnson is a milder form of toxic epidermal necrolysis (TEN), with <10% body surface area involvement.

This clinical picture most likely reflects TEN (diagnosis of which based on clinical presentation and tissue biopsy), which is a dermatological emergency resulting from an immune reaction, aimed at destruction of keratinocytes expressing foreign antigen. It presents as widespread erythema, necrosis, and bullous detachment of the epidermis and mucous membranes. Drugs are the main precipitating cause (anticonvulsants, antivirals, antibiotics, and anti-inflammatory drugs); however, infection can precipitate TEN, or it may be idiopathic.

There is a severity of illness score which can predict mortality (a point for each criteria).

- Age >40 years
- Heart rate >120 beats per minute
- Cancer or haematologic malignancy
- Involved body surface area >10%
- Blood urea nitrogen level >10mmol/L (28mg/dL)
- Serum bicarbonate level <20mmol/L (20mEq/L)
- Blood glucose level >14mmol/L (252mg/dL)

The number of positive criteria and the corresponding mortality rates are as follows:

- 0: 1 to 3%
- 2: 12%
- 3: 35%
- 4: 58%
- 5 or more, the mortality is >90%

Death is mostly related to sepsis (*Pseudomonas aeruginosa*, *Staphylococcus aureus*, Gram-negative species, and *Candida albicans*) and multiorgan failure. Treatment is supportive and best managed in a burns unit. Measures include isolation, fluid and electrolyte replacement, nutrition, and protective dressings.

Creamer D, Walsh SA, Dziewulski P. UK guidelines for the management of Stevens–Johnson syndrome/toxic epidermal necrolysis in adults 2016. *British Journal of Dermatology* 2016;174:1194–227.

Question 6 T T T T F

Due to the presence of citrate in bags of stored blood, there is chelation of calcium and hence a fall in the ionized calcium levels. Coagulopathy in massive transfusion may be dilutional, with a relative reduction in platelets and clotting factors. Coagulopathy may be consumptive, resulting from disseminated intravascular coagulation secondary to the initial pathology. Hypoxaemia can result from circulatory overload and pulmonary oedema, or transfusion-related acute lung injury (TRALI). Hypothermia can result from the continued transfusion of cold stored packs of blood (red blood cells are stored at 4°C). Hyperthermia can occur as part of an immediate or delayed haemolytic reaction, nonhaemolytic febrile reaction, allergic rection, TRALI, or transfusion-related infection (Gram-negative bacteria such as Pseudomonas proliferate rapidly at 4°C).

Clevenger B, Kelleher A. Hazards of blood transfusion in adults and children. *Continuing Education in Anaesthesia, Critical Care & Pain* 2014;14:112–18.

Question 7 T T T T F

The CURB65 score is used to assess the severity of community-acquired pneumonia. Age of >65 gets a point, as does confusion, as assessed by a mini-mental test score of <8. Quinolones have been shown to increase the risk of healthcare-associated infection such as MRSA. Urine can be used to test for pneumococcal antigen and Legionella antigen. Mycoplasma is detected by polymerase chain reaction (PCR) of respiratory samples, PCR of a throat swab, or serology. Mortality of a CURB65 score 3 pneumonia is approximately 15%, and anyone with a score of 3 and above is considered at high risk of death.

Barlow G, Nathwani D, Davey P. The CURB65 pneumonia severity score outperforms generic sepsis and early warning scores in predicting mortality in community-acquired pneumonia. *Thorax* 2007;62:253–9.

Question 8 T T F T F

High rates of ventilation encourage gas trapping ('stacking'). If gas trapping becomes a significant problem, potentially indicated by a rising plateau pressure in volume controlled ventilation or falling volumes in pressure controlled ventilation, disconnection from the ventilator may help. Ventilator applied PEEP in asthma is contentious but may improve ventilation and should not be considered contraindicated. Set extrinsic PEEP mitigates against alveolar collapse and can counter-balance the effect of intrinsic PEEP by reducing the effort necessary in triggering inspiration during a patient-initiated breath. However it is important to assess intrinsic PEEP and set extrinsic PEEP to no more than 80% of intrinsic PEEP, to prevent gas trapping and the negative effects of dynamic hyperinflation from breath stacking. Permissive hypercapnia is a reasonable strategy as the effects of respiratory acidosis are generally better tolerated than barotrauma. The described I:E ratio would prolong the expiratory phase and thus improve time for complete exhalation, thus preventing progressive hyperinflation.

Stather D, Stewart T. Clinical review: mechanical ventilation in severe asthma. *Critical Care* 2005;9:581–7.

Question 9 F F T T T

Whilst dobutamine is infused for its β_1-adrenergic effects, it is also exhibits weak β_2, and α_1 effects.

Dobutamine increases AV-nodal conduction and can precipitate tachyarrhythmia, particular in atrial fibrillation.

Unlike dopamine, dobutamine has no dopaminergic-receptor effects, and so does not cause noradrenaline release, but can cause hypotension through its β_2-mediated vasodilatation.

Dobutamine infusion is indicated in acute heart failure with shock, and while there is evidence of symptomatic improvement, there is no placebo-controlled data to give weight behind improved survival. Drugs other than beta agonists that can be considered in acute heart failure include phosphodiesterase inhibitors (e.g. milrinone) and calcium sensitizing agents (levosimendan).

Parker K, Brunton L, Goodman LS, Blumenthal D, Buxton I. *Goodman & Gilman's manual of pharmacology and therapeutics.* London: McGraw-Hill Medical, 2008.

ESC Guidelines for the diagnosis and treatment of acute and chronic heart failure. 2012. http://www.bsh.org.uk/resources/guidelines/ [accessed 11 June 2019].

Question 10 F T F T F

The Passy-Muir valve redirects air flow through the vocal cords, mouth, and nose, enabling voice, management of secretions, and improved olfaction. It is a closed-position speaking valve, unlike the Montgomery valve. The Passy-Muir valve is in a closed position until the patient inhales. The valve opens easily and closes at the end of the inspiratory cycle, without patient expiratory effort.

The Passy-Muir valve. http://www.passy-muir.com [accessed 19 September 2019].

Question 11 F F T F T

The apnoea test can be reliably conducted in patients with a chronically elevated pCO_2, for example patients with chronic obstructive pulmonary disease, by ensuring the initial (pretest) pCO_2 is high enough to give a pH of <7.40. Electrolytes should not be grossly deranged but do not necessarily need to be within the normal physiological range. Detailed guidance can be found in 'A code of practice for the diagnosis and confirmation of death'. The apnoea test should always be performed as the final brainstem test; if any of the other brainstem nuclei are found to be intact, then testing should be halted prior to the apnoea test. The preapnoea arterial blood gas should confirm a pCO_2 of at least 6.0kPa and a pH <7.40. CPAP may be utilized if apnoeic oxygenation is problematic.

Academy of Medical Royal Colleges. *A code of practice for the diagnosis and confirmation of death.* 2008. http://www.aomrc.org.uk/doc_view/42-a-code-of-practice-for-the-diagnosis-and-confirmation-of-death [accessed 12 June 2014].

Question 12 F F T F T

The cricoid ring is the narrowest part of a child's upper airway, and indeed the oral cavity is relatively small, with a comparatively larger tongue. Cuffed endotracheal tubes are no longer considered a significant risk and so can be used in children, with measurement of cuff pressure <30mmHg. Due to the relatively large occiput, children are at risk of airway obstruction when lying flat (e.g. on a spinal board). The very short cricothyroid membrane makes needle and surgical cricothyroidotomy extremely difficult in the paediatric patient.

Cardwell M, Walker RWM, Management of the difficult paediatric airway. *BJA CEPD Reviews* 2003;6;167–70.

Question 13 F T T T T

The cricoid cartilage is a signet-ring shaped cartilage which lies level with C6. The trachea is a cartilaginous tube continuous with the larynx inferiorly, and comprises of 16 to 20 C-shaped cartilages connected by fibroelastic connective tissue. The trachea runs midline throughout most of its course until its point of bifurcation when it is slightly displaced rightwards by the arch of the aorta. Posterior relations of the trachea include the oesophagus and the recurrent laryngeal nerve in the tracheoesophageal groove bilaterally. The larynx extends from the root of the tongue superiorly to the cricoid cartilage inferiorly, anteriorly related to C3 to C6. To avoid risk of tracheal stenosis, tracheostomy is most commonly performed at the level of the second and third tracheal rings.

Batuwitage B, Webber S, Glossop A. Percutaneous tracheostomy. *Continuing Education in Anaesthesia, Critical Care & Pain* 2014;14:268–72.

Question 14 F T T T T

All except CMV are routinely screened for in the UK. Donated blood in the UK is routinely screened for: syphilis, Hepatitis B, Hepatitis C, HIV, and HTLV.

NHS Blood and Transplant. https://www.blood.co.uk/the-donation-process/further-information/tests-we-carry-out/ (accessed14 February 2021)

https://www.transfusionguidelines.org/transfusion-handbook/3-providing-safe-blood/3-2-tests-on-blood-donations (accessed 14 February 2021)

Question 15 F F F T T

This situation represents hyperglycaemic hyperosmolar state (HHS), whereby patients are extremely dehydrated and often have very high capillary blood glucose levels and high plasma osmolality. Commonly there is no significant ketosis or acidaemia, although there can be an overlap with an element of ketosis as insulin levels become deficient in the face of glucotoxicity. HHS presents most often in the older type 2 diabetic patient, although may represent a first presentation in a much younger patient. The goal of treatment is to restore fluids, and this is done using 0.9% NaCl. As fluids are replaced, blood glucose levels will naturally fall, and with a decrease in plasma osmolality, water will move back into cells, leading to a risk of hypernatraemia. Potassium is often depleted, but as a result of hyperosmolality and insulin deficiency, potassium levels may be normal or high on presentation. Potassium levels may fall as treatment starts. Use of 0.45% NaCl may only be considered if, despite adequate fluid resuscitation with 0.9% NaCl, osmolality and glucose levels are not falling. Precipitous falls in glucose and osmolality are not recommended (cerebral oedema may occur with rapid changes). A safe fall rate of glucose should be 4–6mmol/hr with an aim of blood glucose 10–15mmol/l. If there is no significant ketonaemia, then there is no requirement to start insulin. If insulin is started, use a fixed rate of 0.05 units/kg/hr Actrapid, as HSS patients tend to be more insulin sensitive. Mortality is higher, and HSS patients are at risk of seizures, central pontine myelinolysis, cerebral oedema, stroke, and myocardial infarction as well as arterial and venous thromboembolism.

Joint British Diabetes Societies Inpatient Care Group. *The management of the hyperosmolar hyperglycaemic state (HHS) in adults with diabetes.* August 2012. https://www.diabetes.org.uk/ Documents/Position%20statements/JBDS-IP-HHS-Adults.pdf (accessed 14 February 2021)

Question 16 F F F T T

A short-necked, obese patient, undergoing rapid sequence induction in unfamiliar circumstances, should raise alarm bells for the potential for less than straightforward airway manipulation, especially given the reduced respiratory reserve.

To increase your chances of success, the patient should be placed in an optimal position, which is neck flexion and head extension ('sniffing the morning air'). Cricoid pressure is initially applied at 10N, which should increase to 30N as the patient is anaesthetized.

As it quickly becomes apparent that intubation is going to be difficult, help should be sought urgently, and there should not be more than three attempts at reposition and intubation. If intubation remains unsuccessful, rescue oxygenation and ventilation should be maintained with bag and mask plus oropharyngeal airway or insertion of second generation supraglottic device, ideally with cricoid pressure maintained. If there is ongoing failure of oxygenation and inability to position the supraglottic device (no more than three attempts) then there needs to be adherence to the 'can't intubate, can't ventilate' algorithm and early preparation for emergency front of neck access.

Difficult Airway Society. *DAS guidelines for management of unanticipated difficult intubation in adults.* 2015. https://www.das.uk.com/guidelines/das_intubation_guidelines [accessed 19 September 2019].

Question 17 F T T F F

Adult haemoglobin contains four globin chains—two α and two β. Each globin chain contains a haem molecule consisting of iron in the ferrous state (Fe^{2+}), and a protoporphyrin ring. The Fe^{2+} ion binds oxygen so that each haemoglobin molecule is capable of carrying four oxygen molecules.

The sigmoid shape of the oxygen haemoglobin curve is due to co-operative binding, as binding one oxygen molecule induces a small conformational change which increases oxygen binding affinity of the other globin chains.

The Haldane effect describes the ability of deoxygenated blood to carry more carbon dioxide than oxygenated blood. As blood passes through a capillary, haemoglobin desaturates, and more carbon dioxide can be carried. In addition, the greater hydrogen ion concentration and fall in pH reduces the affinity of oxygen and increases oxygen release to the tissues (the Bohr effect).

Methaemoglobin occurs when the Fe molecule is in the ferric state (Fe^{3+}) and cannot bind oxygen. In health, normal levels are <1%.

Hall J, Hall M. *Guyton and Hall Textbook of medical physiology*. Philadelphia: Elsevier, 2016.

Question 18 F T T F F

Digoxin is a glycoside that is widely used to control the rate in atrial flutter or fibrillation. It inhibits Na^+/K^+ ATPase, which leads to an increase in inotropy as a result of increased intracellular calcium, and it slows conduction by increasing acetylcholine at the muscarinic receptors. The toxic profile of digoxin is potentiated by hypokalaemia, although hyperkalaemia will develop as a result of toxicity. Toxic side-effects can occur at plasma levels >2.5µg/l. Severe digoxin toxicity (plasma levels >20µg/l) require the use of digoxin-specific antibody fragments.

Adenosine can differentiate between supraventricular SVT (rate transiently slowed) and ventricular VT (rate does not slow). If the SVT is due to a re-entry circuit involving the AV node, adenosine may convert the rhythm to sinus. Atrial flutter or fibrillation are not generated by re-entry circuits.

Peck T, Hill S, Williams M. *Pharmacology for anaesthesia and intensive care*, 2nd edition. London: Greenwich Medical Media, 2003.

Question 19 F T F T T

Vasopressin (antidiuretic hormone) is an endogenous hormone produced by the supraoptic nuclei of hypothalamus and then transported to the posterior pituitary. It has numerous roles including modulation of plasma volume and osmolality, as well as neurotransmission and regulation of platelet binding during bleeding.

Vasopressin is released in response to reduced plasma volume, increased plasma osmolality, nausea, pain, hypoxia, and numerous chemical mediators including noradrenaline (noradrenaline may also inhibit release).

Vasopressin acts on a variety of receptors: V1 are found on the vascular smooth muscle of the systemic, splanchnic, renal, and coronary circulations. The primary result is vasoconstriction (although vasodilation occurs in the pulmonary circulation). V2 receptors are found in the distal tubule and cortical collecting duct. V3 receptors are found within the pituitary. Vasopressin also acts on oxytocin-type receptors, and their presence in vascular smooth muscle may increase nitric oxide.

Vasopressin has a number of medical used including management of cranial diabetes insipidus (lithium toxicity results in nephrogenic diabetes insipidus).

Sharman A, Low J. Vasopressin and its role in critical care. *Continuing Education in Anaesthesia, Critical Care & Pain* 2008;8:134–7.

Question 20 F F F F F

Temperatures in the ideal gas equation must be converted to Kelvin (Celsius + 273). An increase from 20°C to 40°C results in a 7% decrease in density.

Laminar flow is proportional to the fourth power of the internal radius; resistance is the inverse.

A Venturi mask operates on an 'entrainment ratio' so increasing the flow of oxygen will result in increased gas delivery, but the oxygen concentration will not change. However, reducing it may result in a total flow below the patient's peak inspiratory flow which will cause air to be entrained and reduce the delivered oxygen concentration.

Heliox has a reduced gas density, but this affects turbulent flow which is present in the large airways.

In laminar flow, gas particles along a single streamline must flow at the same speed, but streamlines move differently—those at the centre of the tube move fastest; in theory those at the edge have a speed of zero. This model ignores the random 'Brownian' motion of individual gas particles.

Lumb AB. *Nunn's applied respiratory physiology.* Edinburgh: Churchill Livingstone/Elsevier, 2010.

Question 21 T T F F F

Glutamine has been shown to reduce infection rates and possibly mortality in burns patients. High-fat, low-carbohydrate diets are of benefit in ARDS by altering the respiratory quotient, thereby reducing carbon dioxide production and ventilatory demand. Studies of arginine supplementation show an increase in mortality in severe sepsis. Enteral feeding in pancreatitis has been shown to reduce complications and organ failure compared to the parenteral route. There is some weak evidence of mortality benefit in sepsis with selenium supplementation; however, the Surviving Sepsis 2016 guidelines recommend against the use of it.

Waldmann C, Soni N, Rhodes A (eds). *Oxford desk reference: critical care*, 1st edition. Oxford: Oxford University Press, 2008.

Garrel D, et al. Decreased mortality and infectious morbidity in adult burn patients given enteral glutamine supplements: a prospective, controlled, randomized clinical trial. *Critical Care Medicine* 2003 Oct;31(10):2444–9.

Kalil AC, Danner RL. L-Arginine supplementation in sepsis: beneficial or harmful? *Current Opinions in Critical Care* 2006 Aug;12(4):303–8.

Alhazzani W, et al. The effect of selenium therapy on mortality in patients with sepsis syndrome: a systematic review and meta-analysis of randomized controlled trials. *Critical Care Medicine* 2013 June;41(6):1555–64.

Dellinger RP, et al. Surviving Sepsis Campaign: international guidelines for management of severe sepsis and septic shock. *Critical Care Medicine* 2017;45:580–637.

Question 22 T F F F F

Blood pressure measurement is part of the minimum standard of patient monitoring, and continuous invasive arterial pressure is used commonly on the ICU. Conventionally blood pressure is measured in millimetres of mercury (mmHg).

Auscultation over the brachial artery was first used in 1905, and it is the fifth sound that represents diastolic pressure.

Automatic intermittent noninvasive blood pressure systems are oscillometers, which use one cuff to occlude and sense. Systolic pressure is recognized at the point at which the rate of increase in the size of oscillation is maximal.

Continuous invasive arterial measurement requires an intra-arterial cannula, tubing with an infusion system, a transducer, and a microprocessor and display screen. Each system has a natural frequency, and if this coincides with the fundamental frequency of the arterial waveform, distortion of the signal will occur. Thus the natural frequency of the system should be >40Hz above that of the arterial waveform frequencies.

Damping is inherent within a system, and the amount is indicated by the damping factor. Optimal damping (the system responds rapidly to a change in signal with only a small amount of overshoot) occurs with a damping factor 0.7.

Ward M, Langton J. Blood pressure measurement. *Continuing Education in Anaesthesia, Critical Care & Pain* 2007;7:122–6.

Question 23 F F F F T

Fondaparinux is a synthetic direct Xa-inhibitor, with no antithrombin activity. Similarly Rivaroxaban also has direct Xa inhibitory effects. Low molecular weight heparin activity is reported in anti-Xa units per ml. As anti-Xa activity declines rapidly in vitro, samples must be rapidly transported to the laboratory for analysis, and causes for subtherapeutic anti-Xa levels include prolonged specimen transport time. Renal failure will give rise to supratherapeutic anti-Xa levels if the low molecular weight heparain (LMWH dose) is not appropriately adjusted.

Bauer K. Pros and cons of new oral anticoagulants. *ASH Education Book* 2013;1:464–70.

Question 24 T F T T T

R-time (reaction time): Time from initiation to a 2mm amplitude. Prolonged by anticoagulants (warfarin, heparin), factor deficiencies, and severe hypofibrinogenaemia. If shortened, it indicates the presence of hypercoagulability.

K-time (clot formation time): Time from R-time to a TEG amplitude of 20mm representing clot formation kinetics. Prolonged by anticoagulants, hypofibrinogenaemia, and thrombocytopaenia. Reduced by increased fibrinogen levels or platelet function.

Alpha angle: This is the angle between the middle of the TEG and the K inclination (see Figure 4.1). It indicates the rate at which clot is formed and is thus increased by increased fibrinogen levels or platelet function and decreased by anticoagulants, hypofibrinogenaemia, and thrombocytopaenia.

MA (maximum amplitude): MA is the greatest diameter of the clot and a measure of its strength. It relies fundamentally on the interaction of fibrin and platelets, with the latter exerting the most influence. It is decreased by deficiencies or medications which affect either of these.

LY30 (lysis 30 minutes after MA): This measures percent lysis at 30 minutes reflecting fibrinolysis. If significantly raised, primary and/or secondary hyperfibrinolysis must be considered.

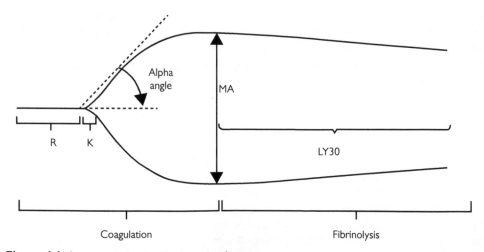

Figure 4.1 Annotated sketch of a thromboelastogram

Sira J, Eyre L. Physiology of haemostasis. *Anaesthesia and Intensive Care Medicine* 2016;17:79–82.

Question 25 F T F F F

When a chest radiograph is taken, the equivalent exposure of background natural radiation is approximately that of 28 days. That of an abdominal computer tomogram (CT) is approximately equivalent to 4 years' worth of background natural radiation.

The diaphragm is seen at the level of eighth through tenth posterior ribs with good inspiration. The right lung has three lobes, and the left has two lobes.

The deep sulcus sign is indicative of pneumothorax, but on the supine film. Air collects anteriorly and basally, within the nondependent portions of the pleural space, as opposed to the apex when the patient is upright. The costophrenic angle is abnormally deepened when the pleural air collects laterally, producing the deep sulcus sign.

On average, >150ml must be present for a pleural effusion to be detected on an erect chest x-ray.

Puddy E. Interpretation of the chest radiograph. *Continuing Education in Anaesthesia, Critical Care & Pain* 2007;7:71–5.

Question 26 F F F F F

The Mental Capacity Act (2005), covering England and Wales, provides a statutory framework for providing care to patients who lack capacity. One of the fundamental principles is that all patients must be assumed to have capacity unless it is proved otherwise. Remember capacity can be fluctuant and may not be lacking for all decisions.

As this is not emergency surgery, every effort should be made to support the patients to make their own decisions, and this may require additional resources (e.g. a letter board to communicate decisions).

If patients lack capacity, their best interest cannot be based on their age, appearance, condition, or behaviour. Protection of liability is given only if you have been compliant with the principles of the MCA (i.e. you have carried out an assessment of capacity and you have reasonable belief that the action you have taken is in the patient's best interest). If this has been undertaken and the patient is subsequently anaesthetized for surgery, deprivation of liberty is not applicable where sedating drugs are used to facilitate a treatment. Deprivation of liberty may apply where physical or chemical restraint are used to restrain patients.

Menon D, Chatfield D. Mental Capacity Act 2005 guidance for critical care. *The Intensive Care Society* 2011. https://www.ics.ac.uk/Society/Guidance/PDFs/Deprivation_of_Liberty [accessed 26 July 2021].

Question 27 T T F F F

Only $[H^+]$ and pCO_2 are measure directly. HCO_3^- is derived from the Henderson and Hasselbach equation.

Base excess provides some information regarding the quantitative aspects of the metabolic component of acid-base disorders; however, it does not provide information about the mechanism of the derangement. To maintain electrical neutrality: measured cations + unmeasured cations = measured anions + unmeasured anions.

Routinely measured cations include Na^+ and K^+ (unmeasured cations include Mg, Ca, and lithium), while routinely measured anions include Cl^- and HCO_3^- (unmeasured anions include albumin, phosphate, sulphate, and organic ions such as lactate and ketoacids). The anion gap is mainly due to negative charge of serum proteins and is underestimated in hypoalbuminaemia.

Stewart's strong ion theory states that body fluid acid-base balance depends on carbon dioxide, strong ions, and weak acids. HCO_3^- is not a strong ion.

Badr A, Nightingale P. An alternative approach to acid–base abnormalities in critically ill patients. *Continuing Education in Anaesthesia, Critical Care & Pain* 2007;7:107–11.

Question 28 T F T T F

Universal decolonization reduces MRSA-positive culture rates compared with screening and isolation; it may also reduce MRSA bloodstream infections, although chlorhexidine resistance is gradually being demonstrated in MRSA isolates, due to the qacA and qacB efflux pumps.

Linezolid is associated with better clinical cure and survival rates than vancomycin.

Risk factors for MRSA infection include longer ICU stay, gastrostomy, femoral catheter, antibiotic use (particularly quinolones and glycopeptides), and MRSA nasal colonization.

Huang SS, et al. Targeted versus universal decolonization to prevent ICU infection. *New England Journal of Medicine* 2013;368(24):2255–65.

Kollef MH, Rello J, Cammarata SK, Croos-Dabrera RV, Wunderink RG. Clinical cure and survival in Gram-positive ventilator-associated pneumonia: retrospective analysis of two double-blind studies comparing linezolid with vancomycin. *Intensive Care Medicine* 2004;30(3):388–94.

Tacconelli E, Angelis GD, Cataldo MA, Pozzi E, Cauda R. Does antibiotic exposure increase the risk of methicillin-resistant Staphylococcus aureus (MRSA) isolation? A systematic review and meta-analysis. *Journal of Antimicrobial Chemotherapy* 2008 Jan;61(1):26–38.

Altınbas A, Shorbagi A, Ascıoglu S, Zarakolu P, Cetinkaya-Sardan Y. Risk factors for intensive care unit acquired nasal colonization of MRSA and its impact on MRSA infection. *Journal of Clinical Laboratory Analysis* 2013;27(5):412–17.

Vali L, Davies SE, Lai LL, Dave J, Amyes SG. Frequency of biocide resistance genes, antibiotic resistance and the effect of chlorhexidine exposure on clinical methicillin-resistant Staphylococcus aureus isolates. *Journal of Antimicrobial Chemotherapy* 2008;61(3):524–32.

Question 29 T T T F T

HFNOT has been well-established in neonatal practice and is gaining widespread acceptance in a variety of circumstances for the adult population such as acute respiratory failure (where it has been shown to reduce intubation rates and improve mortality in noncardiogenic respiratory failure with PaO_2/FiO_2 ratios <200mmHg), airway management (it can provide an apnoeic oxygen reservoir), and postoperative extubation.

HFNOT does indeed provide warmed, humidified gases at flow rates of 40–60l/min and, while 'normal' breathing respiratory flow rates are in the order of 15l/min, in acute respiratory distress, flow rates well may increase up to 120l/min. HFNOT provides an anatomical oxygen reservoir within the nasopharynx and oropharynx, by virtue of a CO_2 washout effect due to high oxygen flow. This reduces dead space and work of breathing. The upper airways are distended when HFNOT is used, and this is then transmitted to lower airways to generate PEEP. It does require closed-mouth breathing, and so PEEP can be variable.

Frat JP, Ragot S, Thille AW. High-flow oxygen through nasal cannula in acute hypoxaemic respiratory failure. *New England Journal of Medicine* 2015;372: 2185–96.

Ashraf-Kashani N, Kumar R. High flow nasal oxygen therapy. *British Journal of Anaesthesia Education* 2017;17:57–62.

Question 30 T T F T T

Severe aortic stenosis is defined by a valve area of 0.5–1cm², or a mean gradient of 41–70mmHg across the valve. Tachycardia shortens coronary perfusion time and is poorly tolerated. In the normal heart, 20% of diastolic filling is provided by atrial contraction, but in this may rise to 40% in aortic stenosis. Due to the resistance to ejection from the left ventricle, CPR is often ineffective.

Bonow RO, et al. ACC/AHA 2006 guidelines for the management of patients with valvular heart disease. *Circulation* 2006;114:e84–e231.

paper 5

MCQ QUESTIONS

1. **A 70-year-old man presents with right-sided weakness and slurred speech, and is noted to have a deviant gaze towards his left side. The following statements are true:**
   A. Alteplase needs to be given within 8 hours of a clearly defined onset of ischaemic stroke
   B. Aspirin should be commenced within 48 hours of ischaemic stroke
   C. Blood pressure 205/115mmHg is a contraindication to thrombolysis
   D. Ischaemic stroke accounts for 85% of all strokes
   E. Posterior fossa haemorrhages are an indication for decompressive surgery

2. **The following statements about traumatic brain injury are true**
   A. A single episode of hypotension can lead to unfavourable outcome
   B. Hypertonic saline should be used as the primary resuscitative fluid following traumatic brain injury
   C. It has a bimodal presentation, with males more commonly affected
   D. Mannitol has a greater beneficial effect when given in intermittent boluses as compared to infusion
   E. Mortality is lower in patients who undergo decompressive craniectomy for persistently elevated intracranial pressure refractory to other therapeutic managements, compared to patients who remain on medical management alone

3. **The following are correct regarding the dynamic response testing of an arterial transducer system:**
   A. Air bubbles in the transducer system tend to cause underdamping
   B. Diastolic blood pressure is underestimated in an overdamped system
   C. Systolic blood pressure is overestimated in an underdamped system
   D. The fast-flush test can be used to determine the dynamic response of the system
   E. The natural frequency of a system is increased by reducing the length of the tubing

4. **Regarding botulism, the following statements are correct:**
   A. It is caused by exotoxin released from the bacterium Clostridium botulinum
   B. It causes an ascending motor paralysis
   C. It is often accompanied by fever
   D. Sensory nerve involvement is an early feature
   E. There is associated autonomic nerve involvement

MCQs and SBAs in Intensive Care Medicine. Lorna Eyre and Andrew Bodenham, Oxford University Press. © Oxford University Press 2021.
DOI: 10.1093/oso/9780198753056.003.0005

5. **In the management of acute liver failure (ALF), the following are correct:**
   A. Aggressive fluid resuscitation should be initiated with 5% dextrose to avoid excessive sodium administration
   B. Citrate anticoagulation can be safely used in the context of renal replacement therapy in those ALF patients requiring support for acute kidney injury
   C. Intrapulmonary shunting is uncommon in ALF compared with chronic liver failure
   D. Lactulose should be given to all patients with ALF to help treat the encephalopathy
   E. Prophylactic antibiotics and antifungals should be administered on admission to reduce incidence of infection complications

6. **A fit, healthy 33-year-old woman presents with pyrexia, low blood pressure, and tachycardia. She has a short history of haemoptysis, and there are multilobular infiltrates on the chest radiograph (CXR) with small bilateral effusions. There is ongoing rapid deterioration in her clinical conditions, and she is transferred to the intensive care unit (ICU) for level 3 care. Blood results reveal low white cell count and neutropaenia with very high CRP level 350mg/l.**
   A. Panton-Valentine leukocidin (PVL) is a strain of Staphylococcus aureus
   B. PVL has been associated with community outbreaks
   C. PVL is associated with necrotizing skin infections
   D. PVL pneumonia is most commonly associated with immunocompromised individuals
   E. While the progression of the disease is rapid, the outcome is rarely fatal with a mortality of 20%

7. **The following are true regarding cytomegalovirus (CMV):**
   A. CMV seropositivity is 90% in the > 80 year old population
   B. CMV reactivation occurs only in immunocompromised individuals, and it remains asymptomatic in immunocompetent patients
   C. CMV pneumonia is the CMV presentation most frequently seen in HIV patients
   D. Primary CMV disease is most often asymptomatic
   E. Viral load, as detected by quantitative polymerase chain reaction (PCR), can be used to determine CMV disease

8. **The following patients meet the diagnostic criteria for acute kidney injury:**
   A. A patient weighing 120kg, passing 50mls of urine per hour for 8 hours
   B. A rise in creatinine from 120μmol/l to 170μmol/l over 7 days
   C. A rise in creatinine from 20μmol/l to 48μmol/l over 5 days
   D. A 70kg patient passing 30mls of urine per hour for 4 hours
   E. A rise in creatinine from 80μmol/l to 115μmol/l over 2 days

9. **A patient is transferred to ICU having had a recent allogenic bone marrow transplant for acute myeloid leukaemia. The following are true:**

   A. Between 10%–20% of patients post haemopoietic stem cell transplant need critical care
   B. Graft-vs-disease is highest in mismatched transplants
   C. Survival to hospital discharge following an ICU admission, may occur in up to 40% patients
   D. Severe skin rash with desquamation, severe diarrhoea, abdominal pain, and ileus, in addition to a raised bilirubin >150 mmol/l are common features of sepsis post bone marrow transplant
   E. Tumour lysis syndrome should be treated with rituximab

10. **Is it true that ABO compatibility is essential for the administration of the following?**

    A. Albumin
    B. Factor VIIa
    C. FFP
    D. Platelets
    E. Red cells

11. **Risk factors for refeeding syndrome include:**

    A. Increasing age
    B. Malignancy
    C. Renal failure
    D. Use of antacids
    E. Use of proton pump inhibitors

12. **Concerning gastric motility, the following are true:**

    A. An appropriate dose of erythromycin in promoting gastric motility is 500mg qds intravenously
    B. Erythromycin therapy can be associated with cardiac dysrhythmias
    C. Illness severity correlates with risk of delayed gastric emptying
    D. Metoclopramide therapy is contraindicated in head injury
    E. Metoclopramide therapy reduces the risk of pneumonia

13. **When managing acute pancreatitis, the following are correct:**

    A. Aggressive fluid resuscitation is recommended for the first 48 hours
    B. Crystalloids such as sodium chloride and Ringers lactate are equally efficacious
    C. If starting a prophylactic antibiotic, consider an antifungal agent as well
    D. Pancreatic duct stents with or without rectal indomethacin may have a role in preventing severe post-endoscopic retrograde cholangiopancreatogram (ERCP) pancreatitis in high-risk patients
    E. There is no role for ERCP in the early stages of acute pancreatitis

14. Regarding hypertensive emergency, the following are correct:

A. Hypertensive emergency is severely elevated blood pressure systolic ≥180 and/or diastolic ≥120mmHg, with no signs or symptoms of target organ damage

B. It may occur in pregnant woman and is the leading cause of maternal death

C. It is frequently attributable to aortic dissection, which needs rapid control of blood pressure

D. It is frequently attributable to ischaemic stroke, which needs rapid control of blood pressure

E. When caused by acute left ventricular dysfunction and pulmonary oedema, hypertensive emergency may be treated with a beta blocker

15. A patient has been intubated and ventilated on the ICU for 5 days. Over the last 24 hours, his oxygen requirement has increased and there is now an increased volume of mucky sputum. The following are correct:

A. Diagnosis of ventilator associated pneumonia requires new chest x-ray changes and fever >38°C

B. Likely causative organism is *Pseudomonas aeruginosa*

C. Invasive respiratory sampling techniques are superior to noninvasive techniques

D. Initial appropriate antibiotic management could include cephtazidime

E. Quantitative culture of respiratory secretions leads to reduced mortality and time on the ICU

16. A patient presents with new confusion, an acute kidney injury, low platelets, low haemoglobin, and fever. Otherwise the patient was previously healthy. The following are correct:

A. ADAMTS13 may be high

B. Conjugated bilirubin levels are likely to be high

C. Complement levels will be normal

D. Platelets should be given to ensure platelet count is >50 × 10⁹/l

E. The lactate level will typically be high

17. Regarding donation after brainstem death, the following are correct:

A. Can only proceed if the patient is on the organ donor register (ODR)

B. Donation should occur as soon as possible after coning

C. Donors frequently donate several organs

D. Occurs between the two sets of brainstem death tests

E. Usually provides organs with shorter warm ischaemic times than donation after cardiovascular death (DCD)

18. It is correct that selective decontamination of the digestive tract (SDD) is associated with the following:

A. A lack of useful evidence supporting its place in critical care medicine and hence its use is not widespread throughout ICUs in the UK

B. A regime consisting of parenteral and enteral antimicrobials

C. May be associated with antimicrobial resistance

D. Solely prevents the spread of infection by pathogens acquired during colonization in ICU

E. Surveillance cultures are essential twice weekly during SDD

19. Extracorporeal membrane oxygenation (ECMO) may be used as an alternative to conventional ventilation. The following are true:

A. Arterio-venous (A-V) ECMO is particularly useful in patients with severe hypercapnia, respiratory acidosis, and low cardiac output

B. Best survival rates are seen in those with non necrotizing bacterial pneumonia

C. Patients with prolonged high peak airway pressures may benefit from ECMO

D. The Cesar research trial study demonstrated that patients receiving ECMO had superior outcomes

E. Veno-venous-ECMO has a higher risk of thromboembolic complications

20. Regarding physiology and acid–base status, the following are true:

A. Infusion of large quantities of dextrose containing solutions results in an increased strong ion difference

B. Infusions of Hartmann's solution will increase strong ion difference

C. Normal saline has a strong ion difference (SID) of zero

D. Renal failure results in a raised anion gap metabolic acidosis

E. Type I renal tubular acidosis results from increased chloride loss

21. Pacemakers are classified by the nature of their pacing mode. The code was developed by the North American Society of Pacing and Electrophysiology (NASPE) and the British Pacing and Electrophysiology Group and last revised in 2002. The following are correct:

A. Biventricular devices do not fit into the classification

B. The first letter corresponds to the chamber sensed

C. The fourth letter corresponds to rate modulation function

D. The fifth letter corresponds to programmability

E. The letter 'D' in the first position denotes defibrillator function

22. Concerning deceased organ donation, the following are true:

A. HIV infection is a contraindication to organ donation

B. On average, three people on the transplant waiting list die every day in the UK

C. One deceased donor can transform or save the lives of up to nine other individuals

D. Patients may donate organs after death diagnosed on either brainstem or cardiovascular criteria

E. The number of transplants performed in the UK each year is currently limited by the small number of transplant centres

23. Following the A&E admission of a 12 year old found submerged in a lake, the following are true regarding drowning:

A. By definition there has to be liquid-air interface present at the entrance to the victim's airway

B. Cold water drowning leads to a better outcome because of the neuroprotective effects

C. Morbidity and mortality arise from aspiration of water and impaired gas exchange

D. Prophylactic antibiotics should be given to prevent infection

E. There are no clinical differences if the water is freshwater or saltwater

24. **Outreach services are commonplace in caring for the critically ill. Which statements are true:**
   A. Outreach teams provide an educational role
   B. Outreach teams provide the opportunity for audit
   C. Outreach teams utilize a track and trigger approach
   D. There is conclusive evidence to support the effectiveness of outreach teams
   E. The Department of Health strongly recommend the use of outreach teams

25. **When a patient with heart failure is positively pressure ventilated, the following are true:**
   A. An increase in intrathoracic pressure decreases venous return to the heart
   B. Increases in intrathoracic pressure increase left ventricular afterload
   C. Increases in intrathoracic pressure decrease right ventricular output
   D. Left ventricular afterload is proportional to transmural systolic left ventricular pressure
   E. Oxygen extraction is reduced

26. **Propofol is frequently used in the ICU, and the following statements are true or false?**
   A. It is a weak acid
   B. It can be associated with opisthotonas
   C. Infusion rates are usually >4mg/kg/hour to ensure full sedation in the critically ill patient
   D. Propofol related Infusion syndrome (PRIS) only occurs in children
   E. PRIS can be prevented with early nutrition

27. **Amiodarone 300mg was prescribed for a patient in fast atrial fibrillation, the following statements are correct:**
   A. Amiodarone blocks Na channels
   B. Amiodarone blocks Ca channels
   C. Amiodarone blocks K channels
   D. Amiodarone is a hepatic enzyme inducer
   E. Amiodarone has been associated with blurred vision

28. **A hospitalized 60-year-old patient was started on olanzapine for agitation. Ten days later he became somnolent. On examination, he had a body temperature of 40°C and was markedly rigid in both upper and lower extremities, with bradykinesia. Associated findings may include:**
   A. Clonus
   B. High creatinine kinase
   C. Improvement with dantrolene
   D. Leukocytosis
   E. Marked autonomic instability

29. **The following statements are correct regarding the principles of pulse oximetry:**

    A. Absorbed radiation can be described by Beer's law and Graham's law
    B. Beer's law states that intensity of transmitted light decreases exponentially as concentration of substance increases
    C. The use of spectrophotometric measurements
    D. The isobestic point is the wavelength at which the absorbances of oxyhaemoglobin and deoxyhaemoglobin are identical
    E. The absorbance of oxyhaemoglobin in red light is less than that of deoxyhaemoglobin

30. **The following are associated with ethylene glycol poisoning:**

    A. An increase in osmolar gap
    B. An acidosis in the presence of a normal lactate level
    C. Causes direct toxicity with subsequent neurological damage and death
    D. Causes hypocalcaemia
    E. Toxicity can be managed with alcohol

Question 1 F F T T F

Ischaemic stroke accounts for 85% of all strokes. Around a third of these are caused by large artery thromboembolism and around 25% are caused by cardiac thromboembolism (e.g. atrial fibrillation). There is strong evidence that aspirin given as soon as possible (following stroke diagnosis and exclusion of intracerebral bleed), and certainly within 24 hours, reduces mortality and risk of recurrent stroke. Alteplase (recombinant tissue plasminogen activator) can be given once intracranial haemorrhage has been excluded and within 4.5 hours of onset of stroke symptoms. Blood pressure reduction to 185/110mmHg or lower should be considered in patients who are candidates for thrombolysis, as severe hypertension is a contraindication. Aspirin should not be given in the first 24 hours after thrombolysis with Alteplase. Computed tomography signs of infarct >50% of the middle cerebral artery territory (with or without infarct of the anterior and, or posterior territories of the same side) is an indication for referral for decompressive surgery. Large cerebellar infarctions can cause oedema and compression of the fourth ventricle, with herniation, so should also be referred for neurosurgical input if there is declining level of consciousness.

National Institute for Health and Clinical Excellence (NICE). *Stroke: diagnosis and initial management of acute stroke and transient ischaemic attack (TIA)*. 2008. http://www.nice.org.uk/nicemedia/pdf/CG68NICEGuideline.pdf [accessed 26 July 2021].

Hacke W, et al. Thrombolysis with alteplase 3 to 4.5 hours after acute ischemic stroke. *New England Journal of Medicine* 2008;359(13):1317–29.

Question 2 T F T F T

The incidence of head injury is high, occurring most frequently in teenagers and the elderly. Although the incidence of death from head injury is relatively low, morbidity, however, is high, with almost half of patients followed-up at 1 year postdischarge having some form of life restriction. Traumatic brain injury (TBI) occurs more frequently in men.

According to the Traumatic Coma Data Bank a single pre-hospital systolic blood pressure (BP) <90mmHg was among the most powerful predictors of outcome. Therefore a systolic <90mmHg should be avoided, but there are no studies identifying treatment thresholds or outcomes relating to specific target values. The 2016 Brain Trauma Foundation guidelines suggest that the literature may support a higher level that varies with age.

Hypertonic saline (HS) reduced cerebral water content by osmotically drawing water across an intact blood–brain barrier. Several studies have shown that HS use reduces intracranial pressure (ICP), increases cerebral perfusion pressure, increases BP, and reduces overall fluid resuscitative requirements. However, these studies are small and inconsistent, so there is insufficient data to recommend HS as the primary treatment for trauma-induced intracranial hypertension.

Mannitol works by an immediate plasma-expanding effect followed by its osmotic effect. Little is known about the effects it may have when given for longer, and there was a low level of recommendation for boluses over infusion; however, again, strong evidence is lacking regarding the overall superiority of one form of mannitol over the other.

Decompressive craniectomy in patients with TBI and persistently raised intracranial pressure, after tiered management, was associated with lower mortality than medical management. However, more survivors in the surgical group than in the medical group were dependent on others.

Cooper DJ, et al. Decompressive craniectomy in diffuse traumatic brain injury. *New England Journal of Medicine* 2011;364:1493–502

Hutchinson P, et al. Trial of decompressive craniectomy for traumatic intracranial hypertension. *New England Journal of Medicine* 2016;375:1119–30.

Brain Trauma Foundation. *Guidelines for the management of severe traumatic brain injury.* 2016. https://www.braintrauma.org/uploads/13/06/Guidelines_for_Management_of_Severe_TBI_4th_Edition.pdf [accessed 13 October 2020].

Question 3 F F T T T

The natural pulsatile nature of the arterial waveform is a summation of multiple sine waves, which are displayed on a monitor using Fourier analysis. To accurately display this natural frequency of the arterial system, transducer systems have a degree of 'damping' (due to the fluid column) that prevents any dynamic distortion. A fast-flush test allows determination of this dynamic response and natural frequency of the transducer system. The system is underdamped if the natural frequency of the transducer system is nearer the frequency of the monitored arterial waveform (falsely exaggerating systolic and dampening diastolic pressures). Clots, air bubbles, and partial obstruction due to kinking can all cause the system to be overdamped. Every material has a frequency at which it oscillates freely. This is called its natural frequency. The natural frequency is determined by the properties of the components of the system. It can be increased, for example in the case of the arterial system by:

- Reducing the length of the cannula or tubing
- Reducing the compliance of the cannula or diaphragm
- Reducing the density of the fluid used in the tubing
- Increasing the diameter of the cannula or tubing

Gardner RM. Blood pressure monitoring. In: Webb AR, Shapiro MJ, Singer M, Suter P (eds), *Oxford textbook of critical care.* New York: Oxford University Press, 1999:602–613.

Question 4 T F F F T

Botulism is a toxin-mediated disease caused by the Gram-positive, anaerobic, spore-forming bacterium Clostridium botulinum. The toxin binds to cholinergic neurotransmitter sites, and prevents the release of acetylcholine from the presynaptic terminal. It therefore has effects at the neuromuscular junction as well as in the autonomic nervous system. Cranial nerve involvement marks the onset of symptoms. Descending muscle weakness progresses to the trunk and upper extremities and then lower extremities. Need for intubation and ventilation are common, and weakness may last weeks. Fever is uncommon (although wound botulism may have concurrent bacterial infection by nonclostridial species).

Waldmann C, Soni N, Rhodes A (eds). *Oxford desk reference: critical care,* 1st edition. Oxford: Oxford University Press, 2008.

Question 5 F T T F T

Excessive sodium administration should be avoided in chronic liver disease. However care needs to be taken with excessive use of 5% dextrose, as this can result in severe hyponatraemia, and there is no role for the use of large quantities of 5% dextrose in ALF. Gut decontamination and lactulose have no proven role in the management of ALF encephalopathy. Hepatopulmonary syndrome is most likely due to ineffective clearance of mediators that cause intrapulmonary vasodilatation, leading to arterio-venous shunting and ventilation and perfusion mismatch. It can occasionally occur in noncirrhotic patients and in those with mild liver disease. Renal replacement therapy is required in up to 75% ALF patients due to acute renal failure. We will start a standard citrate anticoagulation protocol for continuous renal replacement therapy. However caution must be exercised if the systemic ionized calcium subsequently becomes low. Prophylactic antimicrobials with broad-spectrum coverage of Gram-positive and Gram-negative activity and including an antifungal should be administered on admission, as this halves the incidence of infective episodes when compared with commencement at the time of suspected infection.

Lai WK, Murphy N. Management of acute liver failure. *Continuing Education in Anaesthesia, Critical Care & Pain* 2004;4(2):40–3.

Question 6 F T T F F

Staphylococcus aureus alone represents a small proportion of community-acquired pneumonias; however, there is an association between necrotizing pneumonia and Panton-Valentine leukocidin-secreting *S. aureus*. PVL is a cytotoxin forming pores in the cell membranes of neutrophils and macrophages, provoking cell lysis and release of inflammatory mediators. It is carried by both methillin- resistant and methillin-sensitive staphylococcal aureus MRSA and MSSA strains and it is mostly associated with community outbreaks, which may consist of skin infections (cellulitis, necrotizing skin infections). PVL-associated necrotizing pneumonia typically presents in previously healthy children or young adults with an influenza-like prodrome and then rapidly progressive septic shock and respiratory failure. Leucopaenia and, or thrombocytopaenia, airway haemorrhage, and pleural effusion are considered highly predictive for fatal outcome, and mortality is 40%–60%. PVL pneumonia needs prompt recognition and treatment (clindamycin, linezolid, rifampicin, and consideration for IV immunoglobulin).

Kreienbuehl L, Charbonney E, Eggimann P. Community-acquired necrotizing pneumonia due to methicillin-sensitive *Staphylococcus aureus* secreting Panton-Valentine leukocidin: a review of case reports. *Annals of Intensive Care* 2011;1:52.

Question 7 T F F T F

CMV is a double-stranded DNA virus, and the incidence of CMV seropositivity increases with age with CMV exposure seen in 90% of 80 year olds. CMV usually causes an asymptomatic infection and then remains latent with potential for reactivation. Clinically significant CMV disease (reactivation or primary disease) mostly occurs in immunocompromised patients (e.g. with solid organ transplant, bone marrow transplants, HIV, steroid use, or systemic lupus erythematosus (SLE) and can manifest as CMV pneumonia, hepatitis, gastritis, colitis, central nervous system (CNS) disease and Guillain Barre Syndrome, nephritis, retinitis, and graft-versus-host disease.

Immunocompetent patients may also be at risk of CMV disease as throughout a critical illness, immunomodulatory cytokines released in response to sepsis can lead to reactivation of CMV. CMV viraemia can be detected by quantitative PCR, and in theory, a viral load below a certain cut-off could distinguish between infection and disease. However in reality the viral load necessary for CMV disease to occur can be variable and may not correlate with clinical findings. Patients with HIV tend to have CMV retinitis as the major reported CMV disease. Regarding solid organ transplants, CMV disease occurs with the highest frequency in donor positive and recipient negative transplants. Treatment of CMV disease includes gancyclovir, valganciclovir, and foscarnet.

Staras SA, Dollard SC, Radford KW, Flanders WD, Pass RF, Cannon MJ. Seroprevalence of cytomegalovirus infection in the United States, 1988–1994. *Clinical Infectious Diseases* 2006;43(9):1143.

Question 8 T F T F T

The 2013 NICE guidelines recognize the following diagnostic criteria for acute kidney injury: rise in serum creatinine of 26μmol/l in 48 hours, 50% rise in serum creatinine in the previous 7 days, and fall in urine output to below 0.5ml/kg/hour for 6 hours.

National Institute for Health and Care Excellence. *Clinical guideline 169. Acute kidney injury: prevention, detection and management of acute kidney injury up to the point of renal replacement therapy.* 2013. https://www.nice.org.uk/guidance/cg169 [accessed 26 July 2021].

Question 9 T T T F F

Approximately 13% of patients who have received a haemopoietic stem cell transplant will require some form of critical care input, while 7% of patients with a haematological malignancy will develop a critical illness. Stem cell transplants can be autologous (no graft-versus-host effect (GVH) but no graft-versus-disease effect (GVD) either) or allogenic (which may be matched or unmatched, related or unrelated). The greater the transplant mismatch, the greater the benefit from a GVD effect. However the risk of GVH is also increased. The latter presents with skin involvement, gastro intestinal (GIT) upset (often diarrhoea), and liver involvement in advanced stages. The peak time for developing GVH is 30–50 days posttransplant and in its severest form has a 100 day mortality in the order of 75%. The signs and symptoms often overlap with other diagnoses, and it may be prudent to obtain a histological diagnosis. Tumour lysis syndrome occurs most often with acute, high-grade haematological malignancy for which treatment has just begun, and results in hyperkalaemia, increased phosphate, low calcium, and high uric acid levels. It can progress to acute kidney injury (AKI). Fluid therapy, management of hyperkalaemia, and rasburicase are the mainstays of treatment.

Been M, Levitt M, Bokhari S. Intensive care management of patients with haematological malignancy. *Continuing Education In Anaesthesia, Critical Care & Pain* 2010;10:167.

Question 10 F F T F T

Red cells contain ABO antigens, and require cross-matching to prevent haemolytic reactions. Fresh frozen plasma may contain ABO antibodies, and, therefore, ABO compatibility is required. Platelets carry a very low risk of haemolytic reactions; transfusions are usually type-specific, but this is not essential. Factor VIIa and albumin do not require computability matching.

Joint United Kingdom (UK) Blood Transfusion and Tissue Transplantation Services Professional Advisory Committee. *The ABO system.* 2014 https://www.transfusionguidelines.org/transfusion-handbook/2-basics-of-blood-groups-and-antibodies/2-4-the-abo-system [accessed 19 January 2019].

Question 11 T T F T F

Specific risk factors for refeeding syndrome include malabsorption syndromes, chronic alcoholism, anorexia, malignancy, long-term diuretic use (electrolyte depletion), long-term antacid use (chelation of phosphate), uncontrolled diabetes, and being elderly. PPI use and renal failure are not specific risk factors.

NICE. *Clinical guideline CG32. Nutrition support in adults.* 2006. https://www.nice.org.uk/guidance/cg32 [accessed 26 March 2019].

Question 12 F T T F

There are several risk factors for delayed gastric emptying, including illness severity, sepsis, burns, trauma, and use of certain drugs (e.g. inotropes, opioids, and PPIs). Metoclopramide may increase ICP, so it is contraindicated in head injury patients. It has been shown to delay the onset of pneumonia but not reduce chance of infection. Erythromycin is used intravenously at a dose of 60–250mg qds. It can cause arrhythmias.

Grant K, Thomas R. Prokinetic drugs in the intensive care unit: reviewing the evidence. *Journal of the Intensive Care Society* Jan 2009;10(1):34–7.

Question 13 F F F T F

Aggressive fluid resuscitation is recommended in the first 12–24 hours, as there is benefit in preventing multiple organ failure (MOF). However continued aggressive fluid resuscitation beyond that may be detrimental. Each individual needs their hydration status evaluated, and persistent hypotension requires admission to the high dependency or intensive care unit. There is a study highlighting the benefit of Ringer's lactate over sodium chloride in preventing systemic inflammatory response syndrome. Prophylactic antibiotics and antifungals should be avoided. Early ERCP is indicated in acute pancreatitis with gallstones and acute cholangitis. Pancreatic duct stents +/− rectal indomethacin may help prevent post-ERCP pancreatitis.

Tenner S, Baillie J, DeWitt J. Management of acute pancreatitis. *American Journal of Gastroenterology* 2013;108:1400–15.

Question 14 F F F F F

Hypertensive emergency can be described as severely elevated BP systolic ≥180mmHg and/or diastolic ≥120mmHg, with ongoing or impending end organ damage. Hypertensive urgency or severe asymptomatic hypertension describes severely elevated BP, with no signs or symptoms or laboratory evidence of end organ damage.

Hypertensive emergencies are relatively uncommon, with cerebral infarction and acute pulmonary oedema and left ventricular dysfunction being the commonest causes of hypertensive emergency. Eclampsia is the least frequent cause, and death from pre-eclampsia or eclampsia in the UK has reduced significantly, with the most common cause of maternal death remaining thromboembolism.

Management of the hypertensive emergency depends on the underlying cause. For example, aortic dissection remains an infrequent cause, but should promote rapid BP lowering in order to reduce aortic shearing forces. Regarding ischaemic stroke as the precipitant for hypertensive emergency, the blood pressure is usually not lowered unless it is ≥185/110mmHg in patients who are candidates for reperfusion therapy or ≥220/120mmHg in patients who are not candidates for reperfusion (thrombolytic) therapy. Drugs such as beta blockers acutely reduce cardiac output and therefore are not ideal for pulmonary oedema and left ventricular dysfunction.

Zampaglione B, Pascale C, Marchisio M, Cavallo-Perin P. Hypertensive urgencies and emergencies. Prevalence and clinical presentation. *Hypertension* Jan 1996;27(1):144–7.

MBRACE-UK. *Saving Lives, improving mothers' care. Surveillance of maternal deaths in the UK 2012–14 and lessons learned to inform maternity care from the UK and Ireland Confidential Enquiries into Maternal Deaths and Morbidity 2009–14.* https://www.npeu.ox.ac.uk/downloads/files/mbrrace-uk/reports/MBRRACE-UK%20Maternal%20Report%202016%20-%20website.pdf [accessed 26 July 2021].

Question 15 F T F T F

The national Centers of Disease Control and Prevention (CDC) states that diagnosis of VAP should be made on:

- Radiological changes
  - (New progressive infiltrate, consolidation, cavitation)
- Clinical signs
  - One of
    - Fever (temperature >38°C with no other recognized cause)
    - Leucocytosis, leucopaenia
    - Adults aged >70 years only—altered mental status
  - And at least two of
    - New or change in purulent sputum
    - Worsening cough/tachypnoea/dyspnoea
    - Bronchial breath sounds
    - Worsening gas exchange
- Microbiological criteria (optional)
  - Positive blood culture and no other source infection
  - Positive growth pleural fluid
  - Positive quantitative culture—bronchoalveolar lavage (≥104 colony forming units/ml) or protected specimen brushing (≥103 colony forming units/ml)
  - 5% or more of cells with intracellular bacteria on direct microscopic examination of Gram-stained bronchoalveolar lavage fluid

Respiratory samples may be obtained by:

- Noninvasive technique (i.e. endotracheal aspirate)
- Invasive techniques
  - Bronchoscopic bronchoalveolar lavage (BAL)
  - Blind BAL
  - Protected specimen brush (PSB)

Once specimens are obtained, Gram stain can provide crucial initial clues to the type of organism(s) and whether or not the material is purulent (defined as ≥25 neutrophils and ≤10 squamous epithelial cells per low power field). Culture can be qualitative (presence or absence pathogens), semiquantitative (i.e. moderate or heavy growth) or quantitative (CDC diagnosis). Cochrane studies have failed to demonstrate the superiority of invasive sampling or the use of qualitative culture values. VAP is defined as *early* (within 4 days) or *late* (>4 days postintubation). Late causes of VAP include *pseudomonas*, MRSA, and *Acinetobacter*, whereas early VAP is caused by *Strep pneumoniae, Haemophilus influenza*, and MSSA. An antipseudomonal cephalosporin may be used in this instance, although individual hospitals will have protocols driven by local microbiological data.

National Healthcare Safety Network (NHSN). CDC/NHSN Protocol clarifications. *Pneumonia (ventilator associated (VAP) and non-ventilator associated pneumonia) event.* http://www.cdc.gov/nhsn/PDFs/pscManual/6pscVAPcurrent.pdf [accessed 26 July 2021].

Question 16 F F T F T

The triad of thrombocytopaenia, acute kidney injury, and neurological involvement should raise the suspicion of thrombotic thrombocytopaenic purpura (TTP). ADAMTS13 is responsible for cleaving von Willebrand factor (vWF), and in TTP, antibodies form against it. This results in large vWF multimers, whereby platelets aggregate and form clots in small vessels. Red blood cells become trapped and fragmented, hence the microangiopathic haemolysis. TTP can be inherited, idiopathic, or secondary to several situations (including pregnancy, malignancy, bone marrow transplant, and several drugs, including clopidogrel and cyclosporine). Patients can present with renal failure, neurological disturbance, fever, and purpura. Gastrointestinal symptoms may also feature, such as pain, nausea, and diarrhoea and vomiting. Investigation will reveal a haemolytic anaemia (high unconjugated bilirubin, high lactate, low haptoglobin, and negative direct antiglobulin Coombs test) and normal complement levels with reduced activity of ADAMTS13 (<10% during an acute episode). In patients with microangiopathic haemolysis and low platelets, consider TTP, even in the absence of organ involvement.

Platelet transfusion is contraindicated, and the mainstay of treatment for TTP is plasma exchange.

Waldmann C, Soni N, Rhodes A (eds). *Oxford desk reference: critical care*, 1st edition. Oxford: Oxford University Press, 2008.

Question 17 F F T F T

Coning causes a 'sympathetic storm' and is therefore heralded by the onset of pronounced hypertension. This outpouring of catecholamines leads to a surge in myocardial oxygen demand, arrhythmias, and vasoconstriction often leading to myocardial ischaemia or infarction and neurogenic pulmonary oedema. After the 'storm' patients become vasodilated and hypotensive. Without balanced resuscitation, organ perfusion may become inadequate, leading, in the case of a donated organ, to impaired function in the recipient. Donor organ function, especially intrathoracic organs, usually benefit from a period of optimization following the diagnosis of brainstem death and before retrieval occurs. Some hearts initially deemed unsuitable for donation have been successfully transplanted after a period of organ optimization. Longer periods of active donor management are associated with improved gas exchange, reduced lung water, and higher lung transplant rates. Donation after brainstem death (DBD) donors donated an average of 3.9 organs in 2012/13, whilst donation after cardiac death (DCD) donors donated an average of 2.6 organs in the same period. Deceased donation can only proceed after the diagnosis of death. Diagnosis of death according to brainstem death criteria requires the completion of two sets of confirmatory brainstem tests, although the time of death is retrospectively recorded as the time the first set of tests were completed. Registration on the ODR is just one way of the patient's desire to donate being communicated to the clinical team. Most patients that donate have not previously registered on the ODR, and consent is provided by family members. National Health Sevice Blood and Transfusion (NHSBT) guidance includes a list of those in a qualifying relationship with the patient who can consent to deceased donation. As of 2020, all adults will be considered an organ donor when they die, unless there is a recorded decision not to donate.

McKeown DW, Bonser RS, Kellum JA. Management of the heartbeating brain-dead organ donor. *British Journal of Anaesthesia* 2012;108(Suppl 1):i96–i107.

Question 18 F T T F T

SDD is a prophylactic measure designed to control primary endogenous infection (pathogens present on admission), secondary endogenous infection (infection caused by pathogens acquired during colonization), and exogenous infection (i.e. pathogens not present on admission and without preceding colonization). SDD is therefore undertaken by parenteral antimicrobial administration (e.g. cefotaxime) to cover the early primary infection by normal pathogenic organisms. Polymixin and tobramycin are then administered enterally as a paste to the oropharynx, and a suspension to the GIT, to eradicate the 'abnormal' pathogens (e.g. pseudomonas), and strict hygiene is used to prevent exogenous infection. There are many studies dedicated to looking at SDD, and a number of randomized controlled trials show benefit; however, reluctance for uptake is mostly related to the potential impact of antimicrobial resistance and the strong lack of evidence supporting SDD in units with high levels of multidrug resistance. Regular surveillance is indicated to monitor efficacy and safety of the regime.

Waldmann C, Soni N, Rhodes A (eds). *Oxford desk reference: critical care*, 1st edition. Oxford: Oxford University Press, 2008.

Question 19 FFFFF

The Cesar trial demonstrated that in patients with early acute respiratory distress syndrome (ARDS), transfer to a facility specializing in ARDS with the ability to initiate ECMO was associated with an improvement in 6-month survival without severe disability. Eligible patients were aged between 18 and 65 years and had severe (Murray score >3 or pH <7.20) but potentially reversible respiratory failure. Patients with peak inspiratory pressures >30 cm H_2O or FiO_2 >80% for more than 7 days were excluded, as were those with a contraindication to anticoagulation.

ECMO circuits can be set up in various ways:

- Veno-arterial (V-A) allows gas exchange and haemodynamic support while blood is pumped from the venous to the arterial side
- Veno-venous (V-V) ECMO improves oxygenation, but there is no haemodynamic support
- Arterio-venous (A-V) utilizes the patient's own arterial pressure to pump the blood from the arterial to the venous side

The aim of V-V ECMO is to provide oxygenation and rest the lungs, which is particularly useful in ARDS where lung compliance is poor. Risk of thromboembolism is reduced compared to V-A ECMO. The best survival rates are observed in patients with non necrotizing viral pneumonia.

Peek GJ, et al. Efficacy and economic assessment of conventional ventilatory support versus extracorporeal membrane oxygenation for severe adult respiratory failure. *Lancet* 2009;374:1351–63.

Martinez G, Vulysteke A. Extracorporeal membrane oxygenation in adults. *Continuing Education In Anaesthesia, Critical Care & Pain* 2012;12:57.

Question 20 F T T T F

Acid–base balance and pH are not only determined by the [H^+] and [$HCO3^-$]. Other Ions in solution also influence pH, and strong ions are those that fully dissociate at the pH of interest of a particular solution (e.g. pH 7.4 for blood). The strong cations are Na^+, K^+, Ca^{2+}, Mg^{2+}, and the strong anions are Cl^- and SO_4^{2-}. SID is the difference between the concentrations of strong cations and strong anions.

$$SID = (Na^+ + K^+ + Ca^{2+} + Mg^{2+}) - (Cl^-, + other strong anions) - 0$$

- the number of positive and negative ions in a solution must be equal
- increased SID (>0) leads to alkalosis (increase in unmeasured anions)
- decreased SID (<0) acidosis

Normal saline does have a SID of zero (154mmol Na and 154mmol Cl). However there is a relative greater effect on body chloride levels and a decrease in plasma SID. Infusion of hypotonic solutions decreases SID and causes a dilutional acidosis through relative decrease in sodium levels. Infusions of Hartmann's solution (which has a SID of 28) will increase SID as lactate is metabolized leaving behind sodium. Renal failure leads to an increased anion gap as there are increased numbers of unmeasured weak anions (e.g. phosphate). Type I renal tubular acidosis occurs because there is failure to excrete chloride.

Badr A, Nightingale P. An alternative approach to acid-base abnormalities in critically ill patients. *Continuing Education In Anaesthesia, Critical Care & Pain* 2007;7:107–11.

Question 21 T F T F F

Table 5.1 The NASPE/BPEG Code

I	II	III	IV	V
Chamber(s) paced	Chamber(s) sensed	Response to sensing	Rate modulation	Multisite pacing
O = none	O = none	O = none	O = none	O = none
A = atrium	A = atrium	T = triggered	R = rate modulation	A = atrium
V = ventricle	V = ventricle	I = inhibited	–	V = ventricle
D = dual (A+V)	D = dual (A+V)	D = dual (T+I)	–	D = dual (A+V)

Biventricular devices do not readily fit into this classification and are referred to as CRT (cardiac resynchronization therapy) devices (see Table 5.1). These may be combined with a defibrillation function, given the designation CRT-D.

Bernstein AD, et al.; North American Society of Pacing and Electrophysiology/British Pacing and Electrophysiology Group. The revised NASPE/BPEG generic code for antibradycardia, adaptive-rate, and multisite pacing. *Pacing Clinical Electrophysiology* 2002;25:260–4.

Question 22 F T T T F

Organ donation may proceed after death diagnosed on either brainstem criteria or cardiovascular criteria. Most patients eligible for deceased donation are critical care patients situated either in critical care or the emergency department. Donation after death diagnosed on cardiovascular criteria (DCD) is usually only practical when a patient's death can be anticipated (e.g. after planned withdrawal of invasive support). Living donor programmes are currently the only alternative source of donor organs. One organ donor can save or transform the lives of up to nine other individuals. Absolute contraindications to organ donation include: Creutzfeldt-Jakob disease, Ebola virus, active cancer and HIV.

Because this list of contraindications has changed over time (e.g. age is no longer a limit for becoming a donor), the final decision on whether to transplant an organ always rests with the transplant surgeon, so critical care staff are encouraged to refer all potential DBD and DCD donors to the specialist nurse for organ donation (SNOD). Early confirmation of a patient's eligibility may avoid offering the option of donation to a family whose loved one would not be a suitable donor. The number of transplants performed in the UK each year is currently limited by the availability of donor organs. On average three people die every day in the UK waiting for an organ.

McKeown DW, Bonser RS, Kellum JA. Management of the heartbeating brain-dead organ donor. *British Journal of Anaesthesia* 2012;108(Suppl 1):i96–i107.

Question 23 T F F F F

Exact definitions regarding drowning have varied widely and have included near-drowning, dry drowning, active drowning, and silent drowning. The most recent definition states that drowning is a process involving primary respiratory impairment from submersion in a liquid medium and that a liquid-air interface is present at the entrance to the victim's airway. There are differences between saltwater and freshwater drowning. For example freshwater is relatively hypotonic, moving rapidly into the microcirculation and disrupting alveolar surfactant. Ingestion of large quantities of freshwater (rather than aspiration) can result in significant hyponatraemia. Saltwater (hypertonic) draws fluid into the alveoli, damaging the alveolar-capillary membrane and resulting in hypoxia.

Warm freshwater is more commonly associated with the development of infection, although pneumonia is rare, and there is no role for prophylactic antibiotics. Not all drowning victims will aspirate fluid. When the airway is below the liquid's surface, involuntary laryngospasm occurs. As hypoxia ensues, laryngospasm breaks, and the victim gasps, aspirating fluid. However 10%–20% of individuals maintain laryngospasm, and these individuals do not aspirate fluid (dry drowning). Neuroprotective effects of cold water (<20°C) drowning remain poorly understood.

Hypothermia reduces cerebral metabolic rate (CMR), but neuroprotective effects occur only if the hypothermia is rapid onset (i.e. temperature of the water is <5°C). Most patients in cold water submersion do not develop hypothermia rapidly enough to decrease the CMR before hypoxic damage occurs. Prognosis ultimately is related to length of submersion, and the likelihood of a good prognosis following submersion of greater than 10 minutes is low.

Van Beeck EF, Branche CM, Szpilman D, Modell JH, Bierens JJ. A new definition of drowning: towards documentation and prevention of a global public health problem. *Bulletin World Health Organization* Nov 2005;83(11):853–6.

Question 24 T T T F T

Outreach arose as a result of the Department of Health report 'Comprehensive Critical Care' in 2000. The principles included preventing ICU admission by early identification and intervention, support post ICU recovery on discharge and share their expertise and experience with ward-based staff. Outreach use a track and trigger scoring system such as the National Early Warning Score. Outreach undoubtedly provide support to nursing staff and junior doctors, especially in the face of reduced trainee numbers, and they also provide a means for audit. Outreach teams typically comprise of trained nursing personnel, with medical input from intensivists. There is no strong evidence to suggest that outreach prevent cardiac arrests, ICU admissions, or death, and a Cochrane review reported inconclusive evidence in supporting the effectiveness of outreach. However despite the lack of robust evidence, the Department of Health continues to support their use.

The Cochrane Collaboration. *Outreach and Early Warning Systems (EWS) for the prevention of intensive care admission and death of critically ill adult patients on general hospital wards. 2007* https://www.cochranelibrary.com/cdsr/doi/10.1002/14651858.CD005529.pub2/related-content#guidelines_data [accessed 14 February 2019].

Question 25 T F T T T

Increased intrathoracic pressure changes the pressure gradient for systemic venous return to the right side of the heart, and decreases transmural pressure across the left ventricle. Consequently venous return is reduced, but so is left ventricular afterload. This may unload the heart in cardiac failure. Right ventricular output and pulmonary blood flow are reduced with reduced intrathoracic pressure. Elimination of the workload of spontaneous ventilatory effort will reduce oxygen demands and improve SvO_2.

Soni N, Williams P. Positive pressure ventilation: what is the real cost? *British Journal of Anaesthesia* 2008;101:446–57.

Waldmann C, Soni N, Rhodes A (eds). *Oxford desk reference: critical care*, 1st edition. Oxford: Oxford University Press, 2008.

Question 26 T T F F T

Propofol is a highly lipid-soluble weak acid. Its administration may be associated with CNS excitatory activity including opisthotonas. PRIS was first recognized in children, but adult cases have been subsequently recognized.

PRIS is associated with:

- Unexplained metabolic acidosis
- Arrhythmia, bradycardia, and CVS collapse
- Rhabdomyolysis, AKI, and hyperkalaemia
- Lipaemia
- Hepatomegaly

Risk factors for PRIS include:

- Critical illness
- Propofol dose >4mk/kg/hour
- Propofol infusion >48 hours
- 'Trigger' (e.g. catecholamine infusion)
- Inadequate delivery of carbohydrate

The exact mechanism of PRIS is unknown but may reflect impaired electron transport and metabolic collapse. Propofol increases hepatocellular oxygen uptake and reduces gluconeogenesis. This disrupts free fatty acid utilization and impairs ATP synthesis and cellular oxygen delivery, leading to cell death. In the absence of carbohydrate, lipid metabolism slows, and so it is essential to ensure early provision of carbohydrate and minimize excessive lipid input to prevent PRIS.

Loh N, Nair P. Propofol infusion syndrome. *Continuing Education In Anaesthesia, Critical Care & Pain* 2013;13:200–2.

Question 27 T T T F T

Amiodarone is primarily regarded as a Vaughn-Williams class III antiarrythmic (which increases the repolarization phase by causing potassium channel blockade); however, it also has class I (sodium channel blockade) and class IV (calcium channel blockade) activity. It is a hepatic enzyme inhibitor, potentiating the effects of several drugs, including warfarin, digoxin, and theophylline. Amiodarone, in longer term use, has several side-effects including pulmonary fibrosis, liver and thyroid dysfunction, skin discolouration, and corneal microdeposits which can lead to blurred vision.

Peck T, Hill S, Williams M. *Pharmacology for anaesthesia and intensive care*, 2nd edition. London: Greenwich Medical Media, 2003.

Question 28 F T T T T

Neuroleptic malignant syndrome (NMS) presents with a combination of hyperthermia, muscle rigidity, and autonomic lability. It is related to the use of antipsychotics, including olanzapine, risperidone, and quetiapine, as well as haloperidol, metoclopramide, and prochlorperazine. It is believed to arise as a result of dopamine D2 receptor antagonism, and so may also occur on abrupt withdrawal of Parkinson treatment.

It presents with temperature rise, rigidity, autonomic instability, and changes in affect and, or delirium. Blood results often include a raised creatinine kinase (CK) and leucocytosis.

Management is largely supportive with cooling, antipyretics, and CVS support. Dantrolene, amantadine, and bromocriptine have also been used. Serotonin syndrome may present similarly to NMS (i.e. altered mental state, autonomic dysfunction, and neuromuscular abnormality). The use of selective serotonin reuptake inhibitor (SSRI) is associated with this, and a thorough drug history is required to differentiate the two syndromes. However, NMS presents with marked (lead pipe) rigidity, and does not include clonus, which may be seen in serotonin syndrome.

Waldmann C, Soni N, Rhodes A (eds). *Oxford desk reference: critical care*, 1st edition. Oxford: Oxford University Press, 2008.

Question 29 F T T T T

Pulse oximetry relies on spectrophotometric techniques. Radiation—red light at 660nm and infrared light at 940nm—is passed through a sample of blood, and the quantity of radiation absorbed can be calculated. As deoxyhaemoglobin and oxyhaemoglobin have differing absorbances at these wavelengths; a comparison of radiation absorbed allows the oximeter to identify the relative quantities of the two haemoglobins. This is compared to calibration graphs, compiled from healthy volunteers breathing variable oxygen concentrations.

Beer's law and Lambert's law define the amount of radiation absorbed by a substance. The latter describes how the intensity of light decreases exponentially as distance travelled through the substance increases. Both laws cannot be strictly applied to blood, hence the need for calibration graphs.

The isosbestic points are the wavelengths at which radiation absorbed by oxy- and deoxyhaemoglobin are equal. Oxyhaemoglobin absorbs less radiation than deoxyhaemoglobin within the red light spectra.

Cross, M, Plunkett E. *Physics, pharmacology, and physiology for anaesthetists*. Cambridge: Cambridge University Press, 2014.

Question 30 T F F T T

Ethylene glycol itself is relatively nontoxic, although it can cause CNS effects such as euphoria at lower doses, and depressed consciousness at higher doses. Toxicity is mainly due to metabolites such as glycolic, formic, and oxalic acids. Laboratory findings are of a raised osmolar gap, a high anion gap acidosis, and elevated lactate. In addition ethylene glycol can contribute to a true rise in serum lactate since this is produced as a result of the large amounts of nicotinamide adenine dinucleotide being formed during the breakdown of ethylene glycol and secondary to inhibition of the citric acid cycle by the condensation products of glyoxylate. Hypocalcaemia is seen due to precipitation of oxalate, and hyperkalaemia develops due to acute renal failure.

Waldmann C, Soni N, Rhodes A (eds). *Oxford desk reference: critical care*, 1st edition. Oxford: Oxford University Press, 2008.

paper
6

MCQ QUESTIONS

1. **Regarding pulmonary embolism (PE) and venous thromboembolism, the following are true:**
   A. Cancer is a risk factor for PE, although this risk varies with the type of cancer
   B. D-dimer is useful if the clinical probability of a PE is high and there is no evidence of shock or hypotension
   C. Thrombolysis should be given to patients where PE is likely and there is evidence of right ventricular dysfunction on echo
   D. Thrombolysis should be administered in an arrest situation, even if PE has not been confirmed radiologically
   E. Thrombolysis can be given if there is worsening respiratory failure in a patient who is being anticoagulated for PE

2. **Regarding traumatic spinal injury, the following are true:**
   A. An injury below C5 usually results in no respiratory dysfunction in the acute setting
   B. Approximately 10% of patients with a cervical fracture will also have a second vertebral fracture
   C. Spinal shock presents with bradycardia and hypotension
   D. Shock associated with spinal cord injury can often be managed with fluid resuscitation alone
   E. The pattern of spinal injury most often involves the thoracolumbar region

3. **Regarding the strong ion theory relating to acid–base balance, the following are correct:**
   A. Acid–base status, of a body fluid depends on CO_2, strong ions, and weak acids
   B. Ammonium [$NH4^+$] loss from the kidney results in acidosis
   C. As the strong ion difference decreases (e.g. due to excess chloride), water dissociates
   D. In hypoalbumnaemic states, the strong ion difference increases to maintain electroneutrality
   E. Strong cations outnumber strong anions and this is the strong ion difference

MCQs and SBAs in Intensive Care Medicine. Lorna Eyre and Andrew Bodenham, Oxford University Press. © Oxford University Press 2021.
DOI: 10.1093/oso/9780198753056.003.0006

4. **A 22-year-old male smoker presents to the ED with fever, cough, diarrhoea, and clinical features of a left lower lobe pneumonia. He is newly confused and has a respiratory rate of 35 breaths per minute and systolic blood pressure of 80mmHg. Oxygen saturations are 88% on room air. Blood tests reveal blood urea of 9mmol/l and abnormal liver function tests. The following are true:**

A. A β lactam provides sufficient antimicrobial cover in the first instance

B. His CURB65 score is 3

C. If the patient is penicillin allergic a quinolone such as levofloxacin would be suitable

D. Noninvasive ventilation would be the most appropriate ventilatory support in the face of acute deterioration

E. The most likely causative organism from the clinical scenario, is Legionella rather than Streptococcal pneumonia

5. **A 53-year-old man is found collapsed next to unlabelled bottles. He has a Glasgow Coma Scale (GCS) of E 2, V 1, M 4 on arrival to ED On examination he is tachypnoeic with Kussmaul breathing, and slightly tachycardic with systolic blood pressure >100mm Hg. Computed tomography (CT) of the head reveals no abnormality. Arterial blood gas findings include: pH 7.13, pCO_2 1.8 kPa, pO_2 11 kPa, HCO_3^- 14mmol/l chloride 100mmol/l. Lactate is normal. Sodium and potassium are 135 and 6.0mmol/l, respectively, and blood glucose is 6.5 mmol/l. The following are correct:**

A. A low calcium level is an expected finding

B. Anion gap is calculated by 2 Na + glucose + urea (mmol/l)

C. Ethanol loading should be used as an immediate management

D. Expected finding would include early osmolar gap

E. The anion gap is calculated as 27mmol/l

6. **A patient is admitted to the intensive care unit (ICU) and requires vasopressor therapy. A central venous catheter (CVC) is inserted, and the following are correct:**

A. Catheters should be removed if the causative organism of a catheter-related blood stream infection (CRBSI) is *Staphylococcus aureus*

B. Chlorhexidine 2% solution alone, prior to line CVC line insertion, has reduced the incidence of CRBSI

C. Diagnosis using differential time to positivity has greater sensitivity and specificity that paired quantitative cultures

D. Most common causative organism of CRBSI is *Staphylococcus aureus*

E. Preferred site of insertion should be internal jugular vein

7. **A 45-year-old man presents to the ICU with respiratory failure and has a new incidental finding of HIV, the following are true:**
   A. Current recommendations are that treatment of primary HIV infection with highly active antiretroviral therapy (HAART) should begin as soon as possible in those with CD4 counts of less than 350/μL
   B. HAART should be commenced in all patients presenting to the ICU with HIV infection
   C. Peri-hilar interstitial ground glass shadowing is characteristic of Pneumocystis jirovecii infection
   D. The most common diagnosis for ICU admission remains Pneumocystis pneumonia in HIV-positive patients
   E. The immune reconstitution inflammatory syndrome (IRIS) may occur after withdrawal of HAART

8. **The following substances are removed by haemodiafiltration:**
   A. Amitriptyline
   B. Iron
   C. Lactate
   D. Salicylic acid
   E. Theophylline

9. **A patient has been in hospital for 9 days and has been receiving a course of antibiotics for a community acquired pneumonia. In addition he has received venous thromboembolism (VTE) prophylaxis. Over the last 48 hours, his platelet count has dropped from baseline 160 × 10⁹/L to 75 × 10⁹/L:**
   A. Heparin-induced thrombocytopaenia (HIT) is via an immune-mediated reaction
   B. HIT occurs more frequently in women
   C. If HIT is suspected, heparin should be stopped, and warfarin can be commenced as an alternative
   D. Platelet levels will often return to normal within a few days of stopping heparin
   E. The timing of platelet fall occurs between 5 and 10 days in cases of HIT

10. **The following are correct when considering the average daily nutrition requirements in adults:**
    A. Carbohydrate 3g/kg/day
    B. Magnesium 0.1mmol/kg/day
    C. Phosphorus 0.1mmol/kg/day
    D. Potassium 1.5mmol/kg/day
    E. Protein 2g/kg/day

11. **A 65-year-old woman presents to the ICU with neutropaenic sepsis, following the start of chemotherapy for a recently diagnosed acute myeloid leukaemia. Biochemically she develops the hallmarks of tumour lysis syndrome. Associations with tumour lysis syndrome include:**
   A. Hyperkalaemia, hyperuricaemia, hyperphosphataemia, and hypercalcaemia
   B. It is linked to haematological malignancies and solid tumours
   C. Patients with acute leukaemia and lower white cell counts are at greater risk
   D. Intratubular precipitation of uric acid can be prevented routinely with an alkaline diuresis
   E. Recombinant urate oxidase increases normal intrinsic levels of this enzyme, thus further reducing uric acid levels

12. **A patient on the ICU develops a markedly distended abdomen, stops absorbing their feed, and has a progressive fall in urine output. The following are true:**
   A. Girth measurement is a reasonable indicator for increased abdominal pressure
   B. Intra-abdominal pressure is 5–7mmHg normally
   C. Intra-abdominal pressure ≥25mmHg will result in an increased risk of morbidity
   D. Laparostomy remains the initial treatment of choice for abdominal compartment syndrome
   E. Laparostomy should be performed once pressure ≥20mmHg

13. **Regarding rhabdomyolysis, the following are true:**
   A. Compartment syndrome may be an early or late complication
   B. Fluid resuscitation to achieve high urinary flow rates (50ml/hr) is recommended
   C. Hypocalcaemia is a complication
   D. Hypercalcaemia is a complication
   E. Sodium bicarbonate may be used to maintain urinary pH>6.5

14. **During volume control ventilation, the following are correct:**
   A. Airway pressure is inversely proportional to lung compliance
   B. Driving pressure falls during the inspiratory period
   C. Inspiratory flow is constant
   D. Peak pressures cannot be limited
   E. The switch from inspiration to expiration may be time-cycled

15. **It is correct that the following assessments can be used to indicate likely successful weaning:**
   A. Minute ventilation >10l/min
   B. PaO_2/FIO_2 ratio >20kpa
   C. Respiratory rate/tidal volume <100l
   D. Respiratory frequency <35 breaths per minute
   E. Vital capacity breath >10ml/kg

16. **The Department of Health High Impact Intervention (HII) bundle for central venous catheter (CVC) placement includes:**
    A. Avoidance of femoral catheter placement
    B. A sterile transparent semi-permeable dressing is used
    C. The use of a single lumen catheter unless otherwise indicated
    D. The use of an antimicrobial impregnated catheter if likely to be required for more than 48 hours
    E. Use of ultrasound for catheter placement

17. **In coronary artery bypass surgery (CABG), the following are true:**
    A. Cardiopulmonary bypass is necessary
    B. Cardiopulmonary bypass causes immune activation
    C. Left internal mammary artery grafts are preferred in proximal left coronary artery lesions
    D. Systemic heparinization is reversed by aprotinin
    E. Transoesophageal echocardiography (TOE) leads to a 1 in 1000 incidence of oesophageal perforation

18. **Regarding acute chest pain and type 1 myocardial infarction (MI), the following are true:**
    A. Aspirin should only be given once the diagnosis is made
    B. If a patient has chest pain and ECG changes, ensure they receive oxygen with target saturation 98%–100% to improve myocardial oxygen delivery
    C. If the chest pain is not relieved by GTN, type 1 MI is unlikely
    D. In the presence of persisting ST elevation after fibrinolysis, fibrinolysis can be repeated
    E. Low level of consciousness post cardiac arrest and type 1 MI is a contraindication to coronary angiography and PCI

19. **With regards to the placement of nasogastric tubes for enteral nutrition, the following are correct:**
    A. Analysis of incidents involving placement of NG feeding tubes since 2005 suggested that x-ray misinterpretation was the single largest contributory factor
    B. Correct nasogastric tube tip placement can be confirmed with the whoosh test, which remains a safe and reliable method
    C. Check chest x-ray is necessary to confirm correct placement of nasogastric tube tip
    D. Litmus paper can be used to confirm that the nasogastric tube tip is in the correct position
    E. Misplacement of a nasogastric tube is a never event

20. **In liver transplantation, the following are true:**
    A. Coagulopathy and hypoalbuminaemia should be corrected preoperatively
    B. New proven hepatopulmonary syndrome is a contraindication to liver transplantation
    C. Severe pulmonary hypertension (mean pulmonary artery pressure >50mmHg) is a contraindication to liver transplantation
    D. Significant hyponatraemia should be corrected preoperatively with sodium containing crystalloid
    E. The model for end-stage liver disease (MELD) score used to prioritize patients for liver transplants is based on bilirubin, INR, and albumin

21. **A patient is being weaned from the mechanical ventilator and has an endotracheal tube in situ, the following are correct:**
    A. Intravenous morphine is superior as an analgesic compared to intravenous fentanyl
    B. Hypertension and tachycardia are useful indicators in assessing pain
    C. Minimizing sedation reduces duration of mechanical ventilation
    D. To date, there are no reliable tools for pain assessment within the critical care environment
    E. Use of dexmedetomidine may reduce the risk of delirium compared to midazolam

22. **Regarding the physiology of infants and children, the following are true:**
    A. A heart rate of 60 beats per minute and blood pressure 80/40mmHg are considered acceptable goals during resuscitation of an infant
    B. Blood volume is approximately 80ml/kg in an infant
    C. Infant daily sodium requirements are similar to that of an adult
    D. PaO_2 is lower in an infant compared to a child
    E. The metabolic rate of an infant is nearly twice that of an adult

23. **The following are typically a cause of a raised anion gap acidosis:**
    A. Acute renal failure
    B. Diabetic ketoacidosis
    C. Ethylene glycol poisoning
    D. Methanol poisoning
    E. Type 3 renal tubular acidosis

24. **It is true that the following predict fluid responsiveness:**
    A. A central venous pressure of 6mmHg
    B. A correct flow time of 310ms
    C. Pulse pressure variation of 10%
    D. Stroke volume variation of 12%
    E. Superior vena cava collapsibility index of 40%

25. **Diuretics are commonly used within the ICU. The following are true regarding their use:**
    A. All diuretics result in a metabolic alkalosis
    B. Loop diuretics act at the early segment of the proximal tubule to increase delivery of Na and water to the distal convoluted tubule
    C. Loop diuretics produce arteriolar vasodilatation and reduction in ventricular preload
    D. Thiazide diuretics cause hypokalaemia by direct inhibition of Na^+ K^+ co-transport in the distal convoluted tubule
    E. Spironolactone is used in cirrhotic patients to prevent secondary hyperaldosteronism

26. **Regarding pharmacological principles, the following are correct:**
    A. All drugs undergo phase I metabolism and then phase II
    B. Cimetidine increases oral bioavailability
    C. First pass metabolism is increased by phenytoin
    D. Local anaesthetics with a low pK_a have a faster onset when given via the epidural route compared to those with a higher pK_a
    E. Phase I metabolism is designed to reduce the activity of a drug

27. **Regarding humidification devices used on the ICU, the following are true:**
    A. Conditions in the heated humidification chamber are tightly controlled to prevent the fresh gas flow from becoming fully saturated
    B. During nebulization, smaller droplets enable more efficacious humidification than larger droplets
    C. Passive humidification rather than active humidification within the breathing system is likely to be associated with ventilator associated pneumonia (VAP)
    D. The heating wire in the inspiratory limb of the circuit allows the inspiratory gases to be warmed as they travel through it thereby increasing the relative humidity
    E. There is robust evidence of improved clinical outcome when humidification is used during noninvasive ventilation (NIV)

28. **Following successful endovascular coiling of a ruptured aneurysmal subarachnoid haemorrhage (SAH), it is true that:**
    A. Delayed cerebral ischaemia (DCI) occurs secondary to vasospasm
    B. Hydrocephalus develops in 20%–30% patients
    C. Nimodipine should be prescribed for 21 days
    D. Seizures should be prevented with prophylactic anticonvulsants
    E. Triple H therapy should be used

29. **The following are true regarding high-frequency oscillatory ventilation (HFOV):**
    A. Decrease in frequency on HFOV leads to decreased CO_2 clearance
    B. It relies on the rapid delivery of tidal volumes that are smaller than dead space
    C. It can be used in patients with broncho-pleural fistula
    D. Mean airway pressure is higher in HFOV compared to Conventional Mechanical Ventilation
    E. When compared to conventional ventilation for patients with acute respiratory distress syndrome, HFOV is associated with a reduction in mortality rate

30. **Regarding the APACHE II score, the following are included:**
    A. Glasgow coma scale
    B. Haemoglobin
    C. Heart rate
    D. Respiratory rate
    E. White blood cell count

Question 1 T F F T T

There is an extensive list of predisposing risk factors for VTE, and cancer is included. The risk of VTE does indeed vary with differing malignancies, with haematological, lung, gastrointestinal, pancreatic, and brain carrying the highest risk. Assessment of clinical probability can be done with either the Wells rule or revised Geneva score. D-dimer can be raised in other clinical scenarios, and so its use is best associated with a low clinical probability case, where a normal result (using a high- sensitive assay) can exclude PE. Thrombolysis treatment of acute PE more rapidly restores pulmonary perfusion; however, in the absence of haemodynamic instability, the clinical benefits of thrombolysis remain less clear. The PEITHO trial suggests that in patients with evidence of RV dysfunction, tenecteplase reduced the rate of haemodynamic collapse, but also increased the rate of haemorrhagic stroke. According to European guidelines, if PE is confirmed and there is an intermediate risk of 30-day mortality (according to PE severity index score) and echo and, or CT or biomarker evidence for RV dysfunction, then anticoagulation should be initiated with thrombolysis being used as a rescue reperfusion strategy. If PE is suspected clinically in an acutely deteriorating patient who is too unwell for CT pulmonary angiogram, then echocardiography may identify signs of acute right heart strain suggestive of acute PE. British Thoracic Society guidelines suggest a bolus dose of 50mg alteplase in the peri-arrest or arrest situation; however, if the cause of arrest is unclear, thrombolysis should not be given during cardiopulmonary resuscitation. If a patient with recent acute PE fails anticoagulation treatment and there is worsening cardiovascular instability or respiratory failure, thrombolysis should be considered.

Condliffe R, et al. Management dilemmas in acute pulmonary embolism *Thorax* 2013;69:1–7.

Konstantinides N, et al. ESC guidelines on the diagnosis and management of acute pulmonary embolism. *Heart* 2014;35:3033–73.

Meyer G, et al. Fibrinolysis for patients with intermediate-risk pulmonary embolism. *New England Journal of Medicine* 2014;370(15):1402–11.

Question 2 F T F F F

The vast majority of spinal injuries occur in the cervical region (55%), and approximately 10% of those with a C spine fracture will also have a second vertebral fracture. *Neurogenic shock* describes hypotension and bradycardia secondary to impaired descending sympathetic pathways resulting from lesions in the cervical or upper thoracic cord. There is vasodilation of visceral and lower extremity vessels, resulting is a distributive shock. Hypotension results from a failure to mount a reflex tachycardia or development of bradycardia. *Spinal shock* describes flaccid paralysis and loss of reflexes from acute cord damage, and symptoms can last for variable duration with the development of subsequent spasticity. Neurogenic shock may initially respond to fluid; however, vasopressors and chronotropes are frequently required to ensure prevention of secondary spinal cord injury by maintenance of spinal cord perfusion pressure. Injuries below C5 may preserve diaphragmatic function (C3–C5); however, intercostal function may be impaired in the acute setting, leading to marked ventilatory dysfunction.

ATLS Subcommittee, American College of Surgeons' Committee on Trauma, International ATLS Working Group. Advanced Trauma Life Support (ATLS^R): the 9th edition. *Journal of Trauma and Acute Care Surgery* 2013;74:1363.

Question 3 T F T F T

Stewart's strong ion theory describes how carbon dioxide, strong ions, and weak acids determine body fluid acid–base status. Strong cations do exceed strong anions, and this difference is known as the strong ion difference (SID).

$$SID = [Na^+ + K^+ + Mg^{2+} + Ca^{2+}] - [Cl^- + lactate] = 40\text{-}44 \text{ mmol/l}$$

A decrease in the SID (i.e. by increasing chloride) results in greater water dissociation and release of free H^+ and hence a metabolic acidosis.

To maintain electroneutrality:

$$SID - (carbon\ dioxide + weak\ acids) = 0.$$

When a weak acid, like albumin, decreases, the SID decreases to adjust.

The kidney controls relative concentrations of strong cations and anions. Ammonium is co-excreted with chloride, and ammonium loss results in a larger SID, and alkalosis.

Chawla G, Drummond G. Water, strong ions, and weak ions. *Continuing Education in Anaesthesia, Critical Care & Pain* 2008;8:108.

Question 4 F F T F F

An assessment of severity of pneumonia helps stratify elements of management and allows prognostication. Typically CURB65 is used with points being accrued for confusion; urea >7mmol/l; respiratory rate >30; systolic <90mmHg or diastolic <60mmHg; and age >65. CURB65 score ≥3 has a high mortality and requires a β lactam and a macrolide for empirical cover. Levofloxacin is a suitable alternative for those that are penicillin allergic. *Strep pneumoniae* remains the most common bacterial cause of CAP in most studies; however, the incidence is declining partly due to widespread use of pneumococcal vaccine but also herd immunity. While it is impossible to differentiate causative organisms based on clinical grounds, Legionella tends to affect the younger and smokers and has greater multisystem involvement (confusion, abnormal liver function tests) and be of greater severity. Legionella accounts for 1%–10% of CAP. Among patients admitted to the ICU, the most common organisms include Strep pneumonia, Legionella, and Staph aureus. There is no clear benefit of noninvasive ventilation in acute respiratory failure due to pneumonia, and use may delay definitive management of intubation and ventilation. However, logistically there may be some merit in instituting noninvasive ventilation early while waiting for transfer to a critical care area for ongoing respiratory support, as it may improve gas exchange (although there is no evidence to suggest it improves mortality).

British Thoracic Society guidelines for the management of community Acquired pneumonia in adults, 2009–10. https://www.brit-thoracic.org.uk/quality-improvement/guidelines/pneumonia-adults/ [accessed 27 July 2021].

Musher DM, Abbers MS, Bartlett JG. Evolving understanding of the causes of pneumonia in adults, with special attention to the role of Pneumococcus. *Clinical Infectious Diseases* 2017;65:1736.

Question 5 T F F T T

Collapse with a profound metabolic acidosis with raised anion gap gives rise to the possibility of intoxication with ethanol, ethylene glycol, and methanol. Ethylene glycol is found in radiator fluid and antifreeze. It has a sweet taste but is odourless and colourless. Initial findings often include neurological impairment and dyspnoea from evolving acidosis. There is an early osmolar gap (measure serum osmolarity - calculated osmolality). There is also a raised anion gap (Na + K − (Cl + HCO_3)). Ethylene glycol is relatively harmless in itself, but it is metabolized by alcohol dehydrogenase to a number of metabolites including glycolic acid and oxalate. Calcium oxalate forms and accumulates in blood and tissues, and oxalate crystals in the urine lead to renal insufficiency. Ethanol can be used, as it is preferentially metabolized by alcohol dehydrogenase, but first-line treatment is preferentially with fomepizole, which blocks the action of alcohol dehydrogenase. Fomepizole does not require regular blood concentration monitoring or cause inebriation. Haemodialysis is also often required.

Oostvogels R, Kemperman H, Hubeek I, ter Braak EWMT. The importance of the osmolality gap in ethylene glycol intoxication. *British Medical Journal* 2013;347:f6904.

Question 6 T F F F F

CRBSI causes significant mortality and morbidity, as well as incurring increased cost, and much has been done to reduce it. Bundles of care, when performed together and consistently have significantly helped in reducing CRBSI, and these include CRBSI surveillance and meticulous training, as well as clinical measures (strict asepsis and hand hygiene, use of chlorhexidine skin preparation, subclavian approach, daily line review, and prompt removal when no longer necessary). The most common causative agents of CRBSI are coagulase-negative Staphylococci. Diagnosis can be done with qualitative or quantitative blood culture through the device, paired quantitative analysis, or differential time to positivity. Paired quantitative blood culture has greater sensitivity and specificity than differential time to positivity. Management should include timely appropriate systemic antibiotics and whether the catheter should be removed or salvaged. Guidelines from the Infectious Diseases Society of America (IDSA) recommend the removal of non tunnelled catheters in all complicated infections (e.g. thrombosis, endocarditis, and osteomyelitis) and in all infections caused by S. aureus, Gram-negative bacilli, Enterococcus species, and Candida species. The catheter may be retained with coagulase-negative Staphylococci if systemic antibiotics are given in conjunction with antibiotic lock therapy.

Mermel L, et al. *Clinical practice guidelines for the diagnosis and management of intravascular catheter-related infection: 2009 update by the Infectious Diseases Society of America.* 2009. http://www.idsociety.org/uploadedFiles/IDSA/Guidelines-Patient_Care/PDF_Library/Management%20IV%20Cath.pdf [accessed 27 July 2021].

Question 7 T F T T F

Antiretroviral therapy has increased the life expectancy of patients who are infected with the HIV and has reduced the incidence of illnesses associated with the acquired immunodeficiency syndrome (AIDS). Lower respiratory tract respiratory pathology remains the leading cause of ICU admission in HIV patients, and while Pneumocystis is a less common respiratory pathogen, it still accounts for the majority of respiratory ICU admissions. Pneumocystis infection results in acute interstitial pneumonitis. Symptoms of shortness of breath, dry cough, and fever may be preceded by malaise and weight loss with profound oxygen desaturation on exertion. The chest x-ray may appear normal or show classical peri-hilar interstitial 'ground glass' shadowing. HAART improves immune function; however, its use on the ICU brings about challenges. Firstly many of the preparations come only as oral capsules, and there are numerous drug interactions, which makes practical application difficult. Some HIV-positive patients presenting to the ICU will not be on ART, and starting such drugs should be considered for those patients presenting with an AIDS-associated illness. For those with non-AIDS-related illness, HAART should be deferred, as initiations lead to the risk of IRIS. Those patients already on HAART and with virologic suppression of HIV should have their treatment continued.

Huang L, Quartin A, Jones D. Intensive care of patients with HIV infection. *New England Journal of Medicine* 2006;355:173.

Wittenberg MD, Kaur N, Miller R, Walker DA. The challenges of HIV disease in the intensive care unit. *Journal of the Intensive Care Society* 2010;11:26.

Question 8 F T F T T

Haemodialysis is effective in removing small, water-soluble substances with low protein binding—examples include alcohols, salicylate, and lithium—while haemofiltration effectively clears larger molecules, including theophylline and iron. Lactate and tricyclics are not cleared.

Waldmann C, Soni N, Rhodes A (eds). *Oxford desk reference: critical care,* 1st edition. Oxford: Oxford University Press, 2008.

Ward C, Sair M. Oral poisoning: an update. *Continuing Education in Anaesthesia, Critical Care & Pain* 2010;10:6–11.

Question 9 F T F F T

Both heparin and the low molecular weight heparins may induce thrombocytopaenia by two mechanisms: type 1—direct action of heparin on platelet activity and is non-immune-mediated. Platelet count falls within 2 days exposure of heparin and quickly returns to normal. Type 2 is an immune-mediated prothrombotic reaction, typically occurring 4–10 days after heparin exposure, which can be life- or limb-threating. Antibodies form against the heparin-platelet factor 4 complex. HIT occurs in up to 5% of the US population and is less common in males.

The more serious type 2 form (HIT) is suspected when the platelet count falls >50% of baseline, occurs within the suspected time frame, is associated with new thrombotic events, and there is no other alternative cause of low platelets (pretest scoring system can ascertain likelihood of HIT).

Management includes stopping heparin or LMWH, and avoiding warfarin, which may cause further thrombosis and necrosis. Alternative anticoagulation includes lepirudin (direct activity against thrombin) and danaparoid.

Warkentin TE. Heparin-induced thrombocytopaenia: a ten-year retrospective. *Annual Review of Medicine* 1999;50:129–47.

Question 10 T T F F F

Protein requirement is 1–1.5g/kg/day, although this is raised in severe catabolic states (e.g. burns). Carbohydrate requirement is 3–4g/kg/day, phosphorus 0.4mmol/kg/day, and potassium 0.7–1mmol/kg/day. Higher replacement rates may be required in patients with electrolyte abnormalities, or specific medical conditions.

Waldmann C, Soni N, Rhodes A (eds). *Oxford desk reference: critical care,* 1st edition. Oxford: Oxford University Press, 2008.

Question 11 F T F F F

Tumour lysis syndrome is a metabolic disturbance most often seen 48–72 hours post treatment of bulky, rapidly proliferating, treatment-responsive tumours. It is most often associated with acute leukaemias and high-grade non-Hodgkin lymphoma, but it may also be linked with other haematological malignancies as well as solid tumours such as hepatoblastoma. It occurs secondary to rapid cell turnover and the release of intracellular contents, which results in hyperkalaemia, hyperphosphataemia through direct cell lysis. Hypocalcaemia occurs due to precipitation with phosphate and deposition of calcium phosphate. Nucleic acid purines are released in cell breakdown and are metabolized by hepatic xanthine oxidase (humans do not possess urate oxidase) to uric acid, which in the acidic renal tubule is relatively insoluble. Producing an alkaline diuresis minimizes precipitation of insoluble uric acid in the tubules but shifts ionized calcium to its nonionized form and increases calcium phosphate deposition in the renal tubules so is not routinely used. Supportive care with renal replacement therapy is given if indicated; electrolyte correction and hydration are essential. Rasburicase (recombinant urate oxidase) can be used to further lower uric acid levels. Allopurinol, a xanthine oxidase inhibitor, may also be considered.

Kalemkerian GP, Darwish B, Varterasian ML. Tumor lysis syndrome in small cell carcinoma and other solid tumors. *American Journal of Medicine* Nov 1997;103(5):363–7.

Question 12 F T T F F

Intra-abdominal hypertension is defined as pressure ≥12 or an abdominal perfusion pressure ≤60mmHg. Abdominal compartment syndrome equates to intra-abdominal pressure ≥20mmHg *and* organ system failure not previously present. Critical intra-abdominal pressures are a major cause of morbidity. Mild elevations in intra-abdominal pressure may initially be compensated for. However at pressures ≥25mmHg, significant cardiovascular, renal, and pulmonary dysfunction occurs. Consideration into the underlying cause of the raised intra-abdominal pressure needs to be made to direct the treatment. Management strategies to improve abdominal organ perfusion include adequate sedation, analgesia, and neuromuscular blockade. NGT placement, purgatives, drainage of ascites/collections, fluid balance can also provide relief in pressure. Opening the abdomen reliably reduces intra-abdominal pressure but may not improve associated morbidity and can lead to unwarranted complications such as fistula formation. There are no established cut-off pressures for when surgery is necessary, and it is advised to consider the entire clinical picture, especially if there is evidence of organ dysfunction. Early decompression may lead to improved outcomes, and it may reverse the complications associated with abdominal compartment syndrome. An open abdomen also has implications for the patient. Girth measurement is very inaccurate. Techniques to measure intra-abdominal pressure include indirect pressure transduction (e.g. intravesical pressure or modified gastric tonometer). Ideally a minimum of three readings will confirm diagnosis. Alternatively direct needle puncture into the abdominal cavity at laparoscopy will confirm diagnosis.

Fletcher S, Berry N. Abdominal compartment syndrome. *Continuing Education in Anesthesia, Critical Care & Pain* 2012;12:110.

Question 13 T F T T T

Hypocalcaemia results from a rise in cellular cytosolic calcium in the initial phase. As muscle injury progresses, potassium, myoglobin, and creatinine kinase leak into the circulation. Calcium that has accumulated in muscle at the time of necrosis is then later released, resulting in hypercalcaemia during the recovery phase. Compartment syndrome can occur at any stage, with fluid sequestration and oedema resulting in high muscle compartment pressures. Pressures >30 mmHg, can lead to muscle ischaemia and further rhabdomyolysis. Fluid resuscitation with 0.9% sodium chloride is preferred at a rate of 10–15ml/kg/hr to achieve high urinary flow rates (>300ml/hr or 3 ml/kg/ hr), with the cautious addition of sodium bicarbonate 1.4% to maintain urinary pH >6.5.

Sever MS, Vanholder R, Lameire N. Management of crush related injuries after disasters. *New England Journal of Medicine* 2006;354:1052–63.

Question 14 T F T F T

Volume controlled ventilation (VCV) is characterized by constant flow and an increasing pressure as the inspiratory period progresses. Increased compliance results in lower required pressures. VCV may be time-cycled. Pressure limits can still be set.

Bersten AD, Soni N. *Oh's intensive care manual*, 6th edition. London: Butterworth Heinemann, 2009.

Question 15 F F T T T

Spontaneous respiratory rate less than 35, PaO_2/FIO_2 ratio >26.3kpa; MV <10l/min; vital capacity breath >10ml/kg; and respiratory rate/tidal volume <100l are all indicative of likely successful weaning.

Lermitte J, Garfield MJ. Weaning from mechanical ventilation. *Continuing Education in Anesthesia, Critical Care & Pain* 2005;5:113–17.

Question 16 T T T F F

The HII bundle recommends the placement of a single lumen catheter in the subclavian or internal jugular vein. An antimicrobial impregnated catheter is recommended if it will be in place for 1–3 weeks and the risk of CRBSI is felt to be high. The site must be inspected daily for signs of infection, using a transparent dressing. The use of ultrasound is not mentioned in the setting of infection control.

Department of Health. *Saving lives: reducing infection, delivering clean and safe care. High impact intervention no.1 central venous catheter care bundle*. 2011. http://webarchive.nationalarchives.gov. uk/20120118164404/hcai.dh.gov.uk/files/2011/03/2011-03-14-HII-Central-Venous-Catheter-Care-Bundle-FINAL.pdf [accessed 27 July 2021].

Question 17 F T T F F

Modern CABG may be performed with both on-pump and off-pump techniques. Transoesophageal echocardiography is associated with a British Society of Echocardiography quoted risk of 1 in 10, 000 of oesophageal perforation. Systemic heparinization is reversed using protamine. Cardiopulmonary bypass causes profound immune activation, leading to a sepsis-like state. Left internal mammary artery grafts demonstrate lesser need for future intervention, and suffer fewer morbid events, with higher long-term graft patency rates.

Lytle BW, Loop FD, Cosgrove FD, Ratliff NB, Easley K, Taylor PC. Long-term (5–12 years) serial studies of internal mammary artery and saphenous vein coronary bypass grafts. *Journal of Thoracic and Cardiovascular Surgery* 1985;89:248–58.

Hett D. Anaesthesia for off-pump coronary artery surgery. *Continuing Education in Anesthesia, Critical Care & Pain* 2006;6:60–2.

Question 18 F F F F F

PCI is the preferred option in treatment of STEMI unless contraindicated or unavailable within 120 minutes, in which case fibrinolytic (thrombolysis) therapy should be considered. Low levels of consciousness or cardiac arrest are not contraindications to patients with MI as the causative factor, undergoing PCI. If ST elevation persists or recurs following fibrinolysis, repeat fibrinolytic therapy is contraindicated, and rescue-PCI should be offered. Antiplatelet agents are indicated in the form of aspirin as soon as the diagnosis is made or suspected (it is often given pre-hospital arrival). Aspirin should be used in combination with other agents. The response to GTN should not be used to make or exclude a diagnosis of acute coronary syndrome in patients with recent-onset chest pain. Routine supplemental oxygen should not be given to patients with new-onset chest pain unless pulse oximetry demonstrates oxygen saturation <94%.

NICE. *NICE Guideline CG167. Myocardial infarction with ST-segment elevation: the acute management of myocardial infarction with ST-segment elevation.* 2013.https://www.nice.org.uk/guidance/cg167 [accessed 27 July 2021].

NICE. *NICE Guideline CG95. Chest pain of recent onset: assessment and diagnosis.* https://www.nice.org.uk/guidance/cg95/resources/chest-pain-of-recent-onset-assessment-and-diagnosis-975751036117 [accessed 27 July 2021].

Question 19 T F F F F

The National Patient Safety Agency has issued guidance for the safe placement and position checking of nasogastric tubes. It was reported that the single greatest cause of harm was the result of misinterpretation of chest x-ray images, which represented 45 serious incidents, including 12 deaths.

The 2005 guidance highlighted the unreliability of the 'whoosh' test (listening over the stomach for bubbling sounds following forced air entry down the nasogastric tube). Testing for the acidity of nasogastric aspirate with litmus paper is also unreliable, and testing with pH indicator paper should be considered the first-line check for correct NG placement. Radiographic demonstration of tube position should be reserved as a second-line check.

The failure to detect a misplaced nasogastric tube prior to starting feeding, flushing, or drug administration is a preventable cause of harm, and this failure to detect the incorrect placement is a 'never event', not the actual misplacement (with the best will in the world NG tubes still end up in the wrong place!).

Lamont T, et al. Checking placement of nasogastric feeding tubes in adults (interpretation of x-ray images): summary of a safety report from the National Patient Safety Agency. *British Medical Journal* 2011;342:d2586.

Question 20 F F T F F

The MELD score is a numerical scale based on the risk of the patient dying while awaiting transplantation. It is based on bilirubin, INR, and creatinine only.

Pulmonary hypertension is not a contraindication per se; however, mortality risk approaches 100% with severe pulmonary hypertension (mean pulmonary artery pressure >50 mm Hg). New proven hepatopulmonary syndrome (triad of liver disease, hypoxaemia on room air, and pulmonary vascular dilatation) is not a contraindication to liver transplantation as it may resolve after successful grafting. Hypoalbuminaemia and coagulopathy tend not to be corrected preoperatively, unless there is active bleeding, and there tends to be little trend between intraoperative blood loss and coagulopathy. Hyponatraemia is a poor prognostic indicator and should be corrected preoperatively with fluid restriction, aldosterone antagonist diuretics (e.g. spironolactone), and in some instances renal replacement therapy.

Fabbroni D, Bellamy M. Anaesthesia for hepatic transplantation. *Continuing Education in Anaesthesia, Critical Care & Pain* 2006;6(5):171–5.

Question 21 F F T F T

Physiological indicators such as hypertension and tachycardia correlate poorly with more valid measures of pain, such as the Critical Care Pain Observation Tool. This has been shown to be valid and reproducible. It scores facial expression, body movement, compliance with the ventilator (if intubated), vocalization (if extubated) and muscle tension, with a score out of 8. Evidence from randomized controlled trials consistently supports the use of the minimum possible level of sedation. Further support comes from a prospective, multicenter, longitudinal cohort study showing that depth of sedation was independently associated with duration of mechanical ventilation, in-hospital mortality, and rates of death within 180 days. Dexmedetomidine may have advantages over benzodiazepines by producing analgesia, less respiratory depression, and seemingly greater patient compliance. As compared with lorazepam and midazolam, dexmedetomidine results in less delirium and a shorter duration of mechanical ventilation but not a reduction in ICU or hospital stay. All available IV opioids when titrated to similar pain-intensity endpoints, are equally effective.

Shehabi Y, et al. Early intensive care sedation predicts long-term mortality in ventilated critically ill patients. *American Journal of Respiratory and Critical Care Medicine* 2012;186:724–31.

Reade M, Finfer S. Sedation and delirium in the intensive care unit. *New England Journal of Medicine* 2014;370:444.

Society of Critical Care Medicine. Clinical practice guidelines for the management of pain, agitation, and delirium in adult patients in the intensive care unit. *Critical Care Medicine* 2013;41:263.

Question 22 F T F T T

Lung compliance is poor in small children (reduced elasticity of lungs), and airway closure may occur during normal tidal volume breathing. This may result in an increase in alveolar-arterial oxygen tension difference, and it explains why PaO_2 is lower in an infant compared to a child. The metabolic rate of an infant is nearly twice that of an adult, which explains why desaturation occurs rapidly in smaller children. Blood volume at birth is approximately 90ml/kg, and this decreases to 80ml/kg in the infant and young child. By 6–8 years, this falls further to the adult level of 75ml/kg.

The high metabolic rate dictates that the cardiac output of infants and small children is high. A heart rate of 60 beats per minute in an infant is considered a cardiac arrest, and blood pressure aim should be in the order of 90/60mmHg. Glomerular filtration rate does not reach adult levels until about the age of 8 years old, and therefore sodium and water handling in the child are inferior. The normal infant requires 3–5mmol/kg per day to maintain electrolyte balance (adult daily requirement of 1mmol/kg).

Aitkenhead A, Moppett I, Thompson J. *Smith and Aitkenhead's textbook of anaesthesia,* 6th edition. London: Churchill Livingstone, 2013.

Question 23 F T T T F

Anion gap is calculated by $(Na^+ + K^+) - (Cl^- + HCO_3^-)$. Normal is 8–12 mmol/l. A raised anion gap acidosis is caused by the presence of unmeasured anions such as lactate. Non-anion gap acidosis is caused by abnormalities in chloride control, for example acute renal failure and renal tubular acidosis.

Waldmann C, Soni N, Rhodes A (eds). *Oxford desk reference: critical care,* 1st edition. Oxford: Oxford University Press, 2008.

Question 24 F T F T T

The expected haemodynamic response to volume expansion is an increase in stroke volume and, therefore, cardiac output; however, this increase in cardiac output is also dependent on ventricular function, and therefore, not all patients will respond to a fluid bolus. Identifying fluid responsiveness is therefore important, and dynamic parameters, which use the predictable heart-lung interactions during positive pressure ventilation can be used to distinguish which patients will continue to benefit from fluid boluses. Dynamic parameters are measured using a wide variety of continuous beat-to-beat cardiac output monitoring devices.

Stroke volume variation of >9.5% is felt to be a likely indicator of fluid responsiveness. For pulse pressure variation the reference value is >13%. Superior vena cava collapsibility index, as assessed by transthoracic echo, of greater than 36%, and a correct flow time (FTc) of <320ms both also correlate with fluid responsiveness. All of these dynamic parameters are generally considered superior to static parameters such as CVP. A CVP of 6mmHg does not accurately predict fluid response.

Eyre L, Breen A. Optimal volaemic status and predicting fluid responsiveness. *Continuing Education in Anesthesia, Critical Care & Pain* 2010;10(2).

Question 25 F F T F T

Loop diuretics act by inhibiting the Na$^+$ K$^+$ 2Cl$^-$ co-transporter in the ascending loop of Henle. This results is more Na and water delivery to the distal convoluted tubule (Na may be exchanged for K, leading to hypokalaemia), and it reduces the renal medullary concentration gradient and amount of water that can be absorbed by the collecting duct. Oxygen consumption in the loop of Henle is reduced, and loop diuretics can be used to convert an oliguric renal failure to a nonoliguric state. Loop diuretics are effective in pulmonary oedema because they reduce ventricular preload. Thiazide diuretics work at the early distal convoluted tubule and exert their action via inhibition of Na$^+$ Cl$^-$ co-transport. As more Na is delivered to the distal convoluted tubule, preferential exchange occurs for potassium, leading to greater potassium excretion and hypokalaemia. Chloride loss results in hypochloraemic alkalosis, which occurs with the vast majority of diuretics, except carbonic anhydrase inhibitors, which result in a metabolic acidosis. Liver cirrhosis results in an effective reduction in circulating volume due to increased systemic vasodilatation. The rennin-angiotensin-aldosterone system is switched on with retention of Na and water. Along with sodium restriction, spironolactone is often used to help control ascites and hyponatraemia.

Peck T, Hill S, Williams M. *Pharmacology for anaesthesia and intensive care,* 2nd edition. London: Greenwich Medical Media, 2003.

Question 26 F T T T F

Drugs absorbed via the GIT pass to the portal vein, undergo an element of metabolism (first pass) within the liver, and then enter the circulation via the hepatic vein and inferior vena cava (IVC) (see Table 6.1). Some drugs induce hepatic enzymes; other drugs inhibit them, which will then increase the oral bioavailability. Metabolism of a drug will often reduce the activity of a drug; however, some drugs are manufactured as prodrugs (e.g. diamorphine), and it is the metabolite that confers the effect. Alternatively some metabolites have equal activity to the parent compound. Phase I metabolism encompass oxidation, reduction, and hydrolysis, while phase II include glucuronidation, acetylation, and methylation. Although most drugs are initially metabolized by phase I and then II, some drugs may undergo only phase II metabolism. Local anaesthetics are weak bases and, therefore, at physiological pH, remain mostly ionized as their pK$_a$ (pH at which 50% unionized) tends to be higher. Therefore local anaesthetics with lower pK$_a$ will work faster as a greater proportion of the drug will be unionized at physiological pH.

Table 6.1 Some common drugs that induce and inhibit hepatic enzymes

Inducers	Inhibitors
Phenytoin	Omeprazole
Carbamazine	Amiodarone
Barbiturates	Disulfiram
Rifampicin	Erythromycin
Alcohol—chronic	Valproate
Sulphonylureas	Isoniazid
	Cimetdine
	Ethanol—acute
	Sulphonamides

Peck T, Hill S, Williams M. *Pharmacology for anaesthesia and intensive care,* 2nd edition. London: Greenwich Medical Media, 2003.

Question 27 F F F F F

Some studies suggest a role of HME for preventing VAP over other methods of humidification. A recent Cochrane review comparing heated humidifiers with HMEs concluded that hydrophobic HMEs may reduce the risk of pneumonia. The conditions within the humidification chamber are tightly controlled to ensure the fresh gas flow is saturated with water vapour before it leaves the chamber. Relative humidity is the absolute humidity divided by the amount present when the gas is fully saturated at the same temperature and pressure. Warmer gas can contain more water vapour, and so warming the inspired gases after the humidification chamber would decrease the relative humidity. Ideal droplet size should be 2–5μm. Any smaller and there may be deposition of droplets within the alveoli, or they may simply be washed away with expiration. Larger droplets may be deposited within the main airways, resulting in increased airway resistance. Comfort scores (scale of mucosal dryness) are demonstrably worse when NIV is used in the absence of humidification. However there are no studies demonstrating clear clinical benefits with the use of humidification and NIV.

Mcnulty G, Eyre L. Humidification in anaesthesia and critical care. *British Journal of Anaesthesia Education* 2015;15(3):131.

Question 28 F T T F F

Hydrocephalus develops in 20%–30% patients, usually within the first 3 days, and risk is increased with poor grade and large amounts of subarachnoid blood. Suspect if deterioration in neurological status and refer for external ventricular drain (EVD), as necessary. Clinical seizures are fairly uncommon, but require prompt treatment. Prophylactic anticonvulsants after SAH are associated with a worse outcome. Prevention of delayed neurological deficit is paramount in the management of SAH. DCI and vasospasm are common, and risk is greatest between days 4 and 10. DCI may occur in the absence of vasospasm, and up to 70% have vasospasm on angiography with 30% being symptomatic. Again those with poor grade SAH and, or large blood load and smokers are at risk. Nimodipine has been shown to reduce cerebral infarction and poor outcome, and it should be started at diagnosis for 21 days. Hypertension, hypervolaemia, and haemodilution (triple H) was advocated to reduce vasospasm; however, there now seems to be limited evidence supporting hypertension (hypotension and cerebral perfusion pressure <70mmHg should be avoided). Hypervolaemia increases cerebral blood flow, but may cause other nonneurological complications such as pulmonary oedema, so euvolaemia is the recommended target. Haemodilution is associated with improved blood rheology but reduced oxygen delivery.

Waldmann C, Soni N, Rhodes A (eds). *Oxford desk reference: critical care*, 1st edition. Oxford: Oxford University Press, 2008.

Question 29 F T T T F

HFOV is an alternative form of mechanical ventilation, which has been used in the past for acute respiratory distress syndrome (ARDS). The OSCAR trial, which compared HFOV in patients with ARDS to controlled mandatory ventilation, did not demonstrate an improvement in mortality or length of stay compared to conventional, low tidal volume mechanical ventilation. Subsequently its use has fallen out of favour. Unlike conventional ventilation, HFOV relies on the rapid delivery of tidal volumes that are smaller than dead space. Typical tidal volumes on HFOV are 1–3ml/kg. The key features of HFOV are small tidal volumes, low peak pressure, and higher mean airway pressures. Weavind and Wenker described various ways of gas transport on HFOV, which include bulk and co-axial flow, molecular diffusion, Taylor dispersion, turbulence, and Pendelluft.

During conventional ventilation, CO_2 removal is dependent on minute volume; however, a decrease in frequency on HFOV leads to larger tidal volumes and subsequent increased CO_2 clearance.

Sud S, et al. High-frequency ventilation versus conventional ventilation for treatment of acute lung injury and acute respiratory distress syndrome. *Cochrane Database Systems Review* Feb 2013;2:CD004085.

Ferguson ND, et al; The OSCILLATE Trial Investigators and the Canadian Critical Care Trials Group. High-frequency oscillation in early acute respiratory distress syndrome. *New England Journal of Medicine* 2013;368:795–805.

Young D, et al; OSCAR Study Group. High-frequency oscillation for acute respiratory distress syndrome. *New England Journal of Medicine* Feb 2013;368(9):806–13.

Question 30 T F T T T

Haematocrit is include. A score ranging from 0 to 71 is calculated from the patient's age and 12 physiological variables, as below:

PaO_2

Temperature

Mean arterial pressure

Arterial pH

Heart rate

Respiratory rate

Serum sodium

Serum potassium

Creatinine

Haematocrit

White blood cell count

Glasgow coma scale

Bouch M, Thompson J. Severity scoring systems in the critically ill. *Continuing Education in Anaesthesia, Critical Care & Pain* 2008;8:181–5.

1. **A 5-year-old patient is brought by paramedics to your Accident & Emergency (A&E) department. The patient has obvious partial and complete burns over his body namely face, chest, and abdomen. Regarding management the following are correct:**
   A. If the burn involves the face, chest, and abdomen, then this equates to approximately 20% body surface area of the 5-year-old patient
   B. If the burn surface area is 25% or greater total body surface area, this represents a severe burn in this situation
   C. Intubation with a size 5 endotracheal tube is indicated
   D. Resuscitation fluid should be running at approximately 200 ml/hour Ringer's lactate for the first 8 hours from A&E presentation
   E. Transfer to a regional burn unit is warranted

2. **A patient is found to be hypothermic. The following features are true:**
   A. At 28°C is considered moderate hypothermia
   B. At 28°C, profound shivering may occur
   C. At 28°C the pupils may be fixed and dilated
   D. Broad QRS and U waves may be seen on the electrocardiogram (ECG)
   E. Rapid rewarming leads to afterdrop

3. **Regarding interpretation of the chest radiograph, the following are correct:**
   A. Bilateral hilar enlargement can be caused by Streptococcus pneumoniae infection
   B. Right upper lobe collapse is associated with tracheal deviation away from the right and volume loss of the right hemithorax
   C. Right lower lobe collapse is associated with loss of the right heart border
   D. 'Sail' sign is seen in right lower lobe collapse
   E. The left upper lobe collapses anteriorly

4. **Regarding measurements derived from oesophageal Doppler monitoring (ODM) the following are true:**
   A. FTc (corrected systolic flow time) correlates well with afterload
   B. Hypovolaemia causes an increase in corrected flow time (FTc)
   C. In the perioperative setting, use of ODM has shown to improve outcome
   D. Mean acceleration is reduced in left ventricular failure (LVF)
   E. Peak velocity and flow time are both increased in vasoconstricted state

MCQs and SBAs in Intensive Care Medicine. Lorna Eyre and Andrew Bodenham, Oxford University Press. © Oxford University Press 2021.
DOI: 10.1093/oso/9780198753056.003.0007

5. **Regarding management of fungal disease in the critically ill patient, the following are correct:**
   A. Aspergillus infection can be readily seen on chest x-ray
   B. Eichonacandins inhibit ergosterol synthesis
   C. Growth of Candida from respiratory specimens alone should not prompt the use of antifungal therapy in most patients
   D. Galactomannan can be used to detect Candida species
   E. The two most common complications of disseminated Candida include endophthalmitis and pyelonephritis so ophthalmology and renal tract imaging are necessary

6. **A 76-year-old hypertensive man presents with 3-hour sudden history of neurological symptoms. Findings include right-sided hemiparesis, right-sided sensory loss, right homonymous hemianopia, and expressive aphasia. His blood pressure is 175/100. The following are correct:**
   A. Clopidogrel is superior to aspirin as the antiplatelet agent of choice for effective early management of ischaemic stroke
   B. This most likely represents a PACI type of stroke according to Oxford Stroke Classification
   C. The patient's blood pressure should be lowered to more normal levels aiming for systolic 120mmHg
   D. The patient is a candidate for recombinant tissue plasminogen activator (tPA) if there are no contraindications and no haemorrhage on computed tomography (CT)
   E. Therapeutic parenteral anticoagulation remains a useful therapy for patients who cannot have t-PA but have had a large ischaemic stroke

7. **In relation to infective endocarditis (IE), the following are true:**
   A. According to the Duke classification, diagnosis can be confirmed clinically by the presence of one major criteria and two minor criteria
   B. According to the Duke criteria, diagnosis can be confirmed clinically by the presence of five minor criteria
   C. Intravenous drug use is associated with right-sided lesions, which carry the highest mortality
   D. Surgery is indicated in 10% of cases
   E. The majority of IE is caused by Streptococcal infections

8. **Concerning anticoagulation in renal replacement therapy, the following are correct:**
   A. Citrate anticoagulation is associated with hypercalcaemia
   B. Citrate anticoagulation is contraindicated in lactic acidosis
   C. Heparin can be used in conjunction with protamine
   D. Low molecular weight heparin is superior to unfractionated heparin
   E. Prostacyclin can cause hypertension

9. **It is true that the transfusion scenarios are compatible:**
   A. Fresh frozen plasma from an A+ donor to an O+ 50-year-old man
   B. Fresh frozen plasma from an O+ donor to an A– 30-year-old woman
   C. Platelets from an O+ donor to an A+ 20-year-old woman
   D. Red cells from an A + donor to an AB– 20-year-old woman
   E. Red cells from an A + donor to an A– 80-year-old man

10. **The following are correct regarding hepatorenal syndrome (HRS):**
    A. Diagnostic criteria requires a serum creatinine >133μmol/l in a patient with cirrhosis and ascites that persists once all other pathologies have been excluded
    B. HRS type 1 is a rapid and severe progressive renal failure occurring in under 2 weeks
    C. Prognosis of HRS type 1 is better than HRS type 2
    D. Type 1 HRS is more prone to recurrence
    E. Use of terlipressin and albumin improves the chances of reversing HRS

11. **Regarding the diagnosis of tuberculosis (TB), the following are true:**
    A. Confluent tuberculosis bronchopneumonia may mimic ARDS
    B. Hydrocephalus is a common complication of TB meningitis
    C. In the UK, 30% of tuberculosis isolates from culture are resistant to any first-line drug
    D. Serial sputum sampling from expectorating patients provides yields similar to that from bronchoscopic sampling
    E. The finding of acid fast bacillus in a sputum sample is diagnostic

12. **Regarding meningococcal meningitis, the following are true:**
    A. Cefotaxime is first-line management
    B. Close contacts should be treated with rifampicin
    C. It is a notifiable disease
    D. It is most commonly caused by meningococcal type C
    E. Patients with suspected meningitis should be isolated

13. **Fluids are required for resuscitation. The following are true:**
    A. Albumin is superior compared to normal saline in the resuscitation of severe sepsis
    B. Infusion of 1litre NaCl 0.9% contributes approximately 250ml to the plasma volume
    C. NaCl 0.9% is more acidic than Hartmann's solution
    D. There is no clinical outcome difference when 0.9% NaCl is compared with lactated Ringer's solution for resuscitation in all clinical cases
    E. The acidosis related to ongoing infusion of NaCl 0.9% results from a narrowed strong ion difference

14. **In patients with antiphospholipid syndrome, the following are correct:**
    A. Catastrophic antiphospholipid syndrome has a mortality >50%
    B. Clinical and biochemical features can include hyponatraemia, hyperkalaemia, and low blood pressure
    C. Diagnosis relies on an episode of thrombosis and presence of lupus anticoagulant
    D. Presence of antiphospholipid syndrome makes pre-eclampsia more likely in affected pregnant women
    E. Unfractionated heparin can be used in thrombosis and is managed in the standard way

15. **It is correct that the 2016 Surviving Sepsis guidelines recommend the following for the treatment of severe sepsis and septic shock:**
    A. Crystalloids as initial fluid therapy, adding albumin if substantial amounts of volume replacement are required
    B. Intravenous hydrocortisone in all patients who fail an adrenocorticotropic (ACTH) stimulation test
    C. Norepinephrine as a first-choice vasopressor, adding dobutamine when an additional agent is required
    D. Platelets should be supported to achieve a platelet counts $\geq 50 \times 10^9/l$
    E. The use of procalcitonin or similar biomarkers to guide antibiotic discontinuation

16. **The following treatments are suitable for managing a first presentation of C. difficile diarrhoea on ICU:**
    A. Intravenous metronidazole
    B. Infusion of donor faeces into the duodenum
    C. Monoclonal antibodies against A & B toxins
    D. Oral vancomycin
    E. Probiotics (lactobacillus acidophilus)

17. **Regarding tracheostomy, the following are true:**
    A. Fenestrated tubes should not be used initially
    B. Optimal site for tracheostomy insertion is around the first tracheal ring
    C. Significant tracheal stenosis occurs in 10% patients
    D. Tracheotomy tubes without an inner need to be changed every 30 days
    E. Tracheostomy dislodgement is a recognized complication

18. **Concerning the insertion of an intercostal chest drain, the following are true:**
    A. Chest drains that continue to bubble should never be clamped, as this may lead to a potentially fatal tension pneumothorax
    B. Removal of a chest drain should be performed during deep inspiration
    C. Regarding spontaneous pneumothorax, a 60-year-old smoker with a small pneumothorax <2cm and is asymptomatic can be discharged with outpatient follow-up
    D. Re-expansion pulmonary oedema is a common and potentially fatal complication associated with drainage of large spontaneous pneumothorax and rapid evacuation of large pleural effusions
    E. The safe triangle can be described by the anterior border of latissimus dorsi, the lateral border of pectoralis major, inferiorly by a horizontal line at the fifth intercostal space and superiorly by the base of the axilla

19. **A noradrenaline infusion is commenced, and the following are correct:**
    A. It is a mixed α- and β-adrenoceptor agonist
    B. It is inferior to dopamine infusion in maintaining urine output in septic shock
    C. It is superior to dopamine infusion in maintaining mean arterial pressure in septic shock
    D. It increases cardiac preload in septic shock
    E. It can cause profound bradycardia

20. **It is true that the following are features of critical illness weakness:**
    A. Asymmetric weakness predominately of the lower limbs
    B. Demyelination of the motor nerves in critical illness polyneuropathy
    C. Histological evidence of muscle necrosis in critical illness myopathy
    D. Raised levels of creatinine kinase with critical illness polyneuropathy
    E. Reduced nerve conduction velocity in critical illness polyneuropathy

21. **Regarding meningitis, the following are true:**
    A. Corticosteroids reduce the mortality rate in children in high-income countries when *Haemophilus influenzae* is the cause
    B. Cranial CT should be used to decide whether it is safe to perform lumbar puncture
    C. In children >3 months and young people, the most frequent causes of bacterial meningitis include Meningococcus, Pneumococcus, and *Haemophilus influenzae* type b
    D. In neonates, the most common causes of meningitis are group A streptococcus, *E. coli*, Pneumococcus, and *Listeria monocytogenes*
    E. There is no vaccine for serogroup B meningococcus, and this is now the commonest pathogen for bacterial meningitis in children

22. **Regarding the jugular venous waveform, the following are true:**
    A. Cannon a waves occur during ventricular tachycardia
    B. Constrictive pericarditis cause an exaggerated x wave
    C. Elevated a waves are seen in atrial fibrillation
    D. The v wave represents ventricular filling
    E. Tricuspid regurgitation causes elevated v waves

23. Regarding drug-receptor interaction, the following are correct:

A. A partial agonist has full receptor affinity and some intrinsic activity
B. Noncompetitive antagonists can be overcome with increasing the concentration of agonist
C. Inverse agonists have the same effect as a competitive antagonist
D. The Michaelis constant is the concentration of the substrate at which the enzyme is working at half its maximal rate
E. G proteins only act by increasing adenylyl cyclase

24. Regarding hypnotics and anxiolytics, the following are correct:

A. Benzodiazepines modulate the effects of GABA at $GABA_B$ receptors
B. γ-aminobutyric acid (GABA) is the main inhibitory neurotransmitter within the CNS
C. $GABA_A$ is a ligand-gated chloride channel
D. Like the other benzodiazepines, lorazepam is metabolized to active metabolites
E. Midazolam is highly lipid soluble

25. The following are true regarding the use of positive end expiratory pressure (PEEP) in ventilated patients:

A. It has a potential mortality benefit in acute respiratory distress syndrome (ARDS) if set at >12cmH₂0 ('high PEEP') rather than <12cmH₂0
B. It is contraindicated in acute severe asthma
C. It reduces ventilator-associated lung injury
D. It may improve cardiac output via a reduction in left ventricular end systolic volume
E. It is acceptable in patients with traumatic brain injury

26. The Intensive Care National Audit and Research Centre (ICNARC) releases a quarterly quality report to participating units. The following quality indicators are included:

A. Nurse-patient ratio
B. Out-of-hours discharges to the ward
C. Unit-acquired bloodstream infections
D. Unplanned readmissions within 48 hours
E. Unit-acquired MRSA

27. Regarding antifungal therapies, the following are true:

A. Amphotericin B is the preferred antifungal for candidiasis in renal failure
B. Aspergillus hypersensitivity pneumonitis (allergic aspergillosis) should be treated with itraconazole as a first-line treatment
C. C. albicans is normally resistant to fluconazole
D. Caspofungin is a potent inhibitor of the cytochrome P450 system
E. *Pneumocystis jirovecii* pneumonia is normally treated with trimethoprim-sulfamethoxazole

28. **Vasopressin is frequently used in critical care, and the following statements are true:**

A. Based on the Resuscitation Council (UK) guidelines, vasopressin should be considered during cardiac arrest

B. Vasopressin may be superior to adrenaline when used in cardiac arrests precipitated by ventricular fibrillation

C. Vasopressin is used to reduce portal hypertension

D. Vasopressin levels are low in patients with sepsis

E. Vasopressin augments noradrenaline

29. **When using cardiopulmonary bypass (CPB), the following are true:**

A. Anaesthetic vapour may be administered through CPB equipment to maintain anaesthesia

B. Blood is most commonly supplied to the sump from the right atrium

C. CPB may lead to severe hypokalaemia

D. Infusion of cardioplegia into the aortic root is contraindicated in aortic stenosis

E. Protamine administration should precede weaning from CPB

30. **Regarding pharmacokinetics, the following are correct:**

A. A drug with a constant context-sensitive half-time will demonstrate rapid action offset once the infusion has stopped

B. Clearance = volume of distribution divided by time constant

C. The rate of change of plasma drug remains constant in first-order kinetics

D. Time constant is the time for plasma concentration to fall to 50% of its original value

E. Volume of distribution at steady state can exceed total body volume

Question 1 F F T F T

Part of the initial management should include taking an accurate history. Important points include whether the burn occurred inside (inhalational injury, or chemical and plastic involvement) or outside. Was there an explosion and therefore a blast injury, was there any additional traumatic injury (did the patient jump?), and where was the patient found? In children, the face accounts for 9% (rather than the adult 4.5%), while the chest and abdomen account for 18%; therefore, in this case, burn body surface area (TBSA) accounts for 27% approximately. The American Burn Association defines a *severe burn* as 20% or greater TBSA in children younger than 10 years old (and adults >40 years). Given the extensive nature of the burns, the location of the burns (face), and referral to a regional burn unit, the child should be intubated. Size 5 endotracheal tube would be a good starting point, but remember to have additional sizes (4.5, 5.5mm ID) available too. The tube in this instance should be left uncut to allow for further facial swelling. Fluid resuscitation is only a guide. The ultimate goal is to give sufficient fluid to achieve a urine output of 1ml/kg/hr. A formula exists and relates to weight and % body surface burn (e.g. 2–4ml per kg weight per % body surface area, for example in this case: 2–4ml × 18kg × 27% TBSA burn = 970–1940ml in 24 hour period). Half of this is given in the first 8 hours from the **onset** of the burn. In children, glucose containing fluid should also be given in addition as background maintenance. Frequent re-evaluation is necessary. Mortality is high for burns >30% TBSA.

American Burn Association. Hospital and prehospital resources for optimal care of patients with burn injury: guidelines for development and operation of burn centers. *Journal of Burn Care Rehabilitation* 1990;11(2):98.

Question 2 T F T F T

Hypothermia is defined as a core temperature less than 35°C.

- mild: 32–35°C
- moderate: 28–32°C
- severe: <28°C

Shivering is maximal at 35°C, but it decreases as the temperature falls and may be absent at temperatures <32°C. Ventricular fibrillation can occur at <28°C, and asystole may occur at <25°C. Risk of cardiac arrhythmia increases as body temperature falls. Ventricular fibrillation in association with hypothermia is often refractory to defibrillation and cardiac drugs. Bretylium was once advocated as the drug of choice in such circumstances, but evidence regarding its efficacy remains lacking. Pupils may be fixed and dilated at temperatures <30°C. In hypothermia, there is broadened QRS and increases in PR and QT interval and J waves (U waves are related to hypokalaemia).

Passive rewarming is useful in the conscious patient (i.e. aluminium blankets). Peripheral active rewarming (e.g. using forced air warming blankets; 1–2°C per hour) may cause afterdrop if rewarming is rapid: this describes a drop in core body temperature as a consequence of peripheral vasodilation and release of cold peripheral blood to the body core. Central active warming can be done using warmed, humidified gases, warm IV fluids, warm body cavity lavage, renal replacement therapy, and ECMO.

Brown DJ, Brugger H, Boyd J, Paal P. Accidental hypothermia. *New England Journal of Medicine* 2012;367(20):1930–8.

Question 3   F F F F T

Bilateral hilar lymphadenopathy has a variety of causes including sarcoidosis, infection (fungal, TB, mycoplasma), malignancy (lymphoma), and silicosis. Right upper lobe collapse is associated with tracheal deviation to the right and loss of right hemithorax volume. Right lower lobe collapse is associated with loss of the right medial hemidiaphragm, increased (triangular) opacity medial base right lung, and depression of the right hilum. The right heart border remains seen in right lower lobe collapse. 'Sail sign' or the double cardiac contour is seen with left lower lobe collapse. The left upper lobe collapses anteriorly to give a veiling opacity within the left hemithorax as seen on chest x-ray.

Ellis S. *Interpreting chest x-rays*. Banbury: Scion Publishing, 2010.

Question 4   F F T T F

Oesophageal dopplers are noninvasive cardiac output monitors that measure blood flow velocity in the descending aorta using an ultrasound probe in the oesophagus (see Figure 7.1). It uses the Doppler shift principle when the ultrasound wave is reflected back from moving red blood cells, and this shift in frequency is proportional to the velocity of the blood flow. Measurements can be made, assuming the cross-sectional area of the descending aorta. A number of variables are examined including peak velocity (indicating contractility); corrected systolic flow time (FT$_c$), which indicates preload; stroke volume (measured by stroke distance × aortic root diameter); and cardiac output.

In left ventricular failure, the ODM waveform usually appears dome-shaped due to reduced mean acceleration and increased flow time. In vasoconstricted states, the waveforms appear peaked and narrower. In hypovolaemic states, the FTc is reduced, but peak velocity remains normal. Perioperative outcomes have been shown to be better with use of ODM (better gut perfusion, recovery times, and hospital and ICU lengths of stay). However, this has not been shown to improve outcome in ICU patients.

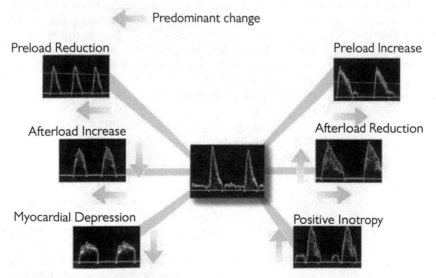

Figure 7.1 Oesophageal Doppler velocity/time graphs

King SL, Lim MST. The use of oesophageal Doppler monitor in intensive care unit. *Critical Care and Resuscitation* 2004;6:113–22.

Question 5 F F T F F

Candida species are often isolated from respiratory tract infections but rarely truly infect the lower respiratory tract. Growth of Candida from respiratory tract secretions should not prompt initial use of antifungals in the majority of cases. Candida in the bloodstream can lead to haematogenous spread to the liver, spleen, brain, eyes, and heart. Aspergillus most commonly affects the lungs and causes nonspecific symptoms with nonspecific chest x-ray changes. CT chest imaging on the other hand may identify specific findings such as 'air crescent' formations and the 'halo' sign. Galactomannan can be used in the diagnosis of Aspergillus. Management of fungal disease includes echinocandins (inhibit glucan cell wall synthesis), polyenes (bind to ergosterol, cell membrane), and imidazoles (prevent ergosterol synthesis, cell membrane). Other treatments include flucytosine (inhibits DNA/RNA synthesis) and griseofulvin (inhibits cell mitosis).

Enoch DA, Ludlam HA, Brown NM. Invasive fungal infections: a review of epidemiology and management options. *Journal of Medical Microbiology* Jul 2006;55(Pt 7):809–18.

Question 6 F F F T F

The signs and symptoms are suggestive of cerebral stroke. Cerebral vascular accident may be caused by intracerebral or subarachnoid haemorrhage or by ischaemia secondary to thrombosis, embolism, or hypoperfusion. Hypertension is a risk factor for ischaemic stroke, and those involving the anterior circulation of the left hemisphere can expect right-sided signs and symptoms as well as language involvement. The symptoms describe a total anterior circulation stroke, as all three of the following are present:

Unilateral weakness (and or sensory deficit), homonymous hemianopia, and higher cerebral dysfunction (aphasia).

Blood pressure (BP) will often elevate during acute stroke, and in the mainstay the consensus is to avoid treating hypertension during the acute stage, unless the systolic is >220mmHg and diastolic >110mmHg. When blood pressure is extreme and may lead to end organ compromise, cautious blood pressure lowering therapy should occur with no more than 15% reducing in BP during the first 24 hours. This patient would be a candidate for thrombolysis unless imaging suggesting haemorrhage or there were other contraindications present. During thrombolysis BP also needs to be managed, and ensure BP <180/105mmHg for at least 24 hours after tPA. Aspirin remains the antiplatelet agent of choice in the early management of ischaemic stroke (ideally give within 48 hours of symptoms or 24 hours after thrombolysis). Parenteral therapeutic anticoagulation is not recommended for use in acute ischaemic stroke in unselected patients, although may be considered for acute cardioembolic ischaemic stroke.

Lansberg MG, et al. Antithrombotic and thrombolytic therapy for ischemic stroke: antithrombotic therapy and prevention of thrombosis, 9th edition. American College of Chest Physicians evidence-based clinical practice guidelines. Chest 2012;141(Suppl 2):e601S.

Question 7 F T F F T

The commonest lesions are those affecting the left side of the heart, with aortic valve lesions representing 55%–60% of cases. However, in IV drug users, right-sided lesions are more common, and these actually have a more favourable prognosis, with a mortality rate of 4%–5% compared with an overall mortality of approximately 20%. The Duke classification is divided into major and minor criteria. Diagnosis can be made by demonstrating the presence of: two major, one major and three minor, or five minor criteria. The majority of cases are indeed caused by streptococcal infections, with S. *viridians*. Staphylococcal infections are more common in IV drug users. IE may also be caused by fungi or indeed be culture negative. Surgery is required in approximately 25%–30% of cases, with indications for surgery including life-threatening congestive cardiac failure, endocarditis in prosthetic heart valves, and in patients with cardiogenic shock.

Thury F, Grisoli D, Collart F, Habib G, Raoult D. Management of infective endocarditis: challenges and perspectives. *Lancet* 2012.

Kang DH, et al. Early surgery versus conventional treatment for infective endocarditis. *New England Journal of Medicine*. Jun 2012;366(26):2466–73.

Question 8 F T T F F

Prostacyclin is an antiplatelet agent that can cause significant hypotension. Citrate chelates calcium to prevent clot formation, and hence requires postfilter calcium replacement to restore normal coagulation. It is contraindicated in severe lactic acidosis. Heparin can be combined with postfilter protamine. While low molecular weight heparins have been used, there is no evidence of superiority, and the lack of reversibility may give a higher bleeding risk.

Hall N, Fox A. Renal replacement therapies in critical care. *Continuing Education in Anaesthesia, Critical Care & Pain* 2006;6:197–202.

Waldmann C, Soni N, Rhodes A (eds). *Oxford desk reference: critical care*, 1st edition. Oxford: Oxford University Press, 2008.

Question 9 T F T F T

Rhesus-negative females with child-bearing potential must be given rhesus-negative red cells and platelets to avoid developing Anti-D. While rhesus compatibility is desirable in other patients, it is not essential. Anti-ABO antibodies are carried in the plasma, so O group donors have anti-A and anti-B, whereas AB donors have no antibodies. Plasma compatibility is therefore the opposite to that for red cells and platelets (i.e. O Is the universal recipient and AB the universal donor; see Table 7.1).

Table 7.1 Compatible Blood Transfusions

			Compatible	Compatible
Patient's ABO Group	Antigen Red Cells	Antibody Serum	Red Blood Cells	Plasma
O	none	Anti-A Anti-B	O	O AB A B
A	A	Anti-B	O A	A AB
B	B	Anti-A	B O	B AB
AB	A and B	none	AB A B O	AB

Joint United Kingdom Blood Transfusion and Tissue Transplantation Services Professional Advisory Committee. http://www.transfusionguidelines.org.uk [accessed 30 July 2021].

Question 10 T T F F T

Hepatorenal syndrome (HRS) is the development of renal failure in those with chronic liver disease or fulminant hepatitis who have portal hypertension and ascites. It results from generalized vasodilation and altered hormone release (renin-angiotensin-aldosterone) and localized vasoconstriction. Risk factors include low mean arterial pressure, dilutional hyponatraemia, and severe urinary sodium retention.

HRS occurs as one of two patterns. HRS type1 is a rapid decline (<2 weeks) in renal function due to precipitating factors such as bleeding, alcoholic hepatitis, or infections. HRS type 2 is a more progressive decline in renal function with refractory ascites as the predominant clinical feature. Once other causes of acute kidney injury have been excluded and if a precipitant can be identified and managed appropriately, HRS should be managed with a combination of terlipressin 0.5mg qds increasing to 2mg qds and IV albumin 20–40g per day. Type 2 HRS is more prone to recurrence and responds less well to albumin and terlipressin therapy, but it has a better prognosis than HRS type 1.

Jackson P, Gleeson D. Alcoholic liver disease. *New England Journal of Medicine* 2010;10:66–71.

Question 11 T T F T F

Acid fast bacillus (AFB) in a sputum sample may be due to a nontuberculous mycobacteria, and correlation with other diagnostic tests is advised. However an AFB-positive specimen in a patient with a suggestive history and clinical findings should be assumed to be TB unless proven otherwise. TB polymerase chain reaction (PCR) may have a role if there is doubt. In the UK, only 8.4% of TB isolates are resistant to any first-line drug, and 1.6% are multidrug resistant. This is lower than some other countries. Hydrocephalus is a common complication of TB meningitis and is present radiologically in about 77% of cases. It is usually due to communicating hydrocephalus associated with tuberculosis exudates in the basal cisterns.

Hagan G, Nathani N. Clinical review: tuberculosis on the intensive care unit. *Critical Care* 2013;17:240.

Zumla A, Raviglione M, Hafner R, and Fordham von Reyn C. Tuberculosis. *New England Journal of Medicine* 2013;368:745–55.

Question 12 T T T F T

Neisseria meningitidis is a Gram-negative diplococcus, with a number of serogroups based on the capsular antigen. In Europe, the most prevalent cause of meningococcal disease is serogroup B. Modes of infection include direct contact or respiratory droplets from infected individuals. Public health should be notified immediately so as to organize contact tracing and antibiotic prophylaxis of close contacts. It is estimated that 5%–10% adults are asymptomatic carriers of meningococci, which reside in the nasopharynx, but this increases in closed populations (e.g. military recruits, university campus). Complications of bacterial meningitis include seizures, cerebral venous thrombosis, sagittal sinus thrombosis, and hydrocephalus, and a high proportion of surviving patients have long-term neurological sequelae. Meningococcal disease (meningitis with nonblanching rash or septicaemia) remains one of the top causes of infection-related death and prompt antibiotics with a third-generation cephalosporin are essential. Babies in the UK currently receive a meningitis B and C vaccine as part of their childhood vaccination programme. Teenagers in the UK get a combined ACWY vaccine.

NICE. *NICE guidelines CG102. Meningitis (bacterial) and meningococcal septicaemia in under 16s: recognition, diagnosis and management.* 2010. https://www.nice.org.uk/guidance/cg102/resources/meningitis-bacterial-and-meningococcal-septicaemia-in-under-16s-recognition-diagnosis-and-management-pdf-35109325611205 [accessed 30 July 2021].

Question 13 F T T F T

NaCl 0.9% has a pH of 5.0, while Hartmann's solution has a pH of 6.5. Albumin has not shown to be vastly superior to resuscitation with NaCl 0.9%, although it is recommended as a fluid for resuscitation in severe sepsis. Some particular clinical instances cite the superiority of one crystalloid over another (e.g. lactated Ringer's solution) better reduces incidence of inflammatory response in acute pancreatitis compared to NaCl 0.9%). There is a reduction in positivity of strong ion difference with prolonged resuscitation of NaCl 0.9% (i.e. the SID is narrowed, and proton generation is an immediate compensatory mechanism). Na and Cl are the principle electrolytes in the extracellular spaces, and since the interstitial space accounts for approximately 70%, exogenously administered NaCl 0.9% will follow the same distribution.

Safe Study Investigators. A comparison of albumin and saline for fluid resuscitation in the intensive care unit. *New England Journal of Medicine* 2004;350:2247.

Wu BU, et al. Lactated Ringer's solution reduces systemic inflammation compared with saline in patients with acute pancreatitis. *Clinical Gastroenterological Hepatology* 2011;9:710–17.

Question 14 T T T T F

Antiphospholipid syndrome (APS) is an autoimmune hypercoagulable state characterized by the presence of antiphospholipid antibodies.

The three major APS antibodies are anticardiolipin, lupus anticoagulant, and anti-beta2-glycoprotein-I. Diagnosis is made in the presence of one or more antibodies in the setting of vascular thrombosis or pregnancy-related morbidity.

APS causes thrombosis in both arteries and veins, and pregnancy-related complications include pre-eclampsia and miscarriage. In addition to vascular thrombosis, other features can include haematological (low platelets and clotting anomalies), pulmonary (pulmonary hypertension), cardiac (endocarditis), as well as cutaneous manifestations and loss of adrenal function, bilateral adrenal vein thrombosis and haemorrhagic infarction.

Lupus anticoagulant (LA) is a common cause of prolonged aPTT in patients without a bleeding history, regardless of whether the patient has a history of thrombosis. LA may function as an inhibitor in vitro by binding to the reagent phospholipid and blocking the phospholipid-dependent reactions of the intrinsic pathway. The net effect is prolongation of the activated partial thromboplastin time (aPTT). In reality thrombosis associated with APS is managed with LMWH and warfarin. There are currently no data on the novel oral anticoagulants, but the RAPS trial (rivaroxaban in APS is currently underway). Other strategies include corticosteroids and rituximab. *Catastrophic antiphospholipid syndrome* (APS) is defined as life-threatening multiorgan thromboses developing simultaneously or over a short period. The survival rate of catastrophic APS is about 50%, but the long-term outcome of patients who survive is unknown.

Erkan D, et al. Long term outcome of catastrophic antiphospholipid syndrome survivors. *Annals of Rheumatic Diseases* 2003;62:530–33.

Question 15 T F F F T

The guidelines recommend crystalloids, and against the use of hydroxyethyl starches. Albumin can be added when patients require 'substantial amounts' of crystalloids.

Noradrenaline (norepinephrine) is the first-choice vasopressor, with adrenaline (epinephrine) or vasopressin added or substituted if required. Dopamine should only be used if there is a low risk of tachyarrhythmias and the patient is bradycardic. Dobutamine should be used when there is persistent hypoperfusion despite adequate fluid loading and the use of vasopressor agents.

Intravenous hydrocortisone (20mg daily) should be used only when fluids and vasopressors are unable to restore haemodynamic stability; the ACTH stimulation test is not recommended.

Procalcitonin or similar biomarkers are recommended to assist the discontinuation of empiric antibiotics.

Prophylactic platelet transfusions should be given when counts are <10 × 10⁹/l in the absence of apparent bleeding or when counts are <20 × 10⁹/l if the patient has a significant risk of bleeding. Higher platelet counts ≥50 × 10⁹/l should be the goal when active bleeding, surgery, or invasive procedures are occurring.

Dellinger RP, et al. Surviving Sepsis Campaign: international guidelines for management of severe sepsis and septic shock. *Critical Care Medicine* 2017;45:580–637.

Question 16 T F F T F

C. difficile is a Gram-positive spore-forming organism, which can cause significant morbidity within the health care setting. Initial treatment should include oral vancomycin and, or IV metronidazole. Oral fidaxomicin can also be used for severe cases in patients with multiple co morbidities. If symptoms are not improving and the patient is deteriorating, further input should be sought from the microbiologists and general surgeons. Consideration can be given to IV immunoglobulin if the patient is worsening and there is evidence of recurrence (especially when there is nutritional failure and low albumin). Donor stool transplant may also be considered for recurrent *C. difficile* infection. Probiotics may be of use for the prevention of *C. difficile* diarrhoea, but there is little evidence to support their use in its treatment.

Van Nood E, et al. Duodenal infusion of donor feces for recurrent Clostridium difficile. *New England Journal of Medicine* 2013;368(5):407–15.

You DM, Franzos MA, Holman RP. Successful treatment of fulminant *Clostridium difficile* infection with fecal bacteriotherapy. *Annals of Internal Medicine* Apr 2008;148(8):632–3.

Lowy I, et al. Treatment with monoclonal antibodies against *Clostridium difficile* toxins. *New England Journal of Medicine* 2010;362(3):197–205.

Question 17 T F F F T

Fenestrated tubes facilitate vocalization, but reduce the diameter of the inner lumen (thus increasing work), and are unsuitable for patients dependent on positive pressure ventilation. Surgical emphysema is a recognized complication when the fenestrations lie within the stoma.

Tracheostomy tubes without an inner cannula need changing every 7–14 days (those with inner can be changed every 30 days). The first change should be at least 7 days after the procedure to allow the stoma to establish.

The National Audit Project 4 highlighted a number of accidental extubations (n = 18, 14 of which with a tracheostomy in situ). Obesity was a risk factor, and again this reflects the need for the appropriate tube size and design.

Clinically significant stenosis occurs when the tracheal diameter is reduced by >50%, incidence of which is quoted <3%. Stomal stenosis can occur secondary to infection and chondritis. Incidence of infra-stomal stenosis has fallen due to the use of high-volume low-pressure cuffs, but caution against over inflation should be noted. Fracture of the first tracheal ring has been associated with stenosis, and ideal placement is between the second and third tracheal rings. Tracheal stenosis may also occur at the distal tip of the tracheal tube.

NAP 4. *Major complications of airway management in the United Kingdom.* http://www.rcoa.ac.uk/system/files/CSQ-NAP4-Full.pdf [accessed 30 July 2021].

Question 18 T F F F T

The 'safe triangle' remains the most logical approach for intercostal chest drain insertion. The safe triangle is the area bordered by the anterior edge of latissimus dorsi, the lateral edge of pectoralis major, inferiorly by a horizontal level at the level of the fifth intercostal space and superiorly with the apex in the base of the axilla. Using this approach minimizes the risk to underlying structures such as the viscera and internal mammary artery, and avoids damage to muscle and breast tissue.

In patients who have a spontaneous primary pneumothorax, which is <2cm, and remain asymptomatic, the British Thoracic Guidelines (BTS) suggest that the patients can be managed without follow-up. However smoking history and age suggest that the pneumothorax is less likely to be primary, and so the patient should be admitted for either oxygen and/or observation, aspiration, or chest drain insertion. Re-expansion pulmonary oedema occurs following drainage of a large pleural effusion or pneumothorax, and the incidence is up to 1%. Symptoms include cough and chest discomfort. The BTS guidelines suggest 1.5 l pleural fluid should be drained at one time, and those at higher risk of re-expansion pulmonary oedema include patients with large pneumothoraxes, young patients, and patients in whom the lung has been down for >7 days. Chest drain removal should occur during expiration.

D Laws, E Neville, J Duffy, on behalf of the British Thoracic Society Pleural Disease Group, a Sub-Group of the British Thoracic Society Standards of care Committee. BTS guidelines for the insertion of a chest drain. *Thorax* 2003;58(Suppl II):ii53–ii59.

British Thoracic Society Pleural Disease Guideline Group. BTS pleural disease guideline. *Thorax* 2010;65(Suppl 2):ii1–ii76.

Elsayed H, Roberts R, Emadi M, Whittle I, Shackcloth M. Chest drain insertion is not a harmless procedure—are we doing it safely? *Oxford Journal of Interactive Cardiovascular and Thoracic Surgery* 2012;11:745–8

Bodenham A, Paramasivam E. Air leaks, pneumothorax, and chest drains. *New England Journal of Medicine* 2008;8:204–9.

Question 19 T F T T T

Noradrenaline, whilst predominantly an α_1- and α_2-adrenoceptor agonist, has minor β adrenoceptor effects. Despite the persisting use of 'renal-dose dopamine', noradrenaline has been shown to be superior in maintaining both urine output and mean arterial pressure in septic shock. Noradrenaline triggers veno- and vasoconstriction, resulting in an increase in cardiac preload. Reflex bradycardia is possible, particularly in overdose or accidental bolus administration.

De Backer D, et al. Comparison of dopamine and norepinephrine in the treatment of shock. *New England Journal of Medicine* 2010;362(9):779–89.

Monnet X, Jabot J, Maizel J, Richard C, Teboul JL. Norepinephrine increases cardiac preload and reduces preload dependency assessed by passive leg raising in septic shock patients. *Critical Care Medicine* 2011;39(4):689–99.

Question 20 F F T F F

Weakness associated with critical illness may be due to differing pathological conditions, often with overlap. Often such weakness is regarded as a polyneuropathy, characterized by primary axonal degeneration (not demyelination) or a myopathy (histological evidence of myosin loss and muscle necrosis). Critical illness polyneuropathy affects the limbs in a symmetric pattern; there is no increase in creatinine kinase, and electrophysiological studies will reveal normal conduction velocity with reduced amplitude of compound muscle action potentials and sensory-nerve action potentials.

Kress J, Hall J. ICU-acquired weakness and recovery from critical illness. *New England Journal of Medicine* 2014;370:1626–35.

Question 21 F F T F F

In children >3 months and younger people, the most frequent causes are *Neisseria meningitides, Streptococcus pneumoniae,* and *Haemophilus influenzae* type b. Following the introduction of Hib, serogroup C meningococcus and some types of pneumococcus vaccines, serogroup B meningococcus is the most common causative pathogen; however, a recent vaccine has been introduced for babies in the UK. In neonates the most common causative pathogens include Group B streptococcus, *E. coli, S. pneumoniae,* and *Listeria monocytogenes.* Lumbar puncture should be performed, unless there are contraindications such as: signs suggestive of raised intracranial pressure, shock, extensive and, or spreading purpura, convulsions, coagulopathy, and respiratory insufficiency. Clinical assessment and not cranial CT should be used to decide the safety of undertaking lumbar puncture. There have been a number of studies looking at the role of corticosteroids in bacterial meningitis, and a recent Cochrane review concluded that there was reduced hearing loss in participants from high-income countries but not low-income countries, and that corticosteroids reduced hearing loss in children when the meningitis was secondary to *Haemophilus influenzae,* but not to other bacteria.

Brouwer M, McIntyre P, Prasad K, Van de Beek D. Corticosteroids for acute bacterial meningitis. *Cochrane Database System Review* Sep 2015;9:CD004405.

NICE. *NICE Guidelines CG102. Meningitis (bacterial) and meningococcal septicaemia in under 16s: recognition, diagnosis and management,* 2010. [accessed 30 July 2021].

Question 22 T T F F T

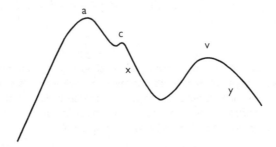

Figure 7.2 JVP waveform

a = atrial contraction

c = ventricular contraction

x = atrial relaxation

v = atrial filling

y = ventricular filling

Elevated a waves are seen in pulmonary hypertension or other causes of resistance to atrial emptying. They are absent in atrial fibrillation. Cannon a waves occur when the right atrium contracts against a closed tricuspid valve, as seen in A-V dissociation or ventricular tachycardia. Exaggerated x waves occur in constrictive pericarditis (Friedrich's sign), while tricuspid regurgitation will elevate the v wave (see Figure 7.2).

Yentis S, Hirsh N, Smith G. *Anaesthesia and intensive care A to Z: an encyclopaedia of principles and practice*. London: Butterworth Heineman, 2003.

Question 23 T F F T F

Partial agonists do have full affinity but only part intrinsic activity. Inverse agonists have high affinity but exert a different pharmacological action compared to the agonist. Competitive antagonists have no pharmacological effect, but prevent the action of the agonist by binding at the receptor site. Antagonism may be reversible or irreversible. Reversible antagonism can be competitive (competition for the same receptor) or noncompetitive, whereby the antagonist binds at a different site but results in a conformational change that hinders the action of the antagonist. This cannot be overcome by further agonist. The Michaelis constant is the concentration of the substrate at which the enzyme is working at half its maximal rate. G proteins are heterotrimeric proteins that facilitate signal amplification when a ligand binds to a G protein coupled receptor. The alpha subunit can stimulate or inhibit adenylyl cyclase to increase or decrease levels of cAMP.

Peck T, Hill S, Williams M. *Pharmacology for anaesthesia and intensive care*, 2nd edition. London: Greenwich Medical Media, 2003.

Question 24 F T T F T

GABA is the main inhibitory transmitter. There are receptor subtypes: $GABA_A$ and $GABA_B$. The latter functions via a G protein or second messenger system, while the former is a ligand-gated chloride channel. Chloride conductance is potentiated by the binding of benzodiazepines to the alpha subunit of the activated receptor complex. Midazolam if lipid soluble at physiological pH, where its ring structure is closed, and it is unionized (at pH<3 it has an open ring structure and is water soluble). The metabolites of lorazepam are inactive.

Peck T, Hill S, Williams M. *Pharmacology for anaesthesia and intensive care*, 2nd edition. London: Greenwich Medical Media, 2003.

Question 25 F F T T

Randomized controlled trials have failed to demonstrate a mortality benefit of 'high' PEEP. Whilst care needs to be taken to avoid stacking, PEEP is not contraindicated in asthma. There has been contradictory evidence on the reduction in ventilator-induced lung injury by PEEP, but current consensus would appear to support the theory. Raised intrathoracic pressure and PEEP may under some circumstances improve cardiac output, with reduction in the LVESV and LV afterload forming part of the postulated mechanism. Whilst significant haemodynamic compromise should be avoided (to maintain cerebral perfusion pressure), the positive effects of PEEP are of value in these patients.

Acute Respiratory Distress Syndrome Network. Higher versus lower positive end-expiratory pressures in patients with the acute respiratory distress syndrome. *New England Journal of Medicine* 2004;351:327–36.

Stather DR, Stewart TE. Clinical review: mechanical ventilation in severe asthma. *Critical Care* 2005;9:581–7.

Pinksy MR. The hemodynamic consequences of mechanical ventilation: an evolving story. *Intensive Care Medicine* 1997;23:493–503.

Question 26 F T T T F

ICNARC promotes local audit of critical care through the provision of comparative data in the Case Mix Programme and it has a well-established research arm. The QQR is the Case Mix Programme (CMP) unit report and is the main product of the CMP. The QQR provides cumulative comparative analysis of individual critical care unit data for local quality improvement initiatives. The quality indicators are presented in funnel plots along with a trend graph and a quarterly results table showing the unit's result for each quarter.

The quality indicators in the QQR are:

- High-risk sepsis admissions
- Unit-acquired infections in the blood
- Out-of-hours discharges to the ward (not delayed)
- Delayed discharges (>8hour delay)
- Nonclinical transfer (out)
- Unplanned readmissions within 48 hours
- Risk-adjusted acute hospital mortality
- Risk-adjusted acute hospital mortality—predicted risk of death <20%

ICNARC. *Quarterly quality report-ICNARC.* https://www.icnarc.org/Our-Audit/Audits/Cmp/Reports/Quarterly-Quality-Report [accessed 1 February 2016].

Question 27 F F F F T

C. albicans is normally sensitive to fluconazole; other candida species may not be. Amphotericin B has many toxic side effects; including renal and liver failure, fever/rigours, hyperkalaemia, and arrhythmias. These may be reduced, by using a lipid formulation. Triazole antifungals (e.g. fluconazole and voriconazole) can inhibit the cytochrome P450 system; this is not a problem with caspofungin. Second-line agents for pneumocystis pneumonia are primaquine-clindamycin, or atovaquone. Patients with moderate to severe pneumonia should also receive corticosteroids.

Aspergillus pneumonitis usually only requires steroid therapy, and so antifungals are not recommended. However, itraconazole has been used as a steroid-sparing agent.

Limper AH, et al. An official American Thoracic Society statement: treatment of fungal infections in adult pulmonary and critical care patients. *American Journal of Respiratory and Critical Care Medicine* 2011;183(1):96–128.

Question 28 F F T T T

Vasopressin has been used in cardiac arrests, and one study has shown it to be superior to adrenaline when used in arrests secondary to asystole. However strong evidence is lacking, and there is no recommendation for its widespread use during arrest. Vasopressin can be used to reduce portal hypertension and has been used to prevent variceal bleeding, although terlipressin, a pro drug of vasopressin, is more commonly used. Vasopressin levels are low in patients with sepsis, and they have greater sensitivity to exogenous vasopressin. Noradrenaline and vasopressin work synergistically, as vasopressin also increases intracellular calcium and vascular tone by blocking potassium-sensitive ATP channels.

Russell JA, Walley KR, Singer J, Gordon AC, Hebert PC, Cooper J. Vasopressin versus norepinephrine infusion in patients with septic shock. *New England Journal of Medicine* 2008;358:877–87.

Wenzel V, Krismer AC, Arntz R, Sitter H, Stadlbauer KH, Linner KH. A comparison of vasopressin and epinephrine for out of hospital cardiopulmonary resuscitation. *New England Journal of Medicine* 2004;350:105–13.

Question 29 T T F F F

Blood is most commonly supplied to the sump from the right atrium, but there may be surgical or anatomic considerations which require alternative venous cannulation sites (e.g. bicaval cannulation, femoral vessels). To optimize surgical conditions, a cross clamp is placed across the ascending aorta, proximal to the aortic cannula. Cardioplegic techniques provide myocardial protection and are administered anterogradely via the aortic root or directly into the coronary ostium or by a retrograde route if the coronary arteries are severely occluded. CPB and the administration of cardioplegia result in hyperkalaemia. Protamine administered before weaning and termination of CPB could lead to potentially fatal pump thrombosis. Anaesthetic vapour is commonly administered through CPB equipment.

Machin D, Allsager C. Principles of cardiopulmonary bypass. *Continuing Education in Anaesthesia, Critical Care & Pain* 2006;6:176–81.

Question 30 T T F F T

Time constant describes the time for plasma concentration to fall to 37% of its original value. *Volume of distribution* is the apparent volume into which the drug disperses. This often reflects several compartments including plasma (infusion and excretion), well-perfused (muscle), and poor-perfused (fat) compartments. There is initial rapid decline with distribution, slower decline due to terminal elimination, and then redistribution. The sum of all these compartments can be described as the volume of distribution at steady state and as it is theoretical, may exceed total body volume. During an infusion of a drug, there is transfer of drug from central to peripheral compartments. For many drugs, the time taken for the plasma concentration to fall to 50% will depend on the duration of infusion (as the drug accumulates in peripheral compartments and then redistributes). Drugs with a constant context-sensitive half-time result a rapid offset of action independent of duration of infusion. Most drugs display first-order kinetics where rate of plasma concentration change is proportional to amount present. Zero order kinetics describe a rate of plasma concentration change that is constant.

Peck T, Hill S, Williams M. *Pharmacology for anaesthesia and intensive care*, 2nd edition. London: Greenwich Medical Media, 2003.

1. **You are asked to review a 65-year-old woman, known to have pulmonary hypertension (PH), and who now is extremely dyspnoeic and hypotensive (BP 87/43mmHg). Select the most relevant stem regarding her condition:**

   A. PH is described as mean pulmonary artery pressure >30mmHg at rest

   B. Peak tricuspid regurgitation velocity (TRV) is used to estimate systolic pulmonary artery pressure

   C. Right heart catheterization is useful in patients with Group 2 PH

   D. There are four World Health Organization (WHO) classifications of PH

   E. The use of nifedipine will help with right ventricular afterload

2. **A 65-year-old woman presents with extensive bruising, jaundice, worsening renal function, and severe neurological impairment. The patient is found to be anaemic (Hb 6.8g/dl) and thrombocytopaenic (platelets 40 × 109/l). The most appropriate next step is (select the best answer):**

   A. Plasmapheresis

   B. Rituximab

   C. Transfusion of 2 units of red packed cells

   D. Transfusion of 2 units of platelets

   E. Transfusion of 4 units of fresh frozen plasma

3. **A 21-year-old man is found collapsed in a nightclub. Other than a history of recreational cocaine abuse, he is otherwise fit and healthy. Findings on examination include reduced conscious level, blood pressure 235/170 mm Hg, and widespread ischaemic changes on his electrocardiogram (ECG). The most appropriate BP-lowering therapy is (select the best answer):**

   A. Amlodipine 10mg

   B. Carvedilol 12.5mg

   C. Glyceryl trinitrate (GTN) infusion

   D. Labetolol 50–100mg IV

   E. Phentolamine 1mg

MCQs and SBAs in Intensive Care Medicine. Lorna Eyre and Andrew Bodenham, Oxford University Press. © Oxford University Press 2021.
DOI: 10.1093/oso/9780198753056.003.0008

4. **A 60-year-old man, with known excess alcohol consumption, is found on the medical admissions unit with a Glasgow Coma Scale (GCS) of 8. He had been admitted a short time ago with headache and subsequent seizure. A cerebrospinal sample taken earlier reveals 50 × 106/l lymphocytes, 500 × 106/l neutrophils, turbid appearance, protein 1.5 g/l, blood glucose <2mmol/l, and 0 red cells. The most appropriate treatment following immediate resuscitation and stabilization is (select best answer):**
    A. Dexamethasone 4mg intravenous
    B. Intravenous acyclovir 10–15mg/kg 8 hourly
    C. Intravenous ceftriaxone 2g
    D. Phenytoin intravenous loading dose
    E. Urgent repeat computed tomography (CT) scan of the head

5. **All the following electrophysiological findings are in keeping with a critical illness myopathy, except one:**
    A. Normal sensory nerve action potential amplitude
    B. Normal nerve conduction velocity
    C. Reduced compound muscle action potential amplitude
    D. Reduced muscle excitability on direct stimulation
    E. Reduced nerve conduction latency

6. **A patient known to have epilepsy is found in status epilepticus and has been fitting for approximately 40 minutes. Currently there is no intravenous access or monitoring on the patient as a result of the continuous generalized seizures. Select the best appropriate management:**
    A. Diazepam 10mg intramuscular (IM)
    B. Leviteracetam 1g intravenous (IV)
    C. Lorazepam 0.1mg/kg initially and then further 4mg lorazepam repeated once only, intraosseous (IO)
    D. Midazolam 10 buccal or IM
    E. Propofol 1–2mg/kg IO

7. **A level 3 patient on the ICU is being treated for *Pneumocystis jireovecii* pneumonia (PCP) with trimethoprim/sulfamethoxazole. On the monitor, her saturations are in the order of 85%, despite arterial blood PaO_2 10.9kPa on a FiO_2 0.45. Select the most appropriate management:**
    A. Add in some loop diuretic (e.g. furosemide 40mg)
    B. Increase the FiO_2
    C. Increase the positive end expiratory pressure (PEEP)
    D. Place the patient in a prone position
    E. Trial of methylene blue 1–2mg/kg

8. **A 60kg 38-week-pregnant woman presents with a blood pressure of 180/ 95mmHg, proteinuria, and ankle oedema. She is started on labetalol and magnesium sulphate; labour is induced, and she has an uneventful vaginal delivery. Postpartum her blood pressure is 140/90mmHg, CVP 8cmH20. She is receiving 80mls/hour of fluid, and her urine output is 10mls per hour for the past 4 hours. Select the most appropriate management:**

    A. Bolus of crystalloid (e.g. 500ml Hartmann's solution)
    B. Bolus dose of human albumin solution (HAS) (e.g. 250ml 4.5% HAS)
    C. Dose of furosemide
    D. Infusion of low dose dopamine
    E. Start haemofiltration

9. **A patient with known alcoholic cirrhosis and ascites is admitted following an acute gastro-intestinal bleed. He is started on terlipressin and an oesophageal varix endoscopically banded. Over the following 2 days, his serum creatinine rises from 50umol/l to 150umol/l, despite fluid resuscitation. There is no sign of ongoing bleeding. The following management is the most appropriate:**

    A. Albumin at a dose of 1g/kg/day (max. 100g)
    B. Bolus of furosemide
    C. Infusion of dopamine
    D. Bolus of crystalloid rather than colloid
    E. Immediate haemofiltration

10. **A 55kg woman, who was being treated for severe gallstone pancreatitis, was intubated for worsening gas exchange. Her chest x-ray revealed extensive bilateral infiltrates. Despite a normal echo, her gas exchange continued to deteriorate. Her ventilator settings included a tidal volume of 500ml, PEEP 7.5cm H_2O, peak plateau pressure of 30cm H_2O. What following intervention is most likely to increase her chance of survival?**

    A. Increasing the PEEP
    B. Prone positioning the patient for 10 hours a day
    C. A tidal volume of 330ml and permissive hypercapnia
    D. Neuromuscular blockade after 72 hours
    E. Early trophic enteral feeding

11. **Regarding the use of the pulse oximeter, select the most relevant correct answer:**

    A. It uses two light emitting diodes (LEDs) emitting monochromatic light at infrared 840nm and red light 660nm wavelengths
    B. Inaccuracy may occur in the presence of fetal haemoglobin
    C. Methaemoglobin may lead to false low readings
    D. Methylene blue can lead to a falsely elevated reading
    E. Polycythaemia leads to a false high reading

12. **A 60-year-old patient develops a left-sided purulent lung abscess, leading to extensive 'white out' of the left hemithorax on the chest x-ray. Due to extensive secretions and risk of soiling, the left lung is isolated with a left-sided double lumen tube (39 Fr Bronchocath). Several hours later the patient develops reduced oxygen saturations and small tidal volumes (below that preset on the ventilator), and alarms are triggered because of high airway pressures. On examination, breath sounds are absent on the right. There is minimal air entry on the left, accompanied by widespread wheeze and crepitations. The trachea is central. The patient's blood pressure falls to 70mmHg systolic; her heart rate falls to 60 beats per minutes; and she desaturates to 80%. Which single manoeuvre should be done now to prevent cardiorespiratory arrest and optimal management?**

A. Bronchial lavage and suction of purulent secretions down the left side of the double lumen tube

B. Increase the FiO_2 to 1.0

C. Needle thoracocentesis of the right side

D. Under direct guidance, deflate both cuffs and pull the tube back and then reinflate

E. Under direct guidance, deflate bronchial and tracheal cuffs and push the tube further in and then reinflate

13. **A 35-year-old woman presents to A&E having taken an overdose of amitriptyline. The toxic effects of this relate to all of the following mechanisms, except:**

A. Anticholinergic action

B. Direct alpha-adrenergic blockade

C. Inhibition of noradrenaline and serotonin uptake 1

D. Inhibition of monoamine oxidase

E. Membrane stabilizing effect via sodium channel blockade

14. **A 77-year-old man presents with hypoxia, tachycardia, and chest pain post a recent long-haul flight. His saturation is 85% despite 15l oxygen via a nonrebreather bag; his systolic blood pressure is 105/75 mm Hg, and he remains stable but looks unwell. His bloods reveal an AKI, creatinine 350µmol/l, and a raised troponin. What is your emergent management strategy?**

A. Immediate CT pulmonary angiography (CTPA)

B. Immediate echo

C. Immediate intubation and ventilation

D. Tinzaparin 175 units/kg actual body weight

E. Thrombolysis with alteplase

15. **A 78-year-old, with known structural heart disease, presents to the emergency department with dyspnoea and a heart rate of 170 beats per minute in new atrial fibrillation. The blood pressure is 72/45mmHg and the patient looks pale and clammy, with widespread ST depression on the 12 lead ECG. Initial management of this patient should include:**

   A. DC cardioversion

   B. Flecainide can be used to pharmacologically cardiovert

   C. Magnesium sulphate 20mmol intravenous

   D. Rate control with digoxin 500mcg intravenous

   E. Rhythm control with amiodarone 300mg

16. **A patient who has been on the intensive care unit deteriorates further, requiring high levels of cardiovascular support and is found to have urosepsis. Microbiology confirms the presence of an extended-spectrum beta-lactamases (ESBL) producing enterobacteria. Select the most appropriate microbial cover includes:**

   A. Ciprofloaxacin

   B. Meropenem

   C. Nitrofurantoin

   D. Tigecycline

   E. Trimethoprim

17. **A young girl has taken a staggered paracetamol overdose. She is somnolent, though can be roused, has a prothrombin time of 110 seconds, and has now developed an acute kidney injury with creatinine 310μmol/l and metabolic acidosis pH 7.24. Select the next most appropriate management:**

   A. Cautious fluid resuscitation with sodium chloride 0.9% and continued N-acetylcysteine infusion

   B. Give fresh frozen plasma and insert an ICP bolt, post intubation and ventilation

   C. High-volume plasma exchange

   D. Initiate renal replacement therapy

   E. List for orthotopic liver transplant

18. **A 77-year-old man on the ICU is 3 days post cardiac arrest. Return of spontaneous circulation occurred after 22 minutes of advanced life support, but there appears to be a 12-minute 'downtime' with no bystander CPR. The patient now remains comatose, despite a lack of sedation. The overall prognosis looks bleak, and decisions regarding withdrawal of care are being considered. Select the best factor below which provides the best prognostic indicator in this circumstance?**

   A. Presence of myoclonic jerks

   B. An abnormal flexor response

   C. Presence of cortical somatosensory evoked potentials

   D. Low levels of neuronal specific enolase

   E. EEG finding of complete generalized suppression

19. **A 55-year-old farmer is brought to the ED with an altered level of consciousness and restlessness and is noted to be tremulous. Further clinical examination reveals a HR of 40 beats per minute, hypotension (BP 85/47mmHg) and widespread wheeze. Prior to admission, the patient had been vomiting, and his partner reports that he is otherwise fit and healthy; however, he has recently been troubled by financial worries. The chest radiology is suggestive of an aspiration pneumonia. What is the next appropriate management?**

A. Atropine 1mg

B. Diazepam 10mg

C. Intubation and ventilation, using rocuronium in reduced dose

D. Metaraminol infusion

E. Pralidoxime 30mg/kg

20. **You are asked to review a young African woman who presents with a recent history of cough and fever and who has now been brought to the Emergency Department with a generalized seizure. She is otherwise previously fit and has returned from sub-Saharan Africa weeks ago. On examination she is febrile, jaundiced with bilateral crackles on respiratory auscultation, and remains postictal, with a GCS of E2 V3 M4. Select the most appropriate immediate management strategy:**

A. Co-amoxiclav + clarithromycin for CAP

B. Intubate and ventilate for CT head

C. HIV test

D. Parenteral artesunate

E. Thick and thin film

21. **A 25-year-old woman has just recently returned to the UK from travelling around the United States. Her family is concerned as she has an altered mental state with change in personality and seems to be weak. On examination, she is pyrexial with a reduced GCS E3 M2 V5. A lumbar puncture has been performed: clear appearance, $200 \times 10^6/l$ lymphocytes, $80 \times 10^6/l$ neutrophils, 0.8g/l protein and a glucose CSF to blood ratio >0.6. What treatment should be given?**

A. IV acyclovir

B. IV cefotaxime

C. IV cefotaxime and IV dexamethasone

D. IV immunoglobulins

E. Nothing other than supportive care, which could include intubation and ventilation

22. **A 53-year-old man was involved in a road traffic accident and is now 72 hours post open reduction and internal fixation of a closed femoral shaft fracture. He is now hypoxaemic on the ward, PaO$_2$ 8.0kPa on 15l per minute oxygen, tachypnoeic >30 breaths per minute, with BP 110/75mmHg, and heart rate 100 beats per minute. There is a petechial rash, and the patient is increasingly agitated, confused, and combative. Select the best following management option:**

   A. Anticoagulate with full dose tinzaparin and organize a CTPA

   B. Intubate and ventilate, with subsequent imaging of chest and head

   C. Loading dose of methylprednisolone and move to critical care for noninvasive ventilation and monitoring

   D. Move to HDU given increased agitation and confusion where high flow oxygen can be given and CXR

   E. Start co-amoxiclav 1.2g IV tds and organize a CT of head and CTPA

23. **Post pneumonectomy, a patient is transferred from the thoracic ward to the ICU for intubation and ventilation secondary to increased oxygen requirements and progressive hypoxia. His remaining lung looks congested on the CXR. He becomes hypotensive with increased noradrenaline requirements, and an echo suggests poor right ventricular function and dilatation, with preservation of left ventricular function. Which of the following would be your next strategy of choice?**

   A. Anticoagulate and organize a CTPA

   B. Further judicious fluid boluses and pulmonary artery catheter

   C. Further judicious fluid boluses and increase in noradrenaline

   D. Levosimendan and noradrenaline

   E. Milrinone and vasopressin

24. **A 45-year-old woman presents with jaundice and anorexia and is found to have tender hepatomegaly. On further questioning, she frequently drinks alcohol and has a 15-year history of >30 units per week in keeping with a presentation of alcoholic hepatitis. Which statement below is most applicable with the clinical situation?**

   A. A high white cell count with predominance of lymphocytes is often seen

   B. An ALT:AST ratio of >2 differentiates alcoholic hepatitis typically

   C. Benefit from steroids only if the Maddrey score ≤32

   D. High AST and ALT enzyme levels would be expected on the blood tests

   E. Pentoxifylline should be started

25. **A 25-year-old woman takes 50 tablets of amitriptyline 50mg (total therefore 2500mg). The patient is approximately 50kg and is currently Glasgow coma scale (GCS) E2 V2 M4. Her ECG reveals sinus tachycardia, with QRS 160ms, and prolonged QT$_c$ 440ms. She is promptly intubated and given sodium bicarbonate. Her pH is now 7.5, but she remains tachycardic, hypotensive, and with a wide QRS. What is the next step?**

    A. Hypertonic sodium chloride (e.g. 100ml bolus 3% saline)
    B. Further sodium bicarbonate bolus 50 ml 8.4%
    C. Magnesium 2g
    D. Lidocaine 1–1.5mg/kg bolus
    E. Lipid emulsion 20% 1–1.5ml/kg

26. **A 60-year-old man, previously fit and healthy is transferred to the ICU for progressive encephalopathy. He has a week-long history of epigastric pain and on examination he is deeply jaundiced. His initial bloods are below. The CT imaging suggests perfusion defects in the right liver, occlusion of the right and middle hepatic veins with patency of the portal vein and hepatic artery.**

Bilirubin 103µmol/L	Hb 191g/L	Na 138mmol/L
ALT 2338iU/L	Wcc 9.9 × 10⁹/L	K 5.1mmol/L
Alk phos 182iU/L	Plts 345 × 10⁹/L	Urea 12.5µmol/L
		Creat 325µmol/L
PT 36 seconds		

What is the next most appropriate management plan?

    A. Aggressive fluid resuscitation
    B. Anticoagulate with tinzaparin 175u/kg
    C. Infusion of N-acetylcysteine
    D. Reversal of coagulopathy in light of needing venous stent
    E. Transjugular intrahepatic portosystemic shunt (TIPSS)

27. **A 23 year old presents to the ED with a 1-month history of weight loss and thirst. This morning the patient's mother was worried as the patient was difficult to rouse. On examination the patient has BP 92/45 and a Glasgow coma scale (GCS) of E3 M6 V3. The blood glucose comes back at 27mmol/l, the urinary ketones are 3+, and the venous bicarbonate is 14mmol/l, while the plasma potassium is 4.5mmol/l. The patient has already had 0.9% NaCl 1 l infused over 1 hour. A fixed-rate insulin infusion is being commenced at 0.1 units/kg/hour. What is the next management strategy?**

    A. A further 1l of 0.9% NaCl infused over 1 hour
    B. A further 1l of 0.9% NaCl with 40mmolKCl infused over 2 hours
    C. A further 1l of 0.9% NaCl with 40mmolKCl over 1 hour
    D. A 100ml bolus of 1.26% sodium bicarbonate run in stat
    E. An increase of insulin infusion by 1 unit/hour if capillary blood glucose has fallen just to 23mmol/l after the first hour

28. **A 75kg, 43-year-old man with a background of type 2 diabetes and hypertension is admitted following entrapment in a house fire. There are two casualties reported at scene, and the man was reported to be intoxicated. On primary assessment, a preliminary figure of 30% total body surface area (TBSA) burn is calculated for resuscitation purposes. He has been intubated as there were related concerns over inhalational injury with a carbon monoxide level of 28% on a co-oximeter. He is currently receiving fluid resuscitation, a FiO_2 1.00 and controlled ventilation with pressure controlled ventilation (PCV). Despite initial resuscitative measures his arterial blood gas (ABG) shows the following:**

pH	7.10
pCO_2	6.0 kPa
pO_2	11.3 kPa
HCO_{3-}	13mmol/L
BE−	15
Lactate	15
Glucose	15

The best initial treatment is:

A. Fixed-rate insulin infusion
B. Hydroxocobalamin
C. Increasing fluid administration to 6mls/kg/% TBSA
D. Reduce the inspired oxygen
E. Renal replacement therapy (RRT)

29. **A 65-year-old woman is admitted to the ICU with signs of bilateral pneumonia. Her FiO_2 requirement has increased significantly, and she is now in atrial fibrillation. The decision is made to perform semi-elective intubation and ventilation. She has a past medical history of heart transplant 4 years ago for end stage cardiac failure secondary to an ischaemic cardiomyopathy. Currently her antirejection medications include cyclosporin and mycophenolate mofetil. Select the drug below which has no physiological response:**

A. Adrenaline
B. Atropine
C. Dobutamine
D. Ephedrine
E. Noradrenaline

30. **A 56-year-old man, who incidentally was found to be HIV positive on admission screening bloods, comes to ICU for progressive type 1 respiratory failure. The CXR shows peri-hilar ground glass shadowing, and the patient receives a course of high-dose co-trimoxazole for presumed PCP pneumonia (*Pneumocystis jirovecci*). Despite treatment for 5 days, there is no improvement in ventilatory parameters, and the patient remains settled but dependent on the noninvasive ventilation and FiO$_2$ 0.7. Select the next best management strategy:**

A. Beta D glucan levels

B. Initiate antiretroviral therapy

C. Intubate and blind bronchoscopic alveolar lavage (BAL)

D. Prednisolone 40mg bd

E. Start clindamycin-primaquine

1. B

PH is defined as mean pulmonary artery pressure >25mmHg at rest and >30mmHg on exercise.

According to the WHO classification, there are five major groups. Patients in Group 1 have pulmonary arterial hypertension (inheritable, drugs, and connective tissue causes); Group 2 have left-sided heart disease; Group 3 have chronic lung disorders and hypoxaemia; Group 4 have pulmonary artery obstruction; and Group 5 have unidentified mechanisms.

Once PH is suspected, transthoracic echo (TTE) is the initial test of choice. TTE can be used to evaluate the probability of PH using TRV, which can also be used to estimate the pulmonary artery systolic pressure. TTE also assesses both right and left ventricles. Right heart catheterization is preserved for Group 1 (pulmonary arterial hypertension) and Group 4 (chronic thromboembolic PH) to assess the severity of haemodynamic impairment and assess potential vasoreactivity.

With the exception of PH associated with lung disease and left-sided heart disease, the condition should be managed in a designated specialist centre. The right ventricle can remodel, and targeted therapies include prostacyclin, sildenafil, and pulmonary endarterectomy. Balloon atrial septostomy and transplantation can also be considered.

The clinical course of PH is one of progressive decline and intermittent episodes of acute decompensation. Mortality of patients, once admitted to the ICU, is high, and strategies should be directed at treating underlying precipitants of acute deterioration (infection, arrythmia), reduction of right ventricular (RV) afterload (nifedipine is a calcium channel blocker that favourably vasodilates in a proportion of patients with pulmonary arterial hypertension, but is not suitable for the vast majority of pulmonary hypertensive patients), improvement of cardiac output with inotropes, fluid balance optimization, and maintenance of systemic blood pressure with vasopressors.

Kiely DG, Elliot CA, Sabroe I, Condliffe R. Pulmonary hypertension: diagnosis and management. *British Medical Journal* 2013;346:31–5.

McLaughlin VV, McGoon MD. Pulmonary arterial hypertension. *Circulation* 2006;114:1417–31.

Galie N, et al. ESC/ERS guidelines for the diagnosis and treatment of pulmonary hypertension: the Joint Task Force for the Diagnosis and Treatment of Pulmonary Hypertension of the European Society of Cardiology (ESC) and the European Respiratory Society (ERS): Endorsed by: Association for European Paediatric and Congenital Cardiology (AEPC), International Society for Heart and Lung Transplantation (ISHLT). *European Heart Journal* 2016;37:67–119.

2. A

This scenario is typical of thrombotic thrombocytopaenic purpura (TTP). TTP arises through inhibition of ADAMTS13, an enzyme responsible for cleaving von Willebrand Factor into smaller units. In the absence of its function, platelet adhesion (and subsequent thrombocytopaenia) increases with generation of thrombi (microangiopathic haemolytic anaemia) leading to neurological symptoms and renal failure.

Plasma exchange is the mainstay of treatment for all patients, as there is removal of autoantibody to ADAMTS13, and replacement of this enzyme in the donor plasma (plasma pheresis with a non-plasma replacement fluid is not an adequate treatment, as there is no enzyme replacement). Glucocorticoids and rituximab may also be given if the disease is sufficiently severe. The latter, a monoclonal antibody, may reduce relapse and may hasten the response to therapy.

Platelet transfusion may be required if there is clinically significant bleeding; however, this is rare. There is an observation that arterial thrombosis may be higher in patients with TTP who received platelets.

Waldmann C, Soni N, Rhodes A (eds). *Oxford desk reference: critical care*, 1st edition. Oxford: Oxford University Press, 2008.

Scully M, et al. Guidelines on the diagnosis and management of thrombotic thrombocytopaenic purpura and other thrombotic microangiopathis. *BJH* 2012;158:323–35.

3. C

The given history suggests cocaine overdose as the most likely cause of hypertensive emergency (although clearly additional history should be sought). Immediate BP-lowering therapy is indicated; however, beta blockade, is generally not recommended because of the theoretical concerns of coronary vasoconstriction and systemic hypertension due to the unopposed alpha-adrenergic stimulation. Labetalol and carvedilol both have alpha-blocking properties; however, in this instance, titration of GTN infusion may be the most efficient option in reducing blood pressure in a timely fashion. Benzodiazepines may also be indicated for any associated agitation. Amlodipine is an oral agent, and phentolamine can be used, but pragmatically may not be as readily available.

Waldmann C, Soni N, Rhodes A (eds). *Oxford desk reference: critical care*, 1st edition. Oxford: Oxford University Press, 2008.

Lange RA, et al. Potentiation of cocaine-induced coronary vasoconstriction by beta-adrenergic blockade. *Annals of Internal Medicine* 1990;112:897.

4. C

The CSF result suggests bacterial meningitis with high neutrophil count, turbid appearance, low glucose, and high protein content. The commonest causes of community acquired bacterial meningitis are *Strep pneumoniae*, *Neisseria meningitidis*, and in those > 50 years, *Listeria monocytogenes*. Given the CSF results, first-line immediate management should include the cephalosporin, and indeed antimicrobial therapy should not be postponed where there is a clinical suspicion and for whatever reason lumbar puncture may be delayed.

Studies have demonstrated that dexamethasone reduces mortality and unfavourable outcome in pneumococcal meningitis. Therefore in the developed world, where bacterial meningitis is suspected and the organism not yet known, dexamethasone 0.15mg/kg should be given before and/or at the time of antibiotics and continued if blood cultures or CSF demonstrate *Strep pneumoniae*.

Waldmann C, Soni N, Rhodes A (eds). *Oxford desk reference: critical care*, 1st edition. Oxford: Oxford University Press, 2008.

McGill F, et al. The UK joint specialist societies on the diagnosis and management of acute meningitis and meningococcal sepsis in immunocompetent adults. *Journal of Infection* 2016;72:405–38.

5. E

ICU-acquired weakness is stratified into those patients who have a critical illness polyneuropathy (CIP), critical illness myopathy (CIM), or critical illness neuromyopathy (CINM).

Those with CIM can be further classified into cachectic myopathy, thick filament myopathy, or necrotizing myopathy.

CIM arises from early initial functional changes (muscle membrane inexcitability, altered sarcoplasmic reticulum, and dysfunctional mitochondria), whereas the later changes result from structural changes and atrophy.

Key findings associated with CIM include: rise in creatine kinase, reduced compound motor action potential amplitude, normal sensory nerve action potential, normal conduction velocity and conduction latency, reduced direct muscle compound muscle action potential amplitude on direct muscle stimulation, and abnormal muscle biopsy.

Appleton R, Kinsella J. Intensive care unit acquired weakness. *CEACCP* 2012;2:62–6.

Waldmann C, Soni N, Rhodes A (eds). *Oxford desk reference: critical care*, 1st edition. Oxford: Oxford University Press, 2008.

6. C

Status epilepticus is defined as continuous seizure activity for 5 minutes or more without return of consciousness or recurrent seizures (two or more) without an intervening period of recovery. Refractory status epilepticus is seizure activity that fails to respond to first-line therapy. Key management goals include terminating seizure activity, preventing secondary brain injury, decreasing cerebral metabolism, and managing any underlying causes (e.g. infection).

Initial treatment should address management of airway, oxygenation and ventilation, and early IV or IO access to attenuate the seizures. Initial therapies can be delivered via the IO route and include consideration of management of hypoglycaemia and life-threatening electrolyte disturbance, that may also contribute to the scenario.

First-line therapies include lorazepam 0.1mg/kg followed by a repeat 4mg dose. Lorazepam is preferred for its longer lasting effects; however, midazolam buccal or IM are alternative. Diazepam can be given IV or PR, but IM is painful.

Second-line therapies may include phenytoin, levetiracetam, and valproate. Usual antiepileptic medication should also be given early and may direct a second-line therapy.

Management of refractory status typically involves intubation and ventilation. Propofol is the usual induction agent, but alternatives may include thiopentone and midazolam, as well as EEG monitoring.

NICE *Clinical Guideline 137. Epilepsies: diagnosis and management* 2012 www.nice.org.uk/guidance/cg137 [accessed 14 March 2021].

7. E

By far the most commonly used antimicrobial for PCP pneumonia remains co-trimoxazole (trimethoprim/ sulfamethoxazole). This is a cause of methaemoglobinaemia (Met Hb), and as there is a clear discrepancy between oxygen content and saturation via the pulse oximeter, consideration of the levels of methaemoglobin via co-oximeter results should be sought. Methylene blue is the treatment of choice initially. Other acquired causes of Met Hb include the use of dapsone and antimalarials.

MetHb occurs when the ferrous iron in haem becomes ferric and the oxygen carrying capacity of haemoglobin is reduced. Normally, levels of Met Hb are kept low at approximately 1% by the red blood cell enzyme cytochrome b5 reductase (congenital causes of Met Hb are caused by a deficiency of this enzyme). MetHb interferes with pulse oximetry as it falsely absorbs light, and hence saturations via pulse oximetry remain at 85%.

Waldmann C, Soni N, Rhodes A (eds). *Oxford desk reference: critical care*, 1st edition. Oxford: Oxford University Press, 2008.

8. C

Pre-eclampsia is a progressive multisystem disorder, characterized by new-onset hypertension and end organ dysfunction in the latter half of pregnancy. Patients are vasoconstricted and fluid deplete; however, there is a significant risk of fluid overload and pulmonary oedema. Therefore excessive fluid administration should be avoided, and a urine output of 80ml per 4 hours is accepted. If this is not achieved, a cautious fluid bolus is acceptable if there is evidence of underfilling. In oliguric euvolaemic patients, furosemide is the drug of choice, and it is prudent to remember that pulmonary oedema can kill, whereas oliguria and acute tubular necrosis does not.

NICE. Clinical guideline 107. *Hypertension in pregnancy*. 2019 https://www.nice.org.uk/guidance/ng133 [accessed 30 July 2021].

9. A

Hepatorenal syndrome is the reduced glomerular filtration and subsequent kidney injury caused by advanced liver disease. Arterial vasodilation in the splanchnic circulation, triggered by portal hypertension seems to play a significant role. Diagnosis is essentially one of exclusion but is in keeping with kidney disease improving global outcomes (KDIGO) kidney injury definitions on the background of cirrhosis, and persisting after all other apparent causes are absent. Hepatorenal syndrome has been classically defined as type 1, which is more acute and severe, and type 2, which tends to have a more insidious course. The outlook of HRS type 1 (acute and rapid progression) is bleak, but consensus treatment is resuscitation with albumin (up to 100g/day) and terlipressin (1–2mg qds). The overall outcome of patients with hepatorenal syndrome and recovery of kidney function ultimately depends on the reversal of the hepatic failure.

Nadim, MK, et al. Hepatorenal syndrome. *Critical Care* 2012;16:23–6.

10. C

The clinical situation would fit with acute respiratory distress syndrome (ARDS). The overall ventilator strategy should include lung protection and lung recruitment. The latter uses PEEP to prevent derecruitment. Several studies have highlighted benefits of PEEP (including the ALVEOLI, LOVS, and EXPRESS trials) but failed to demonstrate a mortality benefit. Proning has recently regained interest following a study which demonstrated impressive mortality benefit with at least 16 hours of proning in severe ARDS. Early trophic feeding has not shown to be of benefit in ARDS (EDEN trial). Early neuromuscular block, within 48 hours, has been shown to improve mortality.

In this particular circumstance the single best answer remains the lung protective strategy and avoidance of excess tidal volume, with peak plateau pressures less than 30cm H_2O.

Silversides JA, Ferguson ND. Clinical review: acute respiratory distress—clinical ventilator management and adjunct therapy. *Critical Care* 2012 17:225.

11. C

Pulse oximeters use two LEDs within the probe that emit monochromatic light at red (660 nm) and infrared (940 nm) wavelengths. Each LED is alternately switched on and off, and a photodiode on the opposite side of the probe detects the transmitted light. The signal is converted to a direct current component, representing tissue background, venous blood, and the constant part of arterial blood flow, while an alternating current component represents pulsatile arterial blood flow. This signal is amplified and averaged over time. Inaccuracy results from presence of carboxyhaemoglobin (false elevation), methaemoglobin (false depression), and methylene blue (temporarily decreased oxygen saturations). Fetal haemoglobin and polycythaemia have no effect on oxygen saturation measurement using pulse oximetry.

Yentis S, Hirsch N, Smith G. *Anaesthesia and Intensive care A-Z: an encyclopaedia of principles and practice.* London: Butterworth Heineman, 2004.

12. E

Double lumen tubes (DLT) are sometimes used to isolate the lung in cases of infection, to prevent contralateral soiling. In this case there are no breath sounds on the 'healthy' side with reduced tidal volumes and increased ventilator pressures. While it is tempting to consider a right pneumothorax, the probability points much more to displacement of the DLT, especially with wheeze and no tracheal changes. Unnecessary needle thoracocentesis of the healthy side will lead to further harm. Increasing the FiO_2 should be done but will not ameliorate the fact that insufficient tidal volume is being achieved, as the right healthy lung is now not being ventilated.

If the left DLT is too far in, then the right lung should still be ventilated through the tracheal lumen, so a drastic drop in oxygen saturation would be less likely. However if the left DLT has migrated caudally, the left bronchial cuff will herniate up and out of the left main bronchus and will obliterate the entire right main bronchus at the carina. In effect the only oxygen now being delivered is to the pathological side, clearly resulting in drastic reduction in tidal volume and gas exchange. The management is to deflate both cuffs and push the DLT tube in further under direct vision.

Brodsky JB, Lung separation and the difficult airway. *British Journal of Anaesthesia* 2009;103:i66–i75.

13. D

Tricyclic antidepressants exert a wide variety of cellular mechanisms, except for monoamine oxidase inhibition. Patients present with a variety of findings, which can include seizures, coma, hypotension, palpitations, dry mouth, and mydriasis. Patients may have a metabolic acidosis, and ECG changes include sinus tachycardia, prolonged QT, and wide QRS, which can develop into a ventricular arrhythmia. Management is supportive with fluid, sodium bicarbonate, intubation if necessary, and control of seizures.

Kerr GW, McGuffie AC, Wilkie S, Tricyclic antidepressant overdose: a review. *Emergency Medicine Journal* 2001:18:236–41.

14. D

Whether a patient should be thrombolysed for a submassive PE remains controversial. *Submassive PE* is defined as evidence of RV dysfunction and, or evidence of myocardial necrosis. Clinical trials have demonstrated more rapid, immediate haemodynamic improvement and clot resolution following thrombolysis, but no clear mortality benefits. Some studies suggest that thrombolysis, in normotensive patients with acute PE, is associated with increased mortality. Validated severity scores such as PE severity index may help identify those patients in whom thrombolysis may be of benefit. Echo of course would be helpful, as would CTPA; however, the clinical symptoms and signs with the history suggest PE and the patient remains hypoxic, so prompt treatment in this instance with low molecular weight heparin is appropriate, prior to imaging.

Meyer G, Vicaut E, Danays T. Fibrinolysis for patients with intermediate-risk pulmonary embolism. *New England Journal of Medicine* 2014;370:1402–11.

Condliffe R, Elliott C, Hughes R. Management dilemmas in acute pulmonary embolism. *Thorax* 2013;69:174–80.

15. A

National Institute for Health and Care Excellence (NICE) guidelines suggest emergency electrical cardioversion, in people with life-threatening haemodynamic instability caused by new-onset atrial fibrillation. In patients with atrial fibrillation presenting acutely without life-threatening haemodynamic instability, rate or rhythm control should be offered if the onset of the arrhythmia is less than 48 hours, and rate control if it is more than 48 hours or is uncertain.

NICE. *NICE guidelines. Atrial fibrillation: the management of atrial fibrillation* 2021 https://www.nice.org.uk/guidance/ng196/resources/atrial-fibrillation-diagnosis-and-management-pdf-66142085507269 [accessed 30 July 2021].

16. B

Carbapenems remain the choice of treatment for ESBL producing bacteria. Tigecycline does have activity against ESBL organisms, but as it is not excreted in urine, it is of limited value in urinary tract sepsis. Nitrofurantoin can be used orally against ESBL producing organisms but is given orally and again is of limited use in associated severe sepsis.

Extended-spectrum beta-lactamases (ESBLs): guidance, data, analysis. 2014. Public Health England www.gov.uk/government/collections/extended-spectrum-beta-lactamases-esbls-guidance-data-analysis [accessed 30 July 2021].

17. E

She meets the King's College Criteria for selection for potential liver transplant. In the context of paracetamol overdose, the following criteria warrant listing, taking into account the background situation and psychiatric history:

* *Either* a pH <7.3, *or*;
* All of the following: prothrombin time > 100 seconds, creatinine >300μmol/l, and grade III encephalopathy

Renal replacement therapy may be required, although AKI associated with paracetamol overdose often rectifies post successful liver graft. At our centre, we have a low threshold for early renal replacement therapy, and in this context, it would be initiated early.

Fresh frozen plasma is not given routinely unless there is significant bleeding, as the prothrombin time gives an indication of the underlying liver function.

Monitoring ICP should be considered; however, there is a lack of evidence to suggest that survival outcomes are improved with ICP monitoring. The benefit of ICP monitoring and guided therapy in managing raised ICP needs to be weighed against the risk of bleeding, and coagulopathy needs to be reversed before insertion of an ICP bolt.

There is emerging evidence that high-volume plasma exchange may attenuate the inflammatory response seen in acute liver failure, and more centres will consider this modality.

Patients with acute liver failure often need aggressive fluid therapy, and the use of sodium containing crystalloid is acceptable.

Lai W, Murphy N. Management of acute liver failure. *Continuing Education In Anaesthesia, Critical Care & Pain* 2004;4:66–7.

Larsen F, Schmidt L, Bernsmeier C. High-volume plasma exchange in patients with acute liver failure: an open randomised controlled trial. *Journal of Hepatology* 2016;64:69–78.

18. E

Prognosis following hypoxic and anoxic brain injury can be difficult and should take into account a number of factors including the circumstances (i.e. duration of circulatory arrest, extent of resuscitation and co-morbidities). The mechanism of the arrest may also influence outcome (e.g. initial rhythm of ventricular tachycardia has a better outcome compared to asystole). Clinical features should also be taken into account. Myoclonic status epilepticus has insufficient negative prognostic power when considered in isolation. It can be difficult to distinguish from tonic-clonic seizures and multifocal myoclonus. Bilaterally absent somatosensory evoked potentials (N20 component of median nerve stimulation) may identify patients with a poor prognosis, but are specific although not sensitive for poor neurologic outcome. Markedly elevated neuronal specific enolase may show promise for predicting poor outcome, but cut-off values and sensitivity need to be defined. Absent motor response and absent pupillary or corneal reflexes are associated with poor outcome, and malignant EEG changes are associated with high mortality, with complete generalized suppression being the most specific for poor outcome.

Wijdicks E, Hijdra A, Young GB. Practice parameter: prediction of outcome in comatose survivors after cardiopulmonary resuscitation (an evidence-based review): report of the Quality Standards Subcommittee of the American Academy of Neurology. *Neurology* 2006;67:203.

Zandbergen EG. Systematic review of prediction of poor outcome in anoxic-ischaemic coma with biochemical markers of brain damage. *Intensive Care Medicine* 2001;27:1661.

19. A

The clinical features and history are suggestive of organophosphate toxicity. Organophosphates have been used in insecticides for more than 50 years, and worldwide, there is significant exposure to these agents. Sarin and other organophosphorus nerve agents have been used in chemical warfare and in acts of terrorism.

Organophosphorus compounds can be absorbed through the skin, lungs, and GIT. They bind to acetylcholinesterase and increase the amounts of acetylcholine at the neuronal synapses and neuromuscular junction. After a period of time, the organophosphate-acetylcholinesterase compound undergoes 'aging', and the enzyme is then irreversibly resistant to reactivation by oxime antidote.

The features of acute cholinergic toxicity include bradycardia, miosis, lacrimation, salivation, bronchospasm, urination, emesis, and diarrhoea. Neck flexion and proximal muscle weakness, as well as cranial nerve abnormalities, can occur as part of an intermediate neurological syndrome, but there can also be a delayed neuropathy.

The management include early intubation and ventilation where there is depressed mental status or respiratory weakness. Non-depolarizing neuromuscular agents can be used, but will be less effective at standard doses due to competitive inhibition at the neuromuscular junction.

Patients with cholinergic toxicity should be treated with atropine initially. Starting with 1–2mg and then doubled every 5 minutes, until respiratory secretions and bronchospasm are cleared. Very large quantities of atropine may be necessary to achieve this. Atropine does not bind to nicotinic receptors and is ineffective in managing the neuromuscular dysfunction. Pralidoxime is a cholinesterase reactivating agent and should be given slowly and early, but not without concurrent atropine. Organophosphate-induced seizures should be treated with diazepam.

Eddleston M, Phillips MR. Self-poisoning with pesticides. *BMJ* 2004;328:42.

20. E

The history is suggestive for malaria, and cerebral malaria is associated with *Plasmodium falciparum*. Classically patients present with cough, malaise, arthralgia, and shaking chills, which may be paroxysmal. Patients may be jaundiced due to haemolysis, and can demonstrate splenomegaly. Severe anaemia, renal failure (black water fever), cerebral, and respiratory symptoms may all be found in severe forms. It may be necessary to intubate and ventilate for a CT of the head if there is continued suppression of GCS and no imminent recovery.

It is important to remember that other pathologies may co-exist, so both HIV tests and lumbar puncture should be undertaken. Thick and thin films can both quantify and qualify the parasitaemia. Treatment of *P. falciparum* is ideally with parenteral artesunate, which is more effective than quinine. However it may be difficult to get hold off, so treatment with quinine should not be delayed. Artemisinin combination treatment should follow on post parenteral artesunate. Bacterial co-infection is relatively common, so a low threshold for starting antibiotics is reasonable.

Marks M, et al. Managing malaria in the intensive care unit. *British Journal of Anaesthesia* 2014;10:910–21.

21. A

The presence of normal brain function can often distinguish between meningitis (often patients are uncomfortable, lethargic, and distracted by headache but with normal cerebral function) and encephalitis (often associated with altered mental state, altered behaviour, motor, and, or sensory deficits and seizures). However the boundaries may overlap with meningoencephalitis, so it is often prudent to cover for both in the early stages.

The clinical history and CSF results are in keeping with a viral CNS infection, rather than bacterial. The commonest cause of viral encephalitis is herpes simplex (HSV) virus type 1, but other viral pathogens include Japanese encephalitis, West Nile (common in the United States and associated with profound weakness and rash), and other arboviruses.

Signs and symptoms of encephalitis include seizures, hemiparesis, cranial nerve palsies, confusion, and agitation.

Findings that are characteristic of the CSF include raised white cell count (usually less than 250/mm^3) with a predominance of lymphocytes compared to neutrophils, elevated protein (although usually less than 1.5g/l) and a normal glucose concentration (>50% of blood value). Diagnosis of HSV is by viral polymerase chain reaction (PCR) on the CSF, and while this is being done, empiric therapy with acyclovir should be started. Serum and CSF IgM antibody can be used to identify West Nile encephalitis, but there is no specific antivirals to treat this.

Whitley RJ, Gnann JW. Viral encephalitis: familiar infections and emerging pathogens. *Lancet* 2002;359:507.

22. B

PE is certainly in the differential diagnosis, but neurological impairment and petechial rash do not make it the most likely cause.

Fat embolism presents with a classic triad of respiratory changes (dyspnoea, tachypnoea, hypoxaemia, and CXR changes), neurological abnormality (acute confusion through to severe seizures), and characteristic petechial rash (conjunctiva, oral mucous membrane, and skin folds of the upper body). Diagnosis is made clinically, and there is a fat embolism index, with scoring assigned to features such as tachycardia, tacypnoea, petechiae, chest xray changes, hypoxaemia and fever.

Fat globules seen in urine, sputum, or serum are not diagnostic. There is no specific treatment and management is supportive, with emphasis on prevention (e.g. orthopaedic techniques). In this instance the patient is unlikely to be managed safely in an HDU environment. Given the reduced GCS, intubation is probably the safest option and would allow a CT of the head to be undertaken to exclude out other causes of neurological impairment. A number of studies have looked at corticosteroids given prophylactically to prevent fat embolism syndrome in patients with long bone fractures. A 2009 Cochrane review of seven trials suggested that corticosteroids may be beneficial in preventing fat embolism syndrome and hypoxia in patients with long bone fractures, although there was no mortality benefit.

Gupta A, Reilly S. Fat embolism. Continuing Education in Anesthesia, Critical Care & Pain 2007;7:(5):148–51. https://doi.org/10.1093/bjaceaccp/mkm027.

The Cochrane Library. Do corticosteroids reduce the risk of fat embolization syndrome in patients with long bone fractures? A meta-analysis. http://onlinelibrary.wiley.com/o/cochrane/cldare/articles/DARE-12010000277/frame.html.

23. E

RV failure may be seen post pneumonectomy in the face of increased pulmonary vascular resistance. Echo is probably sufficient to make the diagnosis, and will help aid the assessment of the patient's response to fluid.

Managing the failing right ventricle means:

1) Optimizing right ventricle preload
   - Closely monitored fluid challenges
   - Possible diuretic/renal replacement therapy if significant tricuspid regurgitation
2) Augment the right ventricle
   - Milrinone strengthens right ventricle contraction and reduces pulmonary vascular resistance
   - Others include dobutamine, adrenaline, and levosimendan

There is a risk of systemic hypotension (and tachycardia/increased myocardial work), so likely noradrenaline or vasopressin will be required.

3) Reduce right ventricle afterload
   - Optimize all factors leading to hypoxic pulmonary vasoconstriction (e.g. acid–base status, CO_2)
   - Inhaled nitric oxide, milrinone (can also be nebulized) and prostacyclin (endothelin receptor antagonists)—in practice these can be difficult to administer
4) Maintain systemic blood pressure and coronary perfusion
   - Noradrenaline
   - Vasopressin, experimentally this may lead to pulmonary vasodilatation (via NO dependent mechanisms) and can improve PVR/SVR ratio

Price LC, Wort SJ, Finney SJ, Marino PS, Brett SJ. Pulmonary vascular and right ventricular dysfunction in adult critical care: current and emerging options for management: a systematic literature review. *Critical Care* 2010;14:R169.

24. E

Hepatic manifestations of excess alcohol include alcoholic fatty liver disease, alcoholic hepatitis, and cirrhosis. The clinical signs of alcoholic hepatitis include jaundice, pyrexia, and tender hepatomegaly, and typical laboratory tests include only moderate elevations in AST and ALT with an AST to ALT ratio ≥2. Bilirubin and gamma-glutamyl transferase are also raised, and there is often a leucocytosis, with a predominate neutrophilia. Medical therapy for alcoholic hepatitis remains controversial, and in severe cases, Maddrey discriminant function score ≥32, prednisolone should be considered. Pentoxyfylline may also be used if steroids are contraindicated. Results of the Steroids or Pentoxifylline for Alcoholic Hepatitis trial involving 1103 subjects showed that treatment with the steroid prednisolone reduced 28-day mortality in patients with severe alcoholic hepatitis, whereas treatment with the oral phosphodiesterase inhibitor pentoxifylline did not. However, the benefit of prednisolone did not extend beyond 28 days, and there was no difference in the mortality rates between the two treatments at 1 year.

Thursz M, et al. Prednisolone or pentoxyfylline for alcoholic hepatitis. *NEJM* 2015;372:1619.

25. B

Amitriptyline is a tricyclic antidepressant, and in overdose, clinical findings are a result of the following:

- Blockade of fast cardiac sodium channels
- Antagonism of central and peripheral muscarinic Ach receptors
- Antagonism of peripheral alpha-1 adrenergic receptors
- Antagonism of histamine 1 receptors
- Antagonism of CNS GABA A receptors.

Thus tachycardia is an issue, as is prolonged QRS and QT_c and risk of arrythmias. There is a CNS depressant effect due to the histamine blockade and a risk of seizures because of the interference with the GABA receptors.

Management should focus on early intubation and ventilation for those with compromised GCS. Hyperventilation will help with the alkalinization. Benzodiazepines may be needed for agitation.

Sodium bicarbonate 1–2mmol/kg is the standard therapy for hypotension, fluid resuscitation, and arrhythmia. The alkalization favours the nonionized form of the drug and makes it less available to bind to sodium channels. The increase in extracellular sodium increases the electrochemical gradient across the cardiac cell membrane. The initial sodium bicarbonate should be as bolus (2–3 prefilled 50ml 8.4% syringes for example). Some suggest an infusion, although boluses may be more efficient in manipulating the amount of free drug available. The goal either way is to achieve a pH of 7.5–7.55. For this reason, another bolus of sodium bicarbonate is not unreasonable in this instance.

Management of refractory toxicity is difficult, but consider hypertonic saline if hypotension persists despite sodium bicarbonate and aggressive fluid resuscitation and vasopressors. Magnesium is not a first-line treatment but can be considered if arrythmia persists despite the sodium bicarbonate. Lidocaine can be used as a second-line therapy for arrythmia, and if there is severe haemodynamic instability and impending cardiac arrest, lipid emulsion has been advocated.

Lynch R. Tricyclic antidepressant overdose. *Emergency Medicine Journal* 2002;19:596.

26. B

This man has polycythaemia and Budd Chiari syndrome leading to acute liver failure. Symptomatic Budd Chiari has a high mortality if left untreated, and the mainstay of therapy focuses on:

- Prevention of propagation of clot, with anticoagulation
- Treatment of underlying precipitant; venesection and rehydration should be instituted to achieve a haematocrit of 0.5
- Restoration of patency of veins (e.g. angioplasty or stent, or thrombolysis)
- Decompression of the congested liver (e.g. TIPSS)
- Management of complications, and this may require liver transplantation in those deemed suitable

Therefore anticoagulation with low molecular weight heparin is the initial treatment unless there are contraindications such as acute bleed. Although stents and TIPSS are undertaken, they can often be procedurally difficult and may result in re-occlusion.

European Association for the study of the liver. EASL clinical practice guidelines: vascular disease of the liver. *Journal of Hepatology* 2016;64:179 202.

27. C

This patient has presented with diabetic ketoacidosis: raised blood glucose >11mmol/l (or known diabetes), and capillary ketones >3 mmol/l (or ketones ≥2+ in urine), and venous pH <7.3 or venous bicarbonate <15mmol/l.

Immediate management is 1l NaCl 0.9 infused over 1 hour, with the addition of up to four repeated 500mL boluses if systolic remains <90mmHg. A fixed-rate insulin infusion should be started 0.1units/kg/hour with the aim of a blood glucose fall of >3 mmol/l/hour until the capillary blood glucose is 14mmol/l. If there is not a fall of >3 mmol/hr, then the insulin infusion can be increased by 1 unit/hour. Sodium bicarbonate is generally not required. Following the essential investigations and critical care review, ongoing fluid therapy is 1l NaCl 0.9% over 1 hour and then followed by two bags of the same, but each of which is infused over 2 hours, and the final 1l bag NaCl 0.9% can be then infused over 4 hours to prevent osmotic shifts and extreme changes in plasma sodium. The addition of potassium should not occur prior to the second intravenous bag unless plasma potassium <3.5mmol/l. If the plasma potassium is 3.5–5.5mmol/l, add 40mmol/l NaCl 0.9% to achieve plasma potassium 4 and 5mmol/L. The peripheral potassium should not be infused at more than 20mmol/hour peripherally.

Joint British Diabetes Societies Inpatient Care Group. *The Management of Diabetic Ketoacidosis in Adults*, 2nd edition. London: Joint British Diabetes Societies Inpatient Care Group for NHS Diabetes, 2013. http:// www.diabetes.org.uk/Documents/About%20Us/What%20we%20say/Mana gement-of-DKA-241013.pdf (accessed 30 July 2021).

28. B

The scenario of major burns provides a number of challenges including trauma-related injuries, underlying co-morbidities, and problems relating to alcohol and drug intoxication, as well as specific issues relating to the burns and inhalational injury. Risk factors for inhalational injury include prolonged entrapment, loss of consciousness, intoxication, head injury, hypoxia, and fatalities at the scene.

Prolonged entrapment leads to increased risk of CO and cyanide poisoning. In those with a persistent metabolic acidosis despite initial resuscitation techniques, a high index of suspicion should remain for the latter. Cyanide toxicity results leads to inactivation of cytochrome oxidase, thus uncoupling mitochondrial oxidative phosphorylation and inhibiting cellular respiration, even in the presence of adequate oxygen stores. Cellular metabolism shifts from aerobic to anaerobic, with the consequent production of lactic acid. There are normal arterial oxygen tensions and abnormally high venous oxygen tensions with a high lactate.

Where cyanide toxicity is suspected, hydroxocobalamin can be given as the antidote. Hydroxocobalamin combines with cyanide to form cyanocobalamin (vitamin B-12), which is renally cleared. Alternatively, cyanocobalamin may dissociate from cyanide at a slow enough rate to allow for cyanide detoxification by the mitochondrial enzyme rhodanese.

Intubation and lung protective ventilation with high inspired oxygen is recommended. Early bronchoscopy and BAL can help with diagnosis and reducing systemic effects of inhaled toxins. Typical inhalational injury protocols suggest nebulized heparin, N-acetylcysteine, and salbutamol with regular bronchoscopic washout.

Bishop S, Maguire S. Anaesthesia and intensive care for major burns. *CEACCP* 2012;3:118.

Gill P, Martin R. Smoke inhalation injury. *CEACCP* 2015;15:143.

29. B

The transplanted heart has no autonomic innervation, and because of the loss of vagal tone, the heart rate rests between 90–100bpm. This leads to large fluctuations in blood pressure during induction of anaesthesia, hypovolaemia, Valsalva, and carotid sinus stimulation. The heart relies on directly acting agents such as catecholamines. Cardiac denervation in the transplanted graft leads to loss of physiological response to certain drugs such as atropine, glycopyrrolate, and digoxin. Conversely denervation supersensitivity is seen with other drugs. Adequate preload is necessary therefore to help counteract the loss of rapid homeostatic heart rate responses seen normally with alterations in vascular resistance, during for example induction of anaesthesia.

Other considerations in this case include risk of atypical infections and the presence of donor coronary artery disease. The recipient patient will not complain of angina because of denervation.

Direct Sympathomimetics
- Adrenaline and Noradrenaline have an augmented inotropic response.
- Dobutamine and Isoprenaline maintain a normal response

Indirect Sympathomimetics
- Ephedrine has a decreased response as there is no catecholamine store in the myocardial neurones.

Parasympathomimetics
- Atropine, Glycopyrrolate and Digoxin have no effect on the transplanted heart

Morgan-Hughes N, Hood G. Anaesthesia for a patient with a cardiac transplant. *CEACCP* 2002;2:74.

30. E

The incidence of PCP (*Pneumocystis jirovecii*, previously named *Pneumocystis carinii*) pneumonia has dramatically declined due to effective antiretroviral therapy (ART) and, to a lesser extent, the use of prophylaxis. Despite this decrease, it remains one of the leading causes of opportunistic infections among HIV-infected persons with low CD4 cell counts, such as those who are unaware of their HIV diagnoses or who are not receiving medical care. Infection results in acute interstitial pneumonitis. Symptoms of shortness of breath, dry cough, and fever may be preceded by malaise and weight loss with profound hypoxia. The chest x-ray may appear normal or show classical peri-hilar interstitial ground glass shadowing.

Despite the reduced incidence, mortality does remain high, and intubation remains a poor prognostic indicator. Targeted BAL may be superior to blind BAL in the context of PCP pneumonia. Beta D glucan levels if high, may indicate infection with PCP; however, high levels are also indicative of aspergillus and histoplasmosis. Corticosteroids given in conjunction with anti-Pneumocystis therapy can decrease the incidence of mortality and respiratory failure associated with PCP and should be given when initial co-trimoxazole treatment is started. The timing of starting antiretroviral therapy is difficult and generally is not commenced until the patient's condition has stabilized, as there is risk of immune reconstitution inflammatory syndrome. In the absence of improvement after 4–8 days, treatment failure may be considered, and a switch to the second-line clindamycin-primaquine in not unreasonable.

Wittenburg MD, Kaur N, Miller RF, Walker DA. The challenges of HIV disease in the intensive care unit. *JICS* 2010;1:26.

Huang L, Quartin A, Jones D, Havlir DV. Intensive care of patients with HIV infection. *NEJM* 2006;355:173.

Benfield T, Atzori C, Miller RF, Helweg-Larsen J. Second-line salvage treatment of AIDS-associated Pneumocystis jirovecii pneumonia: a case series and systematic review. *Journal of Acquired Immune Deficiency Syndrome* 2008;48:63.

1. **A 72-year-old man presents to the Emergency Department (ED) with drowsiness, hypotension, and tachycardia. Initial assessment reveals a blood glucose of 46mmol/l. Urine dip demonstrates nitrites ++, leucocytes +++, and ketones +. The initial blood tests sent come back and Na 155mmol/l, K 5.2mmol/l, urea 27mmol/l, and creatinine 175µmol/l, and bicarbonate 18mmol/l. Select the most appropriate statement below:**
   A. Calculated osmolality is 337mosmol/kg
   B. Change to NaCl 0.45% for fluid resuscitation
   C. Co-amoxiclav should be started for the likely infective precipitant
   D. Commence rehydration with Ringer's lactate solution
   E. Target a fall in glucose level of 5mmol/l per hour

2. **Select the one risk factor below for contrast induced nephropathy:**
   A. Age >65 years
   B. Diabetes with normal renal function
   C. Female
   D. Heart failure
   E. Liver disease

3. **A 35-year-old woman with a history of alcohol excess presents for the first time to hospital and is shortly referred to outreach for low BP and low urine output. She is complaining of diffuse abdominal pain and is found to be confused and pyrexial. She has no other past medical history of note but is allergic to penicillin.**

   Select the most appropriate statement:
   A. A diagnosis of spontaneous bacterial peritonitis (SBP) is made when ascitic fluid neutrophil count is $\geq150/mm^3$
   B. If a coagulase-negative staphylococcus is isolated, commence antibiotics as prompt empirical treatment is necessary
   C. Risk factors for developing SBP include prior episode of SBP, gastro intestinal bleed, and Child-Pugh score
   D. Start the patient on piperacillin with tazobactam, as it covers enterococci, streptococci, and resistant Gram-negative including Pseudomonas
   E. Tigecycline provides adequate cover against enterococci, streptococci, and resistant Gram-negatives including Pseudomonas

MCQs and SBAs in Intensive Care Medicine. Lorna Eyre and Andrew Bodenham, Oxford University Press. © Oxford University Press 2021.
DOI: 10.1093/oso/9780198753056.003.0009

4. **Select the statement that does not accurately reflect the properties of oxygen and gases:**

    A. Dry air at sea level normally contains 20.9% oxygen, equivalent to a partial pressure of 21.2kPa. The partial pressure of oxygen in the alveolar spaces is distinctly lower at 14.7kPa

    B. Inert gases, such as nitrogen and argon, are carried only in the dissolved form in the blood

    C. The partial pressure of oxygen in arterial blood is similar to alveolar partial pressure and the alveolar-arterial gradient of oxygen (normally <1kPa) commonly reflects regional ventilation and perfusion mismatch

    D. The partial pressure of oxygen, at which 50% of haemoglobin is saturated, the P50, is 5.3kPa

    E. The presence of reactive oxygen species increases at higher FiO_2, and damage to respiratory epithelium occurs at FiO_2 >0.6 for ≥24 hours

5. **Regarding intra-abdominal hypertension and abdominal compartment syndrome (ACS), which of the following statements is correct:**

    A. A sustained intra-abdominal pressure of ≥12mmHg defines intra-abdominal hypertension

    B. A sustained intra-abdominal pressure of >25mmHg defines intra-abdominal compartment syndrome

    C. A tensely distended abdomen is a good predictor of the presence of intra-abdominal compartment syndrome

    D. There are five grades of intra-abdominal hypertension

    E. There is strong correlation between bladder pressure and directly measured intra-abdominal pressure

6. **An obese 56-year-old obese man needs intubating on the intensive care unit (ICU) for progressive type 1 respiratory failure. The team members undertake an intubation checklist and continue with induction of anaesthesia using a modified rapid sequence technique. However the intubation proves tricky, and after looking once with direct laryngoscopy using a curved Macintosh size 3 blade you are unable to successfully intubate. Select the next most appropriate management that you would undertake if you were the ICU trainee intubating the patient:**

    A. Exchange the blade 3 for a size 4 blade and have a maximum of no more than three further attempts at intubation, using a bougie and optimizing patient position

    B. Get the front of neck airway set and insert a supraglottic airway in the meantime

    C. Remove cricoid and ensure oxygenation and this may require either two person ventilation or continuous nasal oxygenation

    D. Get a consultant and allow three further attempts with direct or video laryngoscopy

    E. Wake the patient up

7. **A 60-year-old man is admitted to the ICU with pancreatitis and stage 2 AKI.**

   Which of the following best represents stage 2 AKI?

   A. Serum creatinine 1.5 times baseline value
   B. Serum creatinine 3 times baseline value
   C. Serum creatinine 360μmol/l
   D. Urine output <0.5ml/kg/h for 8 hours
   E. Urine output <0.5ml/kg/h for 18 hours

8. **A 56-year-old man with a history of gallstones (confirmed on admission ultrasound), presented 36 hours ago with severe abdominal pain, raised amylase (three times the upper normal limit). He is pyrexial, slightly confused, and with progressive respiratory failure (PaO$_2$ 8.5kPa and FiO$_2$ 0.4). His bloods are slightly deranged with high bilirubin of 89μmol/l, and an elevated creatinine of 150μmol/l. Full blood count parameters are normal. His blood pressure also remains within normal parameters. Select the most appropriate statement regarding this case:**

   A. Fluids should be given IV to maintain the pancreatic microcirculation and compound sodium lactate is best
   B. Given the deterioration, he should be transferred to the ICU and commenced on antibiotics
   C. He should undergo contrast computer tomography of the abdomen to assess for the presence of pancreatic necrosis
   D. Naso-jejunal feeding should be commenced as enteral feeding is paramount
   E. The sequential organ failure assessment score is 7

9. **A 36-year-old man with no past medical history presents with a 5-day history of fever, malaise, and haemoptysis. He is admitted to the respiratory ward and rapidly deteriorates over the next 24 hours to the point of requiring invasive ventilation.**

   Investigations:

Haemoglobin	105g/l	(115–165)
White cell count	6.7 × 10^9/l	(4.0–11.0)
Platelet count	255 × 10^9/l	(150–400)
Prothrombin time	11s	(11.5–15.5)
Activated partial thromboplastin time	32s	(30–40)
Serum creatinine	410μmol/l	(60–110)
Serum albumin	27g/l	(37–49)
Serum CRP	45mg/l	(<10)

   Which of the following is the most appropriate next investigation?

   A. Anti-glomerular basement membrane antibodies
   B. Aspergillus antibodies
   C. Flexible bronchoscopy
   D. High-resolution CT chest
   E. Quantiferon gold testing

10. **A 65-year-old man arrives in ED having had a cardiac arrest at home. Bystander CPR was initiated by his wife, and the ambulance crew continued CPR and administered adrenaline for pulseless electrical activity. After 52 minutes, there was return of spontaneous circulation (ROSC). He is now in the ED intubated (although currently not receiving sedative drugs). His heart rate and blood pressure remain within normal limits. On an initial blood gas, his lactate is very high, with a metabolic acidosis, and his glucose is also very high at 20mmol/l. He is having periodic bursts of myoclonic jerking. The patient's medical background includes: tablet controlled type II diabetes, heavy smoking, and COPD. Choose the most applicable statement:**

A. Post ROSC, aim for oxygen saturations of 98%–100%

B. Post ROSC, aim for blood glucose 4–6mmol/l to improve neurological outcome

C. Post ROSC, avoid core body temperatures of >37°C and aim for a temperature of 33°C to improve neurological outcome

D. Post ROSC, initial lactate concentrations and rate of lactate clearance correlate with survival

E. Post ROSC, isolated myoclonic jerks are an ominous sign

11. **A 64 year-old man weighing 70kg is commenced on chemotherapy for acute myeloid leukaemia. At 48 hours after initiation of treatment you are called to see him and you are asked if you will take him to the ICU for renal replacement therapy. He is currently on no other medication.**

On examination he appears well with clear lung fields on auscultation. Blood pressure is 125/65mmHg. He is receiving intravenous 0.9% NaCl at 150ml/h and is passing between 60 and 80ml/h of urine.

Investigations:

Serum bicarbonate	14mmol/l	(20–28)
Serum creatinine	560µmol/l	(60–110)
Serum potassium	5.9mmol/l	(3.5–4.9)
Serum corrected calcium	1.90mmol/l	(2.20–2.60)
Serum phosphate	3.8mmol/l	(0.8–1.4)

What is the next most appropriate step in management?

A. Allopurinol

B. Haemodialysis

C. Metolazone

D. Rasburicase

E. Sodium bicarbonate 8.4%

12. **A patient who is being ventilated for community-acquired pneumonia has been in the ICU for 48 hours. Select the best correct statement regarding nutrition in this patient:**
    A. Age is not a risk factor for requiring postpyloric feeding
    B. Albumin levels are a good indication of nutritional status
    C. Effectiveness of prokinetics such as erythromycin decreases with time and should be discontinued after a limited number of days
    D. Enteral nutrition is recommended within 48 hours to achieve 100% of resting energy expenditure early
    E. Enteral feeding should be delayed when gastric residual volume is >500ml/3h

13. **Regarding cardio-respiratory physiology throughout the respiratory cycle, select the best most applicable answer:**
    A. During positive pressure ventilation, right ventricle preload increases during the inspiratory phase
    B. During positive pressure ventilation, left ventricular afterload decreases during the inspiratory phase
    C. The blood pressure decreases during spontaneous expiration
    D. The cardiac cycle can be divided into five distinct phases according to ventricular pressure-volume relationships
    E. There is an exaggerated decrease in systolic pressure during expiration in the presence of cardiac tamponade

14. **A 24-year-old man is brought into ED of a major trauma centre. He has a penetrating stab wound to the left anterior chest wall. Findings on examination:**
    A—patent
    B—reduced air entry left side, central trachea, spontaneous ventilatory effort, and saturation 88% on 15l nonrebreather reservoir bag
    C—HR 148bpm, BP 52/28mmHg, raised JVP, and cool peripherally
    D—glucose 7, GCS E1, M3, V, and pupils reactive and equal
    E—stab would site mid clavicular line fifth intercostal space.

    He is promptly intubated, and a left-sided intercostal surgical chest drain is inserted, with no apparent haemothorax but some bubbling when connected to underwater seal. The patient's BP remains extremely low, and there is a marked fall in BP with inspiration. As part of the trauma team, you notice there is now a near-loss of cardiac output. What should be the next management consideration?
    A. Chest compressions as per advanced life support guideline
    B. Combination of vasopressors, adrenaline, tranexamic acid, and supportive measures as per medical guidelines
    C. Decompress the right side of the chest with needle thoracocentesis
    D. Initiate major haemorrhage protocol and start by giving packed red cells initially
    E. Resuscitative emergency thoracotomy

15. **A 75-year-old patient, who is a known drinker of excess alcohol, has been intubated on the ICU for a community-acquired pneumonia. He has subsequently undergone tracheostomy earlier in the day and now on the night shift has become increasingly agitated and is pulling on the tracheotomy and other lines. What should you do to manage this?**

    A. Minimize light and noise
    B. Prevent agitation with regular doses of haloperidol
    C. Treat agitation with dexmedetomidine
    D. Treat with quetiapine
    E. Treat with lorazepam

16. **A 66-year-old woman with a history of depression (normally takes sertraline) and diet-controlled diabetes has just undergone a mastectomy and sentinel lymph node biopsy. Perioperatively she was given fentanyl, propofol, and rocuronium. Anaesthesia was maintained using air and sevoflurane. Methylene blue was used intraoperatively, and neuromuscular blockade was reversed using neostigmine and glycopyrrolate. In recovery, she is referred to ICU because of persistent temperature >40°C, agitation, tremor, diaphoresis, BP 85/51, and a heart rate of 124 sinus tachycardia. On examination she appears to have myoclonus. What is the most likely diagnosis?**

    A. Anticholinergic syndrome
    B. Neuroleptic malignant syndrome
    C. Malignant hyperpyrexia
    D. Perio-operative delirium
    E. Serotonin syndrome

17. **Select the best answer regarding Vitamin C and thiamine:**

    A. A combination of vitamin C, thiamine, and hydrocortisone was shown to improve hospital mortality in septic patients in a multicentre, randomized control trial
    B. Thiamine requires sodium-dependent transporters for enteral absorption
    C. Vitamin C is synthesized, but thiamine requires external supplementation
    D. Vitamin C is a direct free radical scavenger and is a cofactor required for vasopressin and catecholamine synthesis
    E. Vitamin C and thiamine are both lipid soluble

18. **A 54-year-old man, with a history of smoking and high alcohol intake, was initially intubated for severe bronchospasm. His oxygen requirements continued to increase, and chest radiographs demonstrated progressive bilateral pulmonary infiltrates, in keeping with a diagnosis of ARDS. He required some vasopressor, FiO$_2$ 0.8, and was being treated with piperacillin with tazobactam. Renal replacement was necessary for acute kidney injury, and there were high gastric aspirates, attributed to the need for neuromuscular blockade. Both central line and blood cultures subsequently grew a ruminococcus. What should be the next management?**

A. Add in fluconazole

B. Arrange CT of the abdomen

C. Arrange laparotomy

D. Change all invasive lines

E. Change of antimicrobials to improve Gram-negative cover

19. **A fit and healthy 45-year-old man, originally from Zimbabwe, presents with a 2-week history of headache. A head CT demonstrates a ring enhancing cerebral abscess in the frontal lobe and evidence of communicating hydrocephalus. He commences anti-TB drugs only, for presumed TB meningitis in light of a CSF sample that has high protein and high white cell count and is negative for other meningitis pathogens. In addition, a HIV test comes back positive.**

His GCS subsequently drops to 6 and critical care is called. On examination, he has a conjugant gaze to the right and dense left-sided weakness. A repeat CT is ordered. What is the next appropriate management?

A. Transfer to the ICU for intubation and ventilation in light of GCS

B. Start corticosteroids

C. Start antiplatelet therapy

D. Repeat lumbar puncture

E. Refer to neurosurgery

20. **A 30-year-old woman with progressive MS and depression is found by her mother at home collapsed. On arrival, the ambulance personnel find her to be unresponsive (Glasgow coma scale GCS 3), hypotensive (75/34), bradycardic (38 beats per minute), hypothermic (Temp 34°C), and with a reduced respiratory rate (6 breaths per minute). Her blood sugar is normal. Her usual medication include drugs for depression and MS. On examination she is comatose, with bilateral fixed pupils. Brainstem reflexes are absent, and there is a flaccid paralysis with no tendon reflexes. Which of her medications is likely to be responsible?**

A. Amitriptyline

B. Baclofen

C. Diazepam

D. Gabapentin

E. Quetiapine

21. **A 77-year-old hypertensive woman got caught in an acrimonious family feud and was pushed against a radiator by her grandson. She has sustained a number of posterior rib fractures to the left side, involving ribs 3–6. Fractures can also be seen in two places regarding the left ribs 5 and 6. She is transferred to the unit for a rapidly increasing oxygen demand and now has become increasingly agitated and uncooperative. Which of the below statements is most applicable?**

   A. Paracetamol, naproxen, and oxycodone MR are good first-line analgesics in this instance
   B. Serratus anterior plane block is a suitable novel regional technique
   C. Surgical fixation is indicated
   D. This patient likely requires invasive ventilation for underlying pulmonary contusion
   E. There is no validated scoring tool to predict morbidity and mortality

22. **A 70-year-old man presents to the ED with a sudden drop in GCS (E1 V1 M2). He has a history of atrial fibrillation, for which he takes warfarin. He is otherwise fit and well, with a good functional status.**

   The patient was intubated in the pre-hospital setting. On initial assessment, he is mechanically ventilated and sedated. His observations and results are as follows:

BP	198/104 pH 7.38
HR	86 pO_2 24.4kPa
SpO2	97% (FiO_2 0.6) pCO2 5.4kPa
Glucose	13.4mmol/l
Haemoglobin	148g
White cell count	11.5×10^9
Platelets	370×10^9
PT	53s
APTT	36s
Fibrinogen level	2.4mg/dl

   CT head: large right-sided intraparenchymal haematoma

   Which one of the following is the most important immediate next step in treatment?

   A. IV Fresh frozen plasma
   B. IV Insulin infusion
   C. IV Vitamin K
   D. Prothrombin complex concentrate
   E. Surgical evacuation

23. **A 72-year-old woman has been admitted to the ICU due to severe acute pancreatitis. After 7 days she remains mechanically ventilated.**

   Over the last 24 hours, the patient has become increasingly pyrexial. She has required more regular suctioning of respiratory secretions, which are increasingly purulent. CXR shows new pulmonary infiltrates. A broncho-alveolar lavage is performed and is sent for microscopy and culture.

   Which of the following pathogens is most likely to be isolated?

   A. *Escherichia coli*
   B. *Haemophillus influenzae*
   C. *Klebsiella pneumoniae*
   D. *Pseudomonas aeruginosa*
   E. *Streptococcus pneumoniae*

24. **A 76-year-old woman presents to the ED with a 3-week history of cough and increasing shortness of breath. She has a long smoking history and has previously been diagnosed with COPD. She is complaining of a diffuse headache, nausea, and vomiting.**

   On examination she has equal air entry and is saturating at 92% on room air. BP is 120/65mmHg; heart rate is 88 beats per min; and there is no pitting oedema. Capillary refill time is under 2 seconds. Temperature is 37.4°C.

   Blood taken at admission reveals a low serum sodium level with normal renal function. She is admitted to the HDU for monitoring and correction of her electrolyte disturbance.

   Investigations:

Serum potassium	4.0mmol/l	(3.5–4.9)
Serum sodium	118mmol/l	(137–144)
Serum osmolality	240mosmol/kg	(278–300)
Urinary osmolality	550mosmol/kg	(100–1000)
Urinary sodium	46mmol/l	

   What is the most appropriate next step in her management?

   A. 1.5l fluid restriction
   B. 100mg hydrocortisone
   C. 100ml/h 0.9% NaCl
   D. 100ml/h 1.8% NaCl
   E. 150ml 3% NaCl

25. **A 43-year-old man presents to the ED acutely short of breath. He describes a 4-day history of productive cough, fevers, and fatigue. He was prescribed oral antibiotics by his GP. Over the last 4 hours he has rapidly deteriorated and he is now tachypnoeic, cyanotic, and drowsy. He is intubated and ventilated and transferred to the ICU. Chest x-ray shows bilateral diffuse shadowing. No pneumothorax is apparent. An urgent echocardiogram shows only mildly impaired left ventricular (LV) function.**

    His observations after 4 hours are:

PaO_2	8.1kPa (FiO_2 0.8)
RR	22
BP	134/77
HR	110

    Arterial blood gas shows a respiratory acidosis. The patient's ventilatory settings are reviewed and deemed to be appropriate.

    Which of the following is the next most appropriate management option?

    A. Atracurium infusion
    B. Increase FiO_2
    C. Intravenous furosemide
    D. Prone positioning
    E. Recruitment manoeuvre

26. **A 49-year-old woman with a history of myasthenia gravis is under the care of the respiratory team. She was admitted 12 hours earlier with pneumonia. She is on appropriate antibiotics and was initially stable on the ward.**

    Over the course of her admission she has become increasingly tachypnoeic and tachycardic. She has saturations of 94% on 8l oxygen through a face mask. Her respiratory rate is now 24, and she looks distressed. You have been asked to review her regarding the need for respiratory support.

    Which of the following factors is most likely to suggest the need for intubation?

    A. Elevated acetylcholine receptor antibodies
    B. PaCO2 6.3KPa
    C. PaO2 8KPa
    D. Reduced compound action potentials on EMG
    E. Vital capacity 14ml/kg

27. A 38-year-old male presents with shortness of breath, pyrexia, and pleuritic chest pain. He has a history of intravenous drug use. These are his initial observations on attendance to the ED:

SpO2   94% (FiO$_2$ 0.6)
RR   24
HR   115
BP   95/40
Temp   38.8°C

Examination reveals tachypnoea, right-sided crepitations and a large area of erythema in the groin, with associated puncture wounds.

Further investigation results are shown below:

Hb   92g/l
WCC   2.1 × 10^9
Plts   274 × 10^9
Na   131mmol/l
K   4.6mmol/l
Cr   110mmol/l
Ur   9.7mmol/l
CXR   right-sided consolidation with suspected cavitating lesion

Which of the following treatments is least likely to be indicated?

A. Clindamycin
B. Co-amoxiclav
C. Intravenous immunoglobulins
D. Linezolid
E. Rifampicin

28. A 19-year-old man has taken a large paracetamol overdose. He is currently in the ICU and is intubated and mechanically ventilated. After 24 hours, which one of the following factors does not suggest the need for liver transplant?

A. Arterial pH 7.28
B. GCS 8
C. INR 7.1
D. Serum bilirubin 394
E. Serum creatinine 571

29. A 48-year-old woman was admitted to the neuro ICU 6 days ago following a subarachnoid haemorrhage. On admission her Glasgow coma scale GCS was 11. In the subsequent days she has undergone insertion of an external ventricular drain, and radiological coiling of the causative aneurysm. Her renal function was normal on admission.

Over the last 48 hours the patient has become increasingly hypotensive. Initially she responded well to fluid resuscitation but is now requiring vasopressor support. Urine output has increased.

Some blood results from this morning are:

Sodium	121
Potassium	4.4
Creatinine	110
Urea	13.2

Which of the following is least likely to be of benefit?

A. Fludrocortisone

B. Fluid restriction

C. Hypertonic saline

D. Oral sodium supplementation

E. Resuscitation with 0.9% saline

30. **A 38-year-old man is brought to the ED following a large verapamil overdose. He is severely hypotensive, bradycardic, and obtunded. His hypotension is refractory to large volumes of fluid and escalating vasopressor doses. Which of the following is least likely to play a role in his ongoing management?**

A. Calcium

B. Glucagon

C. Insulin

D. Intralipid

E. Renal replacement therapy

1. E

Hyperosmolar hyperglycaemic state (HHS) typically occurs, although not exclusively, in the more elderly patients, and onset is over days with more extreme metabolic disturbance and dehydration compared to diabetic ketoacidosis (DKA). HHS is characterized by hypovolaemia and marked hyperglycaemia (often blood glucose >30mmol/l) without significant hyperketonaemia or acidosis. Osmolality is often >320mosmol/kg. The mortality can be high and so prompt goals of treatment include normalizing the osmolality, replacing fluid and electrolytes, and normalizing blood glucose.

Calculated osmolality: $2Na^+$ glucose + urea = 383mosmol/kg. However some suggest not including urea, as this molecule freely crossed the cell membrane (i.e. urea is an ineffective osmole and plays no role in the distribution of free water in the body).

Effective osmolality: $2Na^+$ glucose = 356mosmol/kg. Effective osmolality gives the tonicity, and this is important in the hyponatraemic state as tonicity indicates the risk of cerebral oedema (i.e. hypo-osmolality). In the hyperosmolar state, calculated osmolality gives the best approximation to measured osmolality, and despite urea being an ineffective osmole, it does provide an indication of severe dehydration.

Initial fluid replacement is with NaCl 0.9%; there is no superiority with Ringer's lactate. There is often a rise initially in plasma sodium, as water shifts into cells as the falling blood glucose reduces the plasma osmolality. This is not an indication to give hypotonic solutions, and a rise in sodium is only a concern if there is no concomitant decrease in plasma osmolality. Rapid changes should be avoided, and a safe fall in glucose is 4–6 mmol/l per hour. A target blood glucose of 10–15mmol/ is the ultimate goal, and fluid rehydration should aim to replace 50% of overall estimated losses within the first 12 hours.

This patient appears to have a urinary tract infection, and as such, IV co-amoxiclav is not usually a first choice for coliforms such as *E. coli*.

JBDS inpatient care group. *The management of the hyperosmolar hyperglycaemic state in adults with diabetes.* 2012 https://abcd.care/sites/abcd.care/files/resources/JBDS_IP_HHS_Adults.pdf [accessed 30 July 2021].

2. D

The 2013 National Institute for Health and Care Excellence (NICE) guidelines highlight several risk factors for CIN. These include chronic kidney disease, diabetes with chronic kidney disease, renal transplant, age >75 years, heart failure, hypovolaemia, increased volume of contrast, and intra-arterial contrast (e.g. angiography). Liver disease is a risk factor for acute kidney injury but not specifically for CIN. There is no difference with gender.

NICE. *Clinical guideline 169.* Acute kidney injury: prevention, detection and management of acute kidney injury up to the point of renal replacement therapy. 2013 http://guidance/nice.org.uk/CG169 [accessed 30 September 2019].

3. C

SBP is the infection of ascitic fluid in the absence of any intra-abdominal, surgically treatable source of infection and in the absence of medical devices such as ventriculoperitoneal shunts or continuous ambulatory peritoneal dialysis catheters. Risk factors for SBP include prior episode, gastro intestinal bleeding, ascitic protein < 1.0g/dl, and Child-Pugh score. The pathogenesis may relate to bacterial translocation or haematogenous spread. Common microorganisms include *E. coli*, Klebsiella, Proteus, Enterococcus, and Pseudomonas. Common symptoms and signs include fever, confusion, and diffuse abdominal pain. An ascitic fluid neutrophil count ≥250mm³ should be considered diagnostic. Tazobactam with piperacillin is a good first-line treatment, although this patient is penicillin allergic. Tigecycline is a viable alternative, but it does not have pseudomonal cover.

Rimola A, et al. Diagnosis, treatment and prophylaxis of spontaneous bacterial peritonitis: a consensus document. *Journal of Hepatology* 2000; 32:142–53.

4. D

The use of oxygen as a therapy is fairly ubiquitous in critical care, and it is important to remember that it can cause harm and therefore should be regarded as any other pharmacological agent.

Successful oxygen uptake depends on the atmospheric barometric pressure, the inspired oxygen concentration (FiO_2), alveolar ventilation, diffusion capacity, and matched ventilation and perfusion. Dry air at sea level normally contains 20.9% oxygen, equivalent to a partial pressure of 21.2kPa. The partial pressure of oxygen in the alveolar spaces is distinctly lower at 14.7kPa, a result of alveolar ventilation and dilution by carbon dioxide, water vapour, and oxygen consumption. Partial pressures of oxygen in arterial blood are similar, and the alveolar-arterial gradient of oxygen (normally <1kPa) commonly reflects regional ventilation and perfusion mismatch rather than diffusion across thin pulmonary capillaries. Further drops in partial pressures of oxygen take place on account of the 'true shunt' mixed venous blood that bypasses the pulmonary capillary bed. Inert gases, such as nitrogen, are carried only in the dissolved form in the blood. Oxygen binds to haemoglobin, and the position of the oxygen-haemoglobin dissociation curve is defined by the P50, the partial pressure of oxygen when 50% of the haemoglobin is saturated, which is 3.5kPa.

At a cellular level there is a balance between oxidant and antioxidant activity, and oxygen can produce reactive oxygen species (ROS) should the antioxidant pathways become overwhelmed, such as in the presence of hyperoxia. This ultimately leads to cellular oxidant stress and damage, and as the lungs are most exposed to higher partial pressures of oxygen, they are more vulnerable to damage. Respiratory epithelial damage does occur when the FiO_2 is >0.6 and for ≥24 hours.

Horncastle E, Lumb A. Hyperoxia in anaesthesia and intensive care. *BJA Education* 2019;19:176.

Taneja R, Vaughn R. Oxygen. *CEACCP* 2001;1:104.

5. A

Intra-abdominal hypertension is defined as sustained intra-abdominal pressures ≥12mmHg. There are four grades: I 12–15mmHg, II 16–20mmHg, III 21–25mmHg, and IV >25mmHg. *Intra-abdominal compartment syndrome* (ACS) is defined as sustained pressure >20mmHg and new organ dysfunction, although clinically, maybe better defined as intra-abdominal hypertension inducing new organ dysfunction. There are numerous causes, and these can be classified as to whether there is an injury or disease of the abdominal pelvic area or whether ACS is due to fluid resuscitation, burns, or other non-abdominal or pelvic pathologies. ACS leads to impaired venous return and cardiac output, reduced mechanical ventilation with higher peak airway pressures and reduced compliance, and reduced renal arterial and venous blood flow. Mesenteric gut flow is also compromised as is the ability of the liver to remove lactic acid. Intra-abdominal pressure can be measured indirectly via the bladder, and this does correlate well with direct pressure measurement. It has the advantages of being simple and noninvasive, although may be inaccurate in the presence of adhesions, pelvic fractures, and abdominal packs. The presence of a tensely distended abdomen does not correlate well with the presence of ACS.

Malbrain ML, et al. Results from the International Conference of Experts on Intra-abdominal Hypertension and Abdominal Compartment Syndrome. *Intensive Care Medicine* 2006;32:1722.

6. C

The necessary steps for intubating a patient on the ICU should include a team brief, allocation of roles and completion of intubation checklist. Once the patient is optimally positioned (ideally allowing for airway assessment and identification of cricothyroid membrane), preoxygenation should be provided either by tight fitting facemask or noninvasive ventilation or nasal oxygen. Monitoring needs to include waveform capnography. If after an unsuccessful first look laryngoscopy, there should only be another two further attempts (i.e. maximum of three attempts), and during this stage consider use of video laryngoscope, bougie, or stylet, as well as removal of cricoid. Maintain oxygenation (continuous nasal or facemask ventilation) between attempts. After the first failed attempt, call for help and get the front of neck airway (FONA) set. If after three attempts, there is still no success, declare a 'failure of intubation.'

The next stage is rescue oxygenation, with a second-generation supraglottic airway device and or two person (+/−adjuncts) facemask ventilation. When the consultant (or someone with more expertise) arrives, allow one more attempt with direct or video laryngoscopy. If this fails but there is success with rescue oxygenation, consider the options. These may include intubating via the supraglottic, FONA, or indeed waking the patient up. This latter option is less frequently a viable choice on the ICU (e.g. by nature of the worsening respiratory failure in this instance).

Should the rescue oxygenation stage fail, then declare a 'can't intubate, can't oxygenate' scenario. Obviously, this is a stressful situation for all team members, but the final plan D is FONA. Once this has been established, it is probably helpful for the team to undertake a debrief.

Higgs A, McGrath B, Goddard C et al. Guidelines for the management of tracheal intubation in critically ill adults. BJA 2018;120:323-352

7. E

Acute kidney injury is common in hospitalized patients and is associated with an increase in patient mortality. Many cases are preventable with the right care and treatment and early recognition.

The Kidney Disease Improving Global Outcomes KDIGO staging system for AKI is widely used across hospitals as part of an alert, in an attempt to identify patients at risk of renal deterioration and to direct medical attention towards these patients. The KDIGO definition of AKI is : an increase in serum creatinine by ≥26.5 μmol/l within 48 hours or; an increase in serum creatinine ≥ 1.5 times baseline which is known (or presumed) to have increased within 7 days or; urine output < 0.5 ml/kg/hr for 6 hours. There are 3 stages of AKI depending on the degree of rise of serum creatinine or the degree of fall in urine output. Stage 2 describes a serum creatinine 2–2.9 times baseline and, or a urine output less than 0.5 ml/kg/h for 12 or more hours.

KDIGO. Staging of AKI. *Kidney International Supplements* 2012;2:8–12.

8. A

Approximately 20%–30% of patients presenting with pancreatitis will develop a severe form. This inflammatory condition of the pancreas is most commonly associated with gallstones or excess alcohol use. The severe form has a mortality of around 15%. Diagnosis requires the presence of at least two out of the following three: abdominal pain consistent with the disease, biochemical evidence (amylase rise of at least three times the upper limit of normal), and characteristic findings from abdominal imaging. The revised Atlanta Classification defines *severe pancreatitis* as the presence of single or multiple organ failure lasting >48 hours. To determine the cause, all patients require an ultrasound on admission, and those patients with severe acute pancreatitis should have contrast enhanced CT at 72–96 hours after onset of symptoms. A CT scan earlier will not identify necrosis, but may well help to define other causes of abdominal pain should the cause be in doubt. Antibiotics should only be started when there is evidence of infected severe acute pancreatitis. Infected necrosis may be identified by an increase in procalcitonin or fine needle aspiration. Unless there is evidence of infected necrosis or other infective sources (e.g. hospital-acquired pneumonia) prophylactic antibiotics should not be commenced.

Early fluid resuscitation is indicated to optimize tissue perfusion targets, without waiting for hemodynamic worsening. Fluid administration should be guided by frequent reassessment of the hemodynamic status since fluid overload is known to have detrimental effects. Isotonic crystalloids are the preferred fluid. The decrease in mortality observed over the last decade might be due to the prevention of pancreatic necrosis by maintenance of microcirculation due to more extensive fluid resuscitation. The SOFA score looks at the PaO_2:FiO_2 ratio, presence of mechanical ventilation, GCS, bilirubin, platelets, creatinine, and blood pressure. Points are scored according to values and mortality can be predicted. Enteral feeding should be commenced, and naso-gastric should be started in the first instance; however, post pyloric enteral feeding may be necessary and indeed may need supplementation with parenteral calories.

Leppaneimi A, et al. WSES guidelines for the management of severe acute pancreatitis. *World Journal of Emergency Surgery* 2019;14:27.

9. A

This patient has rapidly progressive pulmonary and renal disease, and anti-glomerular basement membrane (anti-GBM) disease (formerly known as Goodpasture syndrome) should be considered. In this condition auto-antibodies are formed against type IV collagen found in both the glomerular and alveolar basement membrane. This causes a small vessel vasculitis manifesting as either a rapidly progressive glomerular nephritis, diffuse alveolar haemorrhage, or as in this case, both.

The disease is most common in younger adults (aged 20–30 years) and again in older people (aged 60–70). As well as the lung and renal manifestations, patients can also complain of fever, malaise, and weight loss. Lung involvement is more common in smokers, and smoking is thought to be a trigger for the disease. Like other autoimmune conditions, there appears to be an environmental trigger in patients with genetic susceptibility.

Diagnosis is made with presence of positive immunology and wherever possible a renal biopsy. The treatment involves the rapid initiation of immunosuppression in an attempt to prevent permanent organ damage. Plasma-exchange should be started as soon as possible and is combined with immunosuppressive drugs such as steroids and cyclophosphamide.

Frankel SK, Cosgrove GP, Fischer A, Meehan RT, Brown KK. Update in the diagnosis and management of pulmonary vasculitis. *Chest* 2006;129:452–65.

10. D

Two landmark papers demonstrated the beneficial effects of therapeutic hypothermia in patients who had arrested due to shockable rhythms only. The evidence for therapeutic hypothermia in patients who obtain ROSC post asystole or PEA however has always been lacking. Following another paper 'Targeted Temperature Management at 33°C versus 36°C after Cardiac Arrest', it was found that temperature of 33°C did not confer a benefit, and so now a target temperature of 36°C is widely accepted. Hyperthermia must be avoided following cardiac arrest. Failure to control a patient's core temperature is associated with the development of fever and worse neurologic outcome.

Clearly the deleterious effects of hypoxia need to be avoided in patients who have had recent disruption to their cerebral circulation. Hyperoxaemia seems also to result in poorer outcomes, and, therefore, aims post resuscitation should incorporate normoxaemia. Saturations between 94%–98% with a decrease in FiO_2 as soon as possible should be the goal.

Hyperglycaemia is associated with worse outcome. However the hypoglycaemia associated with 'tight' glucose control is equally deleterious, and again one should aim for normoglycaemia.

Seizure activity and myoclonic jerks are common after cardiac arrest and often are a marker of more severe brain injury. No specific significance has been attributed to isolated myoclonic jerks in patients following cardiac arrest. Conversely, *status myoclonus*, defined as repetitive myoclonic jerks lasting more than 30 minutes, is an ominous sign. Seizure activity needs to be treated promptly, but there is no evidence for prophylactic management.

Initial lactate concentrations and the rate of lactate clearance do correlate with survival.

Bernard SA, et al. Treatment of comatose survivors of out-of- hospital cardiac arrest with induced hypothermia. *New England Journal of Medicine* 2002;346:557–63.

The Hypothermia after Cardiac Arrest Study Group. Mild therapeutic hypothermia to improve the neurologic outcome after cardiac arrest. *New England Journal of Medicine* 2002;346:549–56.

Nielsen N, et al. Targeted temperature management at 33°C versus 36°C after cardiac arrest. *New England Journal of Medicine* 2013;369:2197–206.

Kilgannon JH, et al. Association between arterial hyperoxia following resuscitation from cardiac arrest and in-hospital mortality. *Journal of the American Medical Association* 2010;303:2165–71.

Waldmann C, Soni N, Rhodes A (eds). *Oxford desk reference: critical care*, 1st edition. Oxford: Oxford University Press, 2008.

Donnino MW, et al. Effective lactate clearance is associated with improved outcome in post-cardiac arrest patients. *Resuscitation* 2007;75:229.

11. D

This patient has developed tumour lysis syndrome following the initiation of chemotherapy. The rapid lysis of tumour cells results in the release of intracellular components. This is represented biochemically as hyperuricaemia, hyperkalaemia, hyperphosphataemia, hypocalcaemia, and an acute kidney injury. These abnormalities can rapidly lead to life-threatening manifestations such as tetany, seizures, and cardiac arrhythmias.

Patients identified as being at high risk should be closely monitored and pretreated with intravenous fluids to ensure a urine output of over 100ml/h. This may require the addition of loop diuretics to achieve. Thiazide diuretics (e.g. metolazone) can increase urate levels and should be avoided.

The xanthine oxidase inhibitor allopurinol decreases the production of uric acid and is used to try and prevent renal injury. Rasburicase is a recombinant urate oxidase enzyme and can be used as prevention in high-risk cases or as a treatment measure.

Urinary alkalization is no longer recommended, and haemodialysis is only required in those whose urine output cannot safely be maintained or whose electrolyte disturbance can otherwise not be managed.

Kalemkerian GP, Darwish B, Varterasian ML. Tumor lysis syndrome in small cell carcinoma and other solid tumors. American Journal of Medicine 1997;103(5):363–367.

Howard SC, Trifilio S, Gregory TK, Baxter N, McBride A. Tumor lysis syndrome in the era of novel and targeted agents in patients with hematologic malignancies: a systematic review. *Annals of Hematololgy* 2016;95:563.

12. C

The majority of patients coming through ICU will require some intervention to ensure provision of adequate numbers of calories and nutritional supplementation. Therefore, medical nutrition therapy should be considered for all patients staying in the ICU for more than 48 hours. Gastric access is the standard approach to initiate enteral feeding (where oral intake is not possible), and in patients whereby aspiration is a significant risk, then post pyloric feeding (jejunal) can be performed. The American and European guidelines consider patients at increased risk for aspiration may be identified by a number of factors, including inability to protect the airway, mechanical ventilation, age >70 years, reduced level of consciousness, poor oral care, inadequate nurse-to-patient ratio, supine positioning, neurologic deficits, gastroesophageal reflux, transport out of the ICU, and use of bolus intermittent enteral nutrition. Early enteral nutrition should be initiated within 48 hours, and where there are high gastric residual volumes (e.g. 500ml/6h), enteral feeding may be delayed. Prokinetics should be instituted in the absence of an acute abdominal pathology, and erythromycin +/− metoclopramide can be used; however, the effectiveness of erythromycin or other prokinetics is reduced to one third after 72 hours. An assessment of nutritional status prior to feeding should be done, but albumin is not a good marker of this as it will be low in response to inflammation. Full targeted medical nutrition therapy is considered to achieve more than 70% of the resting energy expenditure, but not more than 100%, and the energy and protein goal should be achieved progressively and not before the first 48 hours to avoid over-nutrition.

Singer P, et al. ESPEN guideline on clinical nutrition in the intensive care unit. *Clinical Nutrition* 2019;38:48–79.

13. B

Spontaneous and positive pressure ventilation produce characteristic changes in the cardiac cycle and hence haemodynamic parameters.

During spontaneous inspiration, intrathoracic pressure decreases, and there is increased right ventricular (RV) venous return and increased RV output. The interventricular septum is pushed across and reduces LV filling. There is pooling of blood in the pulmonary venous vessels, and, therefore, during spontaneous inspiration, there is a decrease in LV output and hence blood pressure. The converse is seen with spontaneous expiration. The normal physiological changes are exaggerated in the instance of cardiac tamponade. So during spontaneous inspiration, the interventricular septum is further pushed towards the left, leading to greater impairment of LV filling and hence a greater fall in arterial pressure with taking a breath in (pulsus paradoxus).

During positive pressure ventilation (PPV), there is an inspiratory reduction in RV preload and hence RV output. However during the inspiratory phase of PPV, there is an increase in LV preload (as blood is squeezed out of the pulmonary vessels with the increased intrathoracic pressure). There is also a reduction in LV afterload during the inspiratory phase of PPV. Therefore during the end of inspiration when PPV is applied, there is an increase in mean arterial pressure. At the end of the expiratory phase of PPV, there is a decrease in LV stroke volume, and mean arterial pressure. The cardiac cycle is divided into isovolumetric contraction, ventricular ejection, isometric relaxation, and diastolic ventricular filling when considering ventricular volume-pressure relationships.

Madhivathanan PR, Corredor C, Smith A. Perioperative implications of pericardial effusions and cardiac tamponade. *BJA Education* 2020;7:226–34.

14. E

Traumatic cardiac arrest is rare and carries a high mortality. While many of the underlying principles of advanced life support apply, TCA is increasingly recognized as a distinct entity. One of the pivotal aspects of managing TCA is recognizing common trauma pathology such as tension pneumothorax, hypoxaemia, hypovolaemia, and cardiac tamponade. Focus should be aimed at interventions which will rapidly manage these conditions.

The effectiveness of chest compressions may be limited, and priority needs to be directed at the cause of the TCA. Chest compressions remain a standard of care, but it is important to consider the mechanism of injury, which will help reveal the underlying pathology (e.g. cardiac tamponade). These pathologies may occur in isolation or may co-exist, and, therefore, a well-briefed trauma team will work simultaneously to manage all of the causes of the TCA (e.g. control of catastrophic external haemorrhage whilst undertaking bilateral chest decompression where necessary).

Of course supportive care in the form of advanced life support will be essential. Consideration of the major haemorrhage protocol, as well as tranexamic acid and ensuring the patient does not become too cold should be standard. But in the case of penetrating or blunt cardiac trauma whereby cardiac tamponade or aortic damage is suspected, resuscitative thoracotomy could be an early option for patient survival. Necessary components to successful resuscitative thoracotomy however, include; an elapsed time of <10 minutes since the arrest, the relevant expertise, equipment, and environment (often performed in ED). Resuscitative emergency thoracotomy is a time-critical event, and survival is improved the earlier the intervention is performed for patients in traumatic cardiac arrest. Resuscitative thoracotomy is ideally performed before cardiac arrest or in the few minutes after it has occurred. The survival rates for blunt trauma are much lower than for penetrating trauma, and blunt traumatic injury may require a higher level of surgical skill to repair. Resuscitative thoracotomy is a fairly dramatic intervention and may not result in a successful outcome, so consider a team debrief in the aftermath.

Paulich S, Lockey D. Resuscitative thoracotomy. *BJA Education* 2020;7:242–8.

15. C

Delirium is common on the ICU, and incidence varies amongst studies. It is characterized by acute onset, fluctuant nature, and inattention with disordered thinking. It occurs as a result of predisposing factors that increase a patient's vulnerability (increased age, cognitive impairment, pre-existing hypertension, nicotine use, and alcohol use) and precipitating factors (acute severe illness, use of benzodiazepines, lack of daylight, and increased noise). The exact pathophysiology of delirium remains unclear. Reduced cerebral perfusion pressure, ischaemia caused by systemic hypotension, hypoxemia, and microcirculatory alterations, as well as reduced neuronal activity involving acetylcholine. Delirium is often described as hyperactive, hypoactive, or mixed, and symptoms fluctuate, often getting worse at night. Several tools have been developed to improve the detection of delirium, of which the Confusion Assessment Method for the ICU (CAM-ICU) is a commonly used example.

Nonpharmacological management strategies seem to work optimally as part of a bundle (e.g. awakening and breathing co-ordination, delirium monitoring and management, and early exercise, mobility and family engagement). Minimizing noise and light is important but is less likely to work as a standalone strategy. Preventative treatments include dexmedetomidine but not haloperidol. The melatonin receptor agonist ramelteon may have an effect on the prevention of delirium also. Benzodiazepines seem to be associated with the development of delirium in the critically ill and are generally avoided. Haloperidol does not seem to influence the duration of delirium but may be used in association with psychosis. Dexmedetomidine, an α_2-agonist, may help with agitation and anxiety. There is limited evidence that atypical antipsychotics have fewer adverse effects than haloperidol.

Van der Boogaard M, Slooter AJC. Delirium in critically ill patients: current knowledge and future perspectives. *BJA Education* 2019;12:398–404.

16. E

Serotonin syndrome (SS) is a potentially life-threatening interaction resulting from excess serotonin activity within the central nervous system. It classically presents as a triad of: change in mental state, neuromuscular abnormality, and autonomic hyperactivity. The variable and nonspecific nature of these presentation, in addition to the absence of a diagnostic test, makes identification of SS challenging. However the presence of altered mental state, neuromuscular abnormality, and autonomic hyperactivity in conjunction with current or previous exposure to a medication with serotonergic activity should prompt consideration of SS as a diagnosis.

Examples of drugs with serotonergic activity include:

- Reuptake inhibition (e.g. SSRI (sertraline), SNRI (venlafaxine), TCA, and ondansetron)
- Direct agonists (e.g. triptans)
- Metabolism alteration (e.g. MAO inhibitors (phenelzine), linezolid, and methylene blue)
- Enhanced release (e.g. opioids, ecstasy, and cocaine)

Differential diagnoses and associated presentations include:

- Anticholinergic syndrome: miosis, bradycardia, bronchoconstriction, salivation, and diarrhoea
- Neuroleptic malignant syndrome: gradual onset, lead-pipe rigidity, and no GIT symptoms
- Malignant hyperpyrexia: hyperthermia >41°C, rigidity, hyporeflexia, and no myoclonus
- Perioperative delirium: inattention, disordered thinking, and altered level of arousal
- Serotonin syndrome: agitation, confusion, clonus, myoclonic jerks, nystagmus, hyperthermia, tachycardia, and diaphoresis

Principles of management include cessation any serotonergic stimulus and provision of supportive treatment. Benzodiazepines and dexmedetomidine can be used for agitation. The latter may help with autonomic instability and myoclonus. Active cooling or sedation, ventilation, and paralysis may be necessary for hyperthermia. Dantrolene does not appear effective. Cyproheptadine, a serotonin antagonist, can also be used for more severe cases.

Bartakke A, Corredor C, van Rensburg A. Serotonin syndrome in the perioperative period. *BJA Education* 2020;20:10–17.

17. D

There are always ongoing studies looking at attenuating the devastating effects of sepsis, and a recent study highlighted the potential benefit of vitamin C and thiamine. The 'Marik' protocol consisted of a combination of vitamin C, thiamine, and hydrocortisone, and it was given to 47 patients with sepsis and high procalcitonin levels. It was a single-centre, retrospective, before-after study. This study demonstrated an impressive reduction in-hospital mortality; however, it was not emulated in a further subsequent multicentre randomized control trial comparing the 'Marik' protocol and hydrocortisone only; therefore, use of hydrocortisone-ascorbic acid-thiamine for sepsis has not been widely adopted.

Vitamin C and thiamine are both water soluble and cannot be synthesized and therefore rely on external supplementation. Vitamin C is absorbed enterally by sodium-dependent transporters, whereas thiamine is absorbed in the jejunum by passive diffusion. Vitamin C is a direct free radical scavenger and reduces the production on ROS. It reduces cytokine release from activated B cells and promotes bacterial killing by neutrophils, as well as lymphocyte proliferation and interferon production. In addition vitamin C is a cofactor for the synthesis of vasopressin and catecholamines and it augments catecholamine sensitivity. Finally it promotes wound healing, protects the endothelial barrier, and maintains microcirculatory patency. Thiamine is a necessary cofactor for the Krebs cycle and is essential in neuronal signalling. It works synergistically with vitamin C and may help offload the risk of oxalate nephropathy which can be seen with prolonged high doses of vitamin C.

Spoelstra-de Man AME, Oudemans-van Straten H, Elbers P. Vitamin C and thiamine in critical illness. *BJA Education* 2019;9.290–6.

Marik PE, et al. Hydrocortisone, vitamin c and thiamine for the treatment of severe sepsis and septic shock: a retrospective before-after study. *Chest* 2016;151(6):1229–38.

Fujii T, et al. Effect of vitamin C, hydrocortisone, and thiamine vs hydrocortisone alone on time alive and free of vasopressor support among patients with septic shock: the VITAMINS randomized clinical trial. *JAMA* 20(323):423–31.

18. B

Ruminococcus are Gram-positive anaerobic cocci, part of the clostridium classification, and they are intrinsic gut pathogens. The presence of which in blood therefore suggests the potential for underlying gut pathology. Further imaging in this case was undertaken, revealing a small bowel perforation, and the patient did subsequently undergo laparotomy. Although surgery was required, it is not the immediate next-line management, as the patient requires high FiO2, renal replacement therapy, and vasopressor, and a trip to theatre is not without risks, which need to be balanced against a potential negative laparotomy finding, had imaging not been performed before. Correct source control of sepsis is vital, and addition or change of antimicrobials may be indicated. Upper GI perforations are often associated with fungal contamination, and consideration should be given to starting antifungal treatment.

Solomkin J, Mazuski J, Baron E. Guidelines for the selection of anti-infective agents for complicated intra-abdominal infections. *Clinical Infectious Diseases* 2003:37:997–1005.

19. B

Tuberculosis remains one of the leading causes of death worldwide, and tuberculous meningitis is one of the most devastating presentations, seen mostly in children and in those with HIV. The outcomes are often poor. Early diagnosis of tuberculous meningitis remains a great challenge because symptoms such as fever, headache, and vomiting are not specific. Since identification of acid-fast bacilli in the cerebrospinal fluid (CSF) and culture of Mycobacterium tuberculosis lack sensitivity, the diagnosis of tuberculous meningitis is often based on clinical suspicion combined with empirical decision-making. Early consideration, prompt antituberculosis treatment and corticosteroids are the main determinants of outcome in tuberculous meningitis. A Cochrane review concluded that steroids reduce deaths in TB meningitis by almost one quarter, and in this scenario, they are an important adjunct. The patient did have antiplatelet therapy started when repeat CT demonstrated a right middle cerebral stroke, and in fact, referral to neurosurgeons resulted in a repeat therapeutic lumbar puncture, to try and alleviate the pressure associated with the hydrocephalus.

Prasad K, Singh M, Ryan H. *Corticosteroids for managing tuberculous meningitis.* 2016. https://doi.org/10.1002/14651858.CD002244.pub4 [accessed 27 September 2020].

20. B

Baclofen in overdose results in rapid onset of delirium, respiratory depression, coma, and seizures. Baclofen is prescribed frequently for MS patients with the aim of reducing painful muscle spasms. It is a synthetic derivative of GABA and not dissimilar to the recreational drug GHB. At a therapeutic dose, it acts on spinal $GABA_b$ receptors, but in overdose, this selectivity is lost, and there is inhibition of excitatory neurotransmitter release in the CNS. Paradoxical seizures occur due to presynaptic inhibition of inhibitory neurones. In large overdose, patients can appear braindead with fixed dilated pupils, hypotonia, and areflexia, including absent brainstem reflexes. Acute ingestion of >200mg can result in significant CNS toxicity. Care is supportive.

Sedation, coma, and seizures can be seen with tricyclic overdose, but there tends to be tachycardia. Similarly benzodiazepine overdose is not associated with loss of reflexes. Quetiapine antagonizes the mesolimbic dopamine (D2), serotonin, histamine the muscarinic M1, and peripheral alpha 1 receptors. This causes an anticholinergic effect (muscarinic receptors) in overdose and drowsiness (histamine receptor blockade). The peripheral alpha blockade is of interest due to the fact that there is paradoxical hypotension if adrenaline is given to these patients.

Leung NY, Whyte IM, Isbister GK. Baclofen overdose: defining the spectrum of toxicity. *Emergency Medicine Australasia* 2006;18:77–82.

21. **A**

In the UK, rib fractures are most commonly associated with blunt trauma, which most often leads to underlying pulmonary contusion. Fractures may also be associated with damage to pleura and intercostal vessels, as well as direct lung damage, so patients can present to critical care with a variety of ventilatory problems. Flail chest is radiologically the presence of fractures in three contiguous ribs in two or more places, and it may present clinically with paradoxical chest movement in a spontaneously breathing patient. Flail chest is associated with higher severity of injury and increased mortality. Other factors associated with worsened outcomes are age >65 years, underlying respiratory or cardiovascular disease, more than three ribs fractured, and development of pneumonia. There are several scoring systems, such as chest trauma score, RibScore, and Study Evaluating the Impact of a Prognostic Model for Management of Blunt Chest Wall Trauma Patients (STUMBL). Management really centres on excellent analgesia, which should be multimodal in approach. Paracetamol, NSAIDs, and opioids should be instituted. Unless contraindicated, NSAIDs should be started, and even in the elderly hypertensive patient, a limited prescription is not unreasonable, as long as there is suitable monitoring of for example renal function and thought for gastric protection. Regional anaesthesia is extremely helpful, and options include thoracic epidural, paravertebral, and more novel techniques such as erector spinae plane blocks and serratus anterior plane blocks, the latter of which help with anterior rib fractures. The only current indication for surgical fixation with a strong evidence base and recommended by NICE is for patients with flail chest injuries requiring mechanical ventilation. If surgery is a valid option, it may be better to undertake this early. Invasive ventilation may ultimately be required for this patient; however, good analgesia, in conjunction with physiotherapy, may stave off the need for this, and in reality, a trial of noninvasive ventilation may be sufficient.

Williams A, Bigham C, Marchbank A. Anaesthetic and surgical management of rib fractures. *BJA Education* 2020;10:332–40.

22. **D**

While all of the steps listed may be necessary in due course, the most important step is reversal of the bleeding tendency with prothrombin complex concentrate. This contains factors II, IX and X at significantly higher levels than fresh frozen plasma. Fresh frozen plasma corrects coagulopathy but takes up to 30 hours and requires significant volumes to be infused, which may be detrimental in certain patients.

Hyperglycaemia is common in haemorrhagic stroke, occurring in approximately 50% of cases. It is associated with worse outcomes, though this may not be a causal relationship. Nevertheless, NICE guidance recommends glucose control with insulin.

The INTERACT2 and ATACH trials showed it was feasible and safe to control blood pressure in haemorrhagic stroke, with improvements in modified Rankin Scale at 90 days. NICE guidance recommends antihypertensive therapy to a systolic blood pressure of less than 140mmHg. The supratentorial lobar intracerebral haematomas (STICH) and STICH II trials looked at early surgical evacuation in intracerebral haemorrhage, and showed no difference in outcome at 6 months. While there may be subgroups in which early surgical intervention may be indicated, reversal of anticoagulation would remain the priority.

Oxygen therapy should of course be titrated appropriately, but this is not an immediate priority. Reversal of anticoagulation is the most important immediate step, as it is likely to reduce haematoma volume. This should be achieved with a combination of intravenous vitamin K and prothrombin complex concentrate. The latter acts most rapidly, while the role of vitamin K is to prevent re-anticoagulation in the subsequent 12–24 hours.

Anderson CS, et al. Rapid blood-pressure lowering in patients with acute intracerebral hemorrhage. *New England Journal of Medicine* 2013;368:2355–65.

Mendelow AD, et al. Early surgery versus initial conservative treatment in patients with spontaneous supratentorial lobar intracerebral haematomas (STICH II): a randomised trial. *Lancet* 2013;382:397–408.

Qureshi AI, et al. Intensive blood-pressure lowering in patients with acute cerebral hemorrhage. *New England Journal of Medicine* 2016;375:1033–43.

Steiner T, et al. Fresh frozen plasma versus prothrombin complex concentrate in patients with intracranial haemorrhage related to vitamin K antagonists (INCH): a randomised trial. *Lancet Neurology* 2016;15:566–73.

Steiner T, et al. ESO guidelines for management of spontaneous intracerebral hemorrhage. *International Journal of Stroke* 2014;9:840–55.

23. D

Ventilator-associated pneumonia (VAP) is defined as any pneumonia that occurs after 48 hours of invasive ventilation. It is a common nosocomial infection, occurring in around 15% of mechanically ventilated patients. It also carries a high mortality of between 25% and 50%.

The main clue here is the period of time that this patient has been ventilated. *Early VAP* is defined by American Thoracic Society guidance as occurring in the first 5 days of ventilation. In these cases, Gram-positive, low-resistance microbes predominate. Late VAP, presenting at later than 5 days, will more likely be caused by multidrug resistant organisms, particularly *Pseudomonas aeruginosa*.

Prevention of VAP has been the focus of a wide range of studies and care bundles. The focus should be on avoiding intubation, early extubation, regular sedation holds, avoiding paralysis, and a 45 degree bed angle.

Kalanuria AA, Ziai W, Mirski M. Ventilator-associated pneumonia in the ICU. *Critical Care* 2014;18:208.

Martin-Loeches I, Rodriguez AH, Torres A. New guidelines for hospital-acquired pneumonia/ventilator-associated pneumonia: USA vs. Europe. *Current Opinion Critical Care* 2018;24:347–52.

24. E

The history and investigations are in keeping with a diagnosis of syndrome of inappropriate antidiuretic hormone (SIADH) from lung pathology; in this case, this may be malignancy or infection. Patients will appear euvolaemic, and clinical dehydration should prompt a search for another cause. Renal, adrenal, and thyroid function should all be checked before the diagnosis can be made. Common causes for this syndrome include major surgery, CNS pathology (e.g. brain injury), malignancy (e.g. lung, pancreas, lymphoma, and prostate), pulmonary infection (e.g. pneumonia, TB, and lung abscess), and drugs (e.g. carbamazepine, SSRIs, and amitriptyline).

The treatment for SIADH is fluid restriction, aiming for a correction in sodium of up to 10mmol in 24 hours. More rapid correct will put the patient at risk of central pontine myelinolysis. In severe cases, medications to decrease ADH production can be given (e.g. demeclocycline or tolvaptan).

The severity of hyponatraemia can be classified as mild: 130–135 mmol/l, moderate: 125–129 mmol/l, or profound <125mmol/l. Severe symptoms include vomiting, cardio-respiratory arrest, seizures, and coma. Moderately severe symptoms are nausea, confusion, and headache.

In this case the patient is symptomatic and requires immediate correction with hypertonic saline as per the European Society of Endocrinology guidelines, aiming to increase the serum sodium concentration by 5mmol/l in the first instance before slowing the correction rate. This is irrespective of the cause of the hyponatraemia.

Hoorne E, Zietse R. Diagnosis and treatment of hyponatremia: compilation of the guidelines. *JASN* 2017;28:1340–9.

25. A

All the steps above can be considered in managing the ARDS patient with refractory hypoxaemia.

Increasing the FiO_2 is a reasonable strategy for transient hypoxaemia, but may increase the risk of atelectasis and is not a viable long-term ventilatory solution. Similarly a recruitment manoeuvre may show transient oxygenation improvement, but the associated increases in pulmonary vascular resistance, right heart strain, and haemodynamic instability mean that a long-term benefit is not seen. Furosemide can be used to help reduce the extravascular lung water volume, but in the presence of a normal echocardiography and no fluid overload, it is unlikely to be of benefit. Prone positioning has been shown to be of benefit in improving hypoxia and has been shown to reduce mortality in ARDS. However, this strategy should probably be considered post neuromuscular blockade.

An atracurium infusion should be the next logical step. This will help improve chest wall compliance, and reduce oxygen consumption, allowing an improvement in ventilation and oxygenation.

The ARDS Definition Task Force. Acute respiratory distress syndrome: the Berlin definition. *JAMA* 2012;12:2526–33.

Griffiths MJD, et al. Guidelines on the management of acute respiratory distress syndrome. *BMJ Open Respiratory Research* 2019;6:e000420.

26. E

Patients presenting with a myasthenic crisis are at high risk of requiring mechanical ventilation. Predicting who will need this, and when, is patient specific. Admission to critical care should be considered in any patient showing increased work of breathing, tachypnoea, and an FVC of under 30ml/kg.

Vital capacity should be monitored regularly, and invasive ventilation considered if below 20ml/kg. Negative inspiratory force of under $30cmH_2O$ is also a useful marker for patients requiring ventilatory support.

Hypoxia and hypercarbia in this case may simply be due to the underlying pathology, and are not useful markers for predicting the need for invasive ventilation. Reduced compound action potentials are seen in myasthenia but are not related to the requirement for critical care admission. The same is true of elevated acetylcholine receptor antibodies.

Jani-Acsadi A, Lisak RP. Myasthenic crisis: guidelines for prevention and treatment. *Journal of Neurological Science* 2007;261:127–33.

27. B

The history and examination in this case are suggestive of necrotizing, cavitating pneumonia. The associated cellulitis, as well as the history of intravenous drug use, suggests a possible *Staphylococcus aureus* infection, and the reduced white cell count should raise suspicion of a Panton-Valentine leukocidin (PVL) producing strain.

The Health Protection Agency has produced guidance on the management of PVL producing *Staph. aureus*. They advise to suspect PVL producing infection in patients with pneumonia and associated skin and soft tissue infections. The recommended antibiotic choices include linezolid and clindamycin, which is used particularly for its direct antitoxin activity.

In severe disease, IVIG and rifampicin are also recommended.

Co-amoxiclav will be of limited benefit in this case.

Health Protection Agency. *Guidance on the diagnosis and management of PVL-associated Staphylococcus aureus infections (PVL-SA) in England,* 2nd edition. 2008.

Shallcross LJ, Fragaszy E, Johnson AM, Hayward AC. The role of the Panton-Valentine leucocidin toxin in staphylococcal disease: a systematic review and meta-analysis. *Lancet Infectious Disease* 2013;13(1):43–54.

28. D

The King's College criteria remains the most commonly used method for predicting survival in acute liver failure, and, therefore, the need for transplant. In paracetamol overdose, an arterial pH of less than 7.3, 24 hours after ingestion, is an indication for transplant. If the arterial pH has normalized, but the patient has a creatinine >300mmol/L, INR >6.5 *and* hepatic encephalopathy grade 3–4 (characterized by somnolence, confusion or reduced GCS), then the patient would still need transplant according to the criteria.

The only factor listed that does not enter the King's College criteria for paracetamol overdose is an elevated bilirubin.

Bernal W, Wendon J. Acute liver failure. *New England Journal of Medicine* 2013;369(26):2525–34.

29. B

Hyponatraemia in the neurosurgical patient can present a difficult clinical dilemma. Close assessment and monitoring of the patient's volaemic status, fluid balance, and biochemistry are required to ascertain the most likely diagnosis, thereby guiding management.

The two primary differentials here are syndrome of inappropriate anti diuretic hormone (SIADH) and cerebral salt wasting syndrome (CSWS). While formal criteria to help differentiate the two are lacking, there are significant differences in presentation. Getting the diagnosis right is essential, as the treatments for each condition are diametrically opposed (fluid restriction versus fluid resuscitation).

CSWS classically presents with diuresis and natriuresis following intracranial pathology. The main factor that discriminates it from SIADH is volaemic status. Presence of haemodynamic instability, raised markers of dehydration, or measurable fluid responsiveness should all be suggestive of CSWS.

Management of CSWS initially involves fluid resuscitation with sodium containing fluids, possibly with high concentrations if the patient has clinical manifestations of hyponatraemia. Long-term sodium supplementation may be required, and fludrocortisone has been used to reduce natriuresis. Fluid restriction does not form part of the treatment of CSWS.

Bradshaw K. Disorders of sodium balance after brain injury. *Continuing Education in Anaesthesia, Critical Care & Pain* Jun 2008:8(4);129–33.

30. E

Calcium channel blocker (CCB) overdose can lead to catastrophic cardiovascular collapse, and a rapid, multifaceted approach is likely required, particularly in patients with refractory hypotension.

CCBs vary in their cardioselectivity. Diltiazem and, in particular, verapamil have potent myocardial depressant activity, and are therefore likely to cause toxicity in overdose. Dihydropyridines such as nifedipine, amlodipine, and felodipine are arterial vasodilators, but with little cardiac depressant activity. As such they are much less likely to cause problems in overdose.

Management of CCB overdose begins with supportive therapy. In severe overdose, hypotension is likely to be refractory to fluids and vasopressors. Activated charcoal may be useful, even in delayed presentation, if a modified release formulation has been ingested.

Glucagon results in an increase in calcium entry into myocytes. This mechanism is separate to adrenergic mechanisms and will therefore act alongside vasopressors to improve blood pressure.

High dose insulin euglycaemic therapy has been shown to be of benefit in animal models and a number of case studies. As well as causing insulin resistance, CCB overdose results in hypoinsulinaemia due to reduced calcium entry into pancreatic islet cells. Insulin therapy counteracts this, resulting in improved glucose uptake, and a resultant improvement in myocardial activity.

Intralipid has been used in a number of case studies with good effect, due to the high lipid solubility of CCBs.

CCBs are highly protein bound, with a large volume of distribution. As such, renal replacement therapy will be of limited benefit in this scenario.

Graudins A, Lee HM, Druda D. Calcium channel antagonist and beta-blocker overdose: antidotes and adjunct therapies. *British Journal of Clinical Pharmacology* 2016;81:453–61.

St-Onge M, et al. Treatment for calcium channel blocker poisoning: a systematic review. *Clinical Toxicology* 2014;52:926–44.

1. A 22-year-old student presents to critical care with hypotension, tachycardia, fever, and a history of sore throat. On insertion of central venous catheter, there is an extensive intraluminal thrombus of the right internal jugular vein and surrounding oedema of the vessel. Clinically the patient has evidence of cervical lymphadenopathy and a moderate effusion on lung ultrasound. What is the most likely diagnosis?

A. Bornholm disease
B. Curtis-Fitz-Hugh syndrome
C. Lemierre syndrome
D. Ludwig angina
E. Waterhouse-Friedrichsen syndrome

2. A previously fit and healthy 59-year-old patient is being managed on the unit for four quadrant peritonitis following perforation of sigmoid colon. Post laparotomy, the patient is hypotensive and tachycardic. The patient is very cool peripherally with delayed capillary refill time. Abdominal examination reveals soft, nondistended abdomen, with minimal output from a Robinson drain. A noradrenaline infusion has been started. Pertinent blood results demonstrate:

Hb	78g/dl	(135–180)
Plts	51 × 10^9/l	(150–400)
PT	29s	(9–14)
APTT	49s	(23.5–37.5)
Fibrinogen	1.0g/l	(1.6–5.9)

What is the most appropriate management in the context of the blood results?

A. Fluid bolus of balanced crystalloid
B. Four units of fresh frozen plasma
C. Four units of platelets
D. Two units of cryoprecipitate
E. Two units of packed red cells

MCQs and SBAs in Intensive Care Medicine. Lorna Eyre and Andrew Bodenham, Oxford University Press. © Oxford University Press 2021.
DOI: 10.1093/oso/9780198753056.003.0010

3. **Select the one statement that is not representative of influenza and its management:**
   A. Clarithromycin has direct antiviral properties
   B. Linezolid is sensible antibacterial cover for post-influenza pneumonia
   C. Naproxen may reduce viral replication
   D. Oseltamivir should be given for a minimum of 3 days
   E. Virus-associated hemophagocytic syndrome (VAHS) occurs with certain strains of influenza

4. **Regarding intravenous fluid management of a 60kg patient in the high dependency unit post emergency laparotomy for duodenal perforation, the patient currently has a systolic blood pressure of 90mmHg, capillary refill time of 2 seconds, heart rate of 90 beats per minute, and no response to passive leg raise. Select the best answer:**
   A. A 500ml bolus of NaCl 0.9% should be given
   B. A 500ml bolus of Hartmann solution should be given
   C. A 500ml bolus of Human albumin solution 5% should be given
   D. Approximately 25–30ml/kg/day of water with1mmol/kg each of potassium, sodium, and chloride should be prescribed
   E. Approximately 300g/kg/day glucose is needed to prevent starvation ketosis

5. **A 45-year-old woman presents to the Emergency Department (ED) with a history of fall and head trauma. Computed tomography (CT) of the head shows nothing abnormal; however, the woman is tremulous, agitated, and acutely confused. In addition, she is combative so cannot safely be discharged to the medical ward. Along with sweatiness and tachycardia, she is jaundiced, with cachexia and nontense ascites. She has several spider naevi and asterixis. What is the next most appropriate management?**
   A. A lumbar puncture
   B. Collateral history and Clinical Institute Withdrawal Assessment for Alcohol (CIWA-Ar) score
   C. Commence piperacillin with tazobactam and perform ascitic tap
   D. Lorazepam 1mg IV initially titrated to effect
   E. Reducing dose chlordiazepoxide

6. **You perform an ultrasound scan of the chest of a patient who is intubated and ventilated for community-acquired pneumonia. They are on co-amoxiclav and apyrexial: however, the CRP remains high after 3 days of treatment, and chest radiograph suggests a pleural effusion. On scanning the patient, you observe a significant amount of pleural fluid, and what looks like echogenic debris and loculations within. You take a pleural sample and on inspection it looks purulent. Select the next most appropriate management step?**
   A. Ascertain pH of the sample and it can be safely performed using a gas analyser
   B. Additional antibiotics for anaerobic cover are indicated
   C. Change antibiotics to piperacillin with tazobactam
   D. Insert a large bore >28 F surgical chest drain and flush every 6 hours
   E. Insert a small bore 10–14 F chest drain and flush every 6 hours

7. A 75-year-old man presents to the neurosurgical intensive care unit
    (ICU) with bilateral subdural haematomas resulting from a fall down the
    stairs. Following surgery, the patient was noted postoperatively to have
    a trend of falling serum sodium. The patient does not normally take any
    drugs, and previous biochemistry, including thyroid function tests, had
    always been within normal limits. You have been called to review and act
    upon the most recent investigations:

Serum sodium	118mmol/l
Serum osmolality	259mOsmol/kg
Urine sodium	232mmol/l
Urine osmolality	825mOsmol/kg

What is your next immediate management?

A. Examine the patient
B. Fluid replacement with 0.9% NaCl
C. Fluid replacement with 1.8%
D. Fluid restriction of I I per day
E. Fludrocortisone 0.2mg/day

8. A 52-year-old man is admitted to the ICU, with fever, hypotension, and
    increasing hypoxaemia. He has been an inpatient for several days and
    has been investigated for haematological malignancy. He started with a
    fever a couple of days ago but has continued to deteriorate despite being
    started on co-amoxiclav + clarithromycin for presumed community-
    acquired pneumonia. Blood culture has been negative, as has urinary
    dip. A high EBV viral titre is the only investigation of note. Currently
    the patient is requiring 0.4mcg/kg/min noradrenaline and needing
    noninvasive ventilation with FiO_2 0.5. Recent new blood trends include:

- Anaemia and thrombocytopaenia
- Lymphopaenia and neutropaenia
- Elevated D-dimer
- Coagulopathy and mildly deranged LFTs
- Very high ferritin
- Low fibrinogen

Select the next most appropriate management strategy:

A. Escalate antibiotics to cover hospital-acquired pathogens
B. Repeat imaging including full body CT scan to exclude PE and investigate pyrexia
C. Start anakinra
D. Start intravenous immunoglobulin
E. Start steroids

9. **A 45-year-old with a body mass index of 45kg/m² is intubated for severe respiratory failure caused by SARS-CoV-2. He is increasingly acutely hypoxic, despite optimizing the ventilator settings and utilizing neuromuscular blockade. Lung ultrasound (LUS) is undertaken. Choose the most appropriate management based on the findings:**

A. C-lines are detected and therefore diuretic should be given

B. Chest radiograph should be ordered as virus tends to affect the terminal alveoli and so LUS may not be that sensitive in picking up Covid lung changes

C. Intercostal drain should be inserted on the left, as there is lung pulse but absent lung sliding detected when scanning the left side of the anterior chest, compared to the right, where lung sliding and pulse are both present

D. Pleural abnormalities and diffuse B-lines bilaterally in the anterior regions suggest a likely response to increase positive end expiratory pressure (PEEP)

E. Subpleural thickening and consolidation on the posterolateral regions, with relative sparing of the anterior regions, suggest a likely response to PEEP

10. **A slim 65-year-old woman presents to the ED with low oxygen saturation of 89% on 15l/min nonrebreather mask and marked dyspnoea. There is no stridor. She is tachycardic and has a slightly low BP. She speaks no English but is accompanied by her daughter who tells you that her mum had radiotherapy to her neck for laryngeal tumour 15 years ago and had been well until recently with what sounds like recurrent chest infections. On examination, marked scarring and deformation is evident on the right side of the neck, with significant distortion of the airways and reduced mouth opening. The chest radiograph is in keeping with right-sided alveolar airspace shadowing. What is your next management strategy?**

A. Commence co-amoxicillin 1.2g 8 hourly and clarithromycin 500mg IV for aspiration pneumonia and start high-flow nasal oxygen therapy

B. Commence piperacillin with tazobactam 4.5g 8 hourly for aspiration pneumonia and start high-flow nasal oxygen therapy

C. Commence noninvasive ventilation to aid work of breathing

D. Prepare for intubation using the difficult airway trolley

E. Prepare for intubation using awake fibreoptic intubation

11. **A 42-year-old with inflammatory bowel disease and myriad complex gastro intestinal surgeries, comes in with low blood pressure, tachycardia, and a history of rigors and fever, which seem to be more marked when the Hickman line is accessed. The patient normally takes steroid for the inflammatory bowel disease. Last surgery was 7 weeks ago, and the patient has been having supplemental home parenteral nutrition via a Hickman line since discharge. Computer tomogram abdomen on admission does not show any new collections, and lung bases are clear; however, inflammatory markers are raised. What should be the next management step?**

    A. Commence piperacillin with tazobactam for intra-abdominal sepsis
    B. Intravascular salvage with antibiotic lock therapy is indicated
    C. Remove the Hickman line if differential time to positivity <2 hours, plus microbiology-guided antimicrobial therapy
    D. Remove the Hickman line if differential time to positivity >2 hours, plus microbiology-guided antimicrobial therapy
    E. Remove the Hickman line, as the likely source of sepsis is a catheter-related blood stream infection, and insert a mid-line for TPN

12. **A patient on the ICU needs intubating as he is becoming increasingly agitated and noncompliant with ICU care, despite multiple sedatives. He was originally admitted with gallstone pancreatitis and is now being treated for sepsis associated with an infected necrotic collection. His chest radiographs have worsened over the last few days with an ARDS-like picture, and he has been needing noninvasive ventilation with FiO_2 of 0.45. Other than BMI of 38 and a history of increased alcohol intake, his medical history is unremarkable. Following induction of anaesthesia and neuromuscular blockade with rocuronium, your colleague fails to secure tracheal intubation with the videolaryngoscope. You take over and attempt intubation with the videolaryngoscope, but you also fail, despite optimal patient positioning and removal of the cricoid. The oxygen saturations are now 82%, and the use of two-person bag mask ventilation is not achieving adequate ventilation and neither is the placement of a supraglottic device. Examination of the front of neck in the extended position reveals no easily identifiable landmarks. What do you do next?**

    A. Call for help, give suggamadex, and allow the patient to breathe and wake back up
    B. Call for help, get the ultrasound to identify the cricothyroid membrane to proceed to front of neck access, and attempt a further intubation while help arrives
    C. Call for help, make a horizonal incision where the cricothyroid membrane is likely to be, using a 'scalpel-bougie-tube' to access the cricothyroid membrane
    D. Call for help, make a vertical long incision, and then use a 'scalpel-bougie-tube' to access the cricothyroid membrane
    E. Call for help, make a vertical long incision, and then use a standard tracheostomy set to access the trachea, and insert a standard tracheostomy

13. **A 27-year-old man, of no fixed abode and known to the hospital with previous substance misuse, presents to the ED with a history of weight loss and fever over the last few weeks. On examination he is febrile, tachypnoeic, has a raised JVP, an apparent new systolic murmur from last ED admission, and marked ankle oedema. He looks unwell and is tachycardic and hypotensive 85/42mmHg. Chest radiograph reveals extensive alveolar airspace shadowing bilaterally. Initial blood tests have been sent including a set of blood cultures. What is your next most appropriate management?**

A. Arrange transthoracic echocardiogram

B. Collect further two sets of blood cultures 6 hours apart and commence flucloxacillin for presumed staphylococcal infective endocarditis

C. Collect two further sets of blood cultures 6 hours apart and hold off antibiotics until the results are known as directed antimicrobial therapy is better

D. Collect a sputum sample for presumed pulmonary TB and liaise with infectious diseases staff regarding appropriate antimicrobial therapy for TB

E. Commence co-amoxiclav and clarithromycin for community-acquired pneumonia

14. **You are called to the ED to see a 67-year-old man who is handed over as being septic, with a high lactate, and is persistently hypotensive despite fluid resuscitation. In fact, when you see the patient, he looks clammy and grey and has a BP 75/44, as well as reduced level of consciousness. An ECG reveals ST elevation in the anterior leads. Which of the following statements is not applicable in this scenario?**

A. Level of consciousness can help make the decision of whether a patient is eligible for percutaneous coronary intervention (PCI)

B. Prescribe 300mg aspirin

C. PCI is the preferred reperfusion strategy as long as it can be delivered within 120 minutes of the time when fibrinolysis could have been given

D. PCI is indicated if presentation is within 12 hours of onset of symptoms

E. Prasugrel as part of dual antiplatelet therapy with aspirin is suitable for patients having primary PCI and who are not already on an anticoagulant

15. **A 77-year-old man with a history of hypertension, angina, and smoking presents to the ED with severe anterior chest pain radiating into the neck, and this has been getting worse over the last few hours. He is noted to have a hoarse voice. Computer tomogram reveals a large thoracic aneurysm, with a tear involving the ascending aorta and affecting all portions of the thoracic aorta. Which of the following statements is not applicable?**

A. Bicuspid aortic valve is a risk factor

B. This is a Stanford type A

C. This is a deBackey type 1

D. Transoesophageal echo can identify causes of hypotension and is superior to transthoracic echo

E. Timely use of aprotonin is required to reverse bleeding after cardiopulmonary bypass

16. You are asked to review a 63-year-old patient who is day 2 post-op oesophagectomy and now has gone into fast atrial fibrillation (AF). He has had a loading dose of digoxin and a couple of subsequent doses. His digoxin level comes back at 1.2 ng/mL. The patient remains in fast AF rate 130 beats per minute, with BP 105/60mmHg. An echo demonstrates moderate to severely impaired left ventricle with ejection fraction 35%. What do you do next?

A. Further 250mcg digoxin dose

B. Further therapy with bisoprolol 2.5mg for rate control

C. Further therapy with diltiazem 15mg

D. Prescribe magnesium sulphate 200mmol over 30 minutes

E. Prescribe 300mg loading dose of amiodarone followed by 900mg over 24 hours

17. A 67-year-old woman with a history of DVT 15 years ago and a stable meningioma, presents to the ED with shortness of breath and is found to be hypoxaemic and hypotensive 98/60mmHg, following an initial fluid bolus of crystalloid. Her echo reveals a dilated right ventricle with paradoxical septal wall motion. There appears to be a mobile worm-like structure in the right atrium, and this is confirmed on CT pulmonary angiography, which also confirms the presence of pulmonary emboli in right and left main pulmonary arteries. Select the best approach to managing this patient?

A. Anticoagulated with low molecular weight heparin

B. Thrombolyse the patient with alteplase

C. Refer the patient to radiology for catheter thrombectomy

D. Refer the patient for surgical embolectomy

E. Refer for IVC filter given the history of meningioma

18. A 46-year-old man is being invasively ventilated on the ICU following admission with severe necrotizing pancreatitis. A recent CT scan revealed ongoing pancreatic inflammation and a peri-pancreatic collection.

On examination he is ventilated with 6ml/kg tidal volumes and peak airway pressures of 30cmH$_2$0. Oxygen saturations are 96% on 50% oxygen. Mean arterial blood pressure is maintained at around 75mmHg with a noradrenaline infusion. Urine outputs over the last 3 hours has been 5ml/15ml/10ml. He is on 20ml/h of nasogastric feed. His last gastric residual volume was 250ml. Intra-abdominal pressure measured indirectly via a urinary catheter is 18mmHg. What is the next most appropriate step in his management?

A. Atracurium infusion

B. Laparostomy

C. Metoclopramide

D. Phosphate enema

E. TPN feeding

19. **A 32-year-old ultramarathon runner is referred to the ICU as he has been brought in midrace complaining of severe chest pain, and he is dyspnoeic. During the race, 2 hours earlier, he stopped to vomit, having just taken a nonsteroidal anti-inflammatory pill. Currently on examination, HR is 77 beats per minute; oxygen saturation on air is 93%; respiratory rate is 22 breaths per minute; and blood pressure is 95/42mmHg following initial fluid bolus. Chest radiograph reveals consolidation at the left lower base. The ECG is unremarkable and d-dimer is raised 620ng/ml. WCC is also raised at 22. CT chest excludes PE but reveals consolidation and effusion. There is also pneumomediastinum and a small left-sided pneumothorax, suggestive of oesophageal perforation and noncontained leak. The patient needs to come to critical care because of sustained low blood pressure and pyrexia. What is the next initial management strategy?**

A. Nil by mouth, intravenous fluids, piperacillin with tazobactam, and prepare patient for primary repair despite the patient's low blood pressure

B. Nil by mouth, intravenous fluids, and urgent oesophagogastroduodenoscopy

C. Nil by mouth, left-sided chest drain, piperacillin with tazobactam and barium oesophagography

D. Nil by mouth, left-sided chest drain, and prepare patient for endoscopic stent repair

E. Nil by mouth, left-sided chest drain, tazobactam with piperacillin, and TPN

20. **A 43-year-old man is admitted to the ICU for respiratory failure. He has a background of HIV and a CD4 + count of 60 cells/ml. He is intubated on day 2 following worsening respiratory failure. Initial bronchoscopic alveolar lavage (BAL) is negative for *Pneumocystis jirovecii*. Day 8 he continues to be febrile, although all blood cultures are negative. A further BAL is performed as the patient has now developed bloody secretions, worsening widespread chest radiograph changes, and an increase in oxygenation requirement. Bronchial washings are positive for CMV. There is no evidence of bacterial or fungal infection, including both *Pneumocystis jirovecii* and herpes. All of the following are true *except*:**

A. CMV is co-isolated with *Pneumocystis jiroveci* approximately 60% of the time in BAL specimens of HIV patients

B. Ganciclovir competitively inhibits the binding of dGTP to DNA polymerase inhibiting viral DNA synthesis

C. In HIV patients, the most common extra pulmonary site for CMV infection is the adrenals, as demonstrated in autopsy studies

D. Routine treatment of CMV isolated from BAL is not recommended

E. The optimal test for detection of CMV from bronchial washings is serology

21. **A 67-year-old with a background of smoking, ischaemic heart disease, and AF, presents to the ED with a large volume haemoptysis. Of note he is on warfarin for the AF. On examination he looks unwell and is still coughing up small amounts of bright red blood, having already had two much large episodes (with approximately 500ml blood loss). His blood pressure is 98/69; heart rate of 130 AF; respiratory rate 28 breaths per minute; and saturations of 93% on oxygen 15l/min via nonrebreather mask. Chest radiograph demonstrates dense opacities in the right mid and lower zone. What is the next most appropriate management strategy?**

   A. Arrange bronchial artery angiography urgently with radiology
   B. Arrange urgent pulmonary computer tomogram (CT) angiogram
   C. Arrange reversal of warfarin with vitamin K 10mg IV and 1g tranexamic acid
   D. Immediate intubation and flexible bronchoscopy
   E. Transfer to theatres for rigid bronchoscopy and double lumen tube to prevent further contamination of the airways

22. **A 62-year-old man is referred to the ICU because of profuse upper GI bleeding. Relevant past medical history includes a left ventricular assist device (LVAD) placed 9 months ago following a myocardial infarction. His medications include aspirin, ramipril, furosemide, and warfarin. He looks unwell, pale, peripherally cool, and shut down. The nurse says she cannot record a blood pressure, and you are unable to feel a radial pulse. Similarly you cannot obtain a saturation reading, and there are no heart sounds, only a hum. From the formal bloods sent, only the clotting has come back and the INR is 3.8. What is your next management strategy in this initial time frame?**

   A. Obtain an ECG and secure femoral arterial line given the lack of radial pulses
   B. Optimize preload with resuscitation fluids and check the LVAD pump speed and flow
   C. Prepare for urgent intubation given the instability of the patient
   D. Reverse the INR to aid resuscitation of the upper GI bleed
   E. Trial of octreotide

23. **A 48-year-old man, known to drink alcohol in excess, presents to the ED with a gastrointestinal bleed. Having had a bleeding duodenal ulcer injected under general anaesthetic, it is difficult to extubate him because of high FiO_2 requirements and bilateral chest radiograph opacities. Over 72 hours he becomes increasingly peripherally oedematous and is started on furosemide 40mg IV once a day to help offset the peripheral and pulmonary oedema. His daily biochemistry shows an upward trend of sodium, and it becomes 160mmol/l despite an improvement in urea and creatinine levels. What is your management strategy?**

   A. Double the dose of the furosemide to 80mg IV once a day
   B. Start intravenous 5% dextrose infusion
   C. Stop the furosemide
   D. Stop the furosemide and start metolozone plus nasogastric water
   E. Use both furosemide and metolozone

24. **A 58-year-old woman, known to have locally advanced cervical cancer, presents to the oncology team with a new AKI. Imaging suggests ureteric involvement, and the patient undergoes bilateral ureteric stent placement. Post procedure she develops very high temperatures on the ward and is managed as a presumed urosepsis with cefuroxime as the antibiotic of choice. Despite initial fluid boluses, totalling 1.5l, she still is pyrexial and hypotensive. Examination has revealed a systolic murmur, and subsequent echo reveals calcified bicuspid aortic valve with a peak velocity of 5.8m/s and gradient of 134mmHg, with preserved left ventricular function. The patient has a BP 85/54mmHg and heart rate 130 beats per minute. ICU staff are called to assess the patient regarding optimizing her management. Prior to this, the patient had been receiving chemotherapy to manage the cancer noncuratively. Select the best option to manage the patient:**

   A. Consider comfort and end of life decisions
   B. Escalate the antibiotics to include gentamicin
   C. Give a stat dose of furosemide 40mg IV
   D. Prescribe a short-acting beta blocker to mitigate the tachycardia
   E. Transfer to the ICU for phenylephrine infusion

25. A 28-year-old garage mechanic is brought to the ED by his co-workers. He initially was acting strangely and appeared drunk, having finished a can of fizzy pop. Over the last hour, he has been vomiting, and they brought him into hospital when he subsequently had an apparent seizure. On examination he is tachypnoeic with respiratory rate 32 breaths per minute, saturation 89% on air, blood pressure 100/89mmHg, and heart rate 120 beats per minute. His GCS is eyes-2, vocalization-1, and motor-5. Arterial blood gas demonstrates pH 7.18; pCO_2 1.8kPa; pO_2 8.5kPa; HCO_3_- 11; Na 131mmol/l; K 3.5mmol/l; Cl 97mmol/l; and lactate 6.4mmol/l. Select the following investigation that is not likely to be helpful in this situation:

A. Serum calcium
B. Serum ethanol
C. Serum ethylene glycol
D. Serum beta-hydroxybutyrate
E. Urinalysis

26. A 30-year-old woman is brought in by ambulance, and ICU staff are asked to see her following a witnessed seizure. The patient is subsequently intubated and ventilated in the ED, and collateral history is taken from her parents, who report that the patient had been complaining of headaches and flu-like symptoms. In addition she had been behaving strangely, talking to herself, exhibiting memory loss, and apparently not turning up for work. There is no significant past medical history and no history of recreational drug use or psychiatric disorder. CT of the head is unremarkable, and CSF results are negative for Gram stain, normal protein, and glucose levels, but a lymphocytic pleocytosis is present. She is commenced on antimicrobials for meningitis and, or Herpes simplex (HSV) encephalitis, but subsequent microbiology results are negative. A magnetic resonance image of her brain is normal, and electroencephalogram (EEG) shows slow wave active, but no epileptic features. What is the next relevant step?

A. Computer tomogram (CT) of the chest, abdomen, and pelvis
B. Commence corticosteroid
C. Continue antimicrobials for a 14-day course
D. Send serum autoantibody screen including antibodies against voltage gated potassium channels and anti-NMDA receptors
E. Wake up and refer to psychiatry

27. **A 47-year-old man presents to the ICU with a type 1 respiratory failure. He has recently been to the United States on a business trip and was staying in a hotel. He has a 2 day history of progressive shortness of breath, wet cough, and diarrhoea. His chest radiograph shows bilateral patchy infiltrates. He is tachypnoeic at 34 breaths per minute, slightly confused, and has developed an acute kidney injury with urea 12mmol/l. He is tachycardic with blood pressure 110/4mmHg. Which statement is most accurate?**

A. Close contacts of patients with Legionnaire disease need tracing

B. Co-amoxiclav 1.2g tds IV is suitable for Legionella pneumonia

C. His CURB-65 score is 4

D. Legionella urine antibody tests should be undertaken in all patients with severe community-acquired pneumonia (CAP)

E. Levofloxacin 500mg PO twice daily is suitable

28. **You are asked to go and see a 56-year-old woman who is known to have multiple sclerosis and is bed bound and hoisted, with carers, 4 times a day. She is currently on the respiratory care unit receiving high-flow oxygen for presumed lower respiratory tract infection. Her oxygen requirements are increasing, and you have been asked to see her. Currently she is receiving co-amoxiclav and clarithromycin for CAP. Looking at her history, you note she has been in hospital multiple times for similar concerns, and her family has been refusing insertion of percutaneous endoscopic gastrostomy (PEG) previously for possible episodes of aspiration. On examination she has saturations of 92% on FiO_2 0.6, with respiratory rate of 24 breaths per minute. On auscultation, there are widespread coarse crepitationss. Not previously documented, she now has a highly active gag reflex, with spastic tongue, no fasciculations, and absent palatal movement. Select the most appropriate management plan:**

A. Change antibiotics to cover aspiration pneumonia and insert nasogastric tube

B. Do not transfer to critical care and keep the patient at a ceiling of ward-based care given the history

C. Keep nil by mouth as she clinically has signs of a bulbar palsy and liaise with her family regarding the risks of aspiration + need for long-term nutrition plan, including PEG

D. Organize a CT of the head for the new cranial nerve findings

E. Transfer to critical care for escalation of respiratory support, initially to noninvasive ventilation

29. An 87-year-old, 45kg, frail woman presents to the orthopaedic department with acute fracture femur. Initially there is a delay in surgery over a mix-up on an echo result and then the arrival of more pressing trauma cases. The patient is inadvertently fasted for 4 days, whilst waiting on the trauma list. ICU are called because the patient looks unwell, and a blood gas is taken by the junior doctor. The patient has normal U&E and FBC. She is being treated with painkillers including paracetamol and codeine.

pH	7.32	(7.35–7.45)
pCO_2	1.6	(4.6–6kPa)
pO_2	11	(10–13.3kPa)
HCO_3-	11	(22–30mmol/l)
BE	−18	(−3-3mmol/l)
Na	141	(135–145mmol/l)
K	4.1	(3.5–5.5mmol/l)
Cl	117	(95–110mmol/l)
Ca	1.16	(1.12–1.30mmol/l)
Glucose	9.5	(3.6–7.7mmol/l)
Lactate	1.9	(0.2–1.8mmol/l)

Select the following stem that is inconsistent with the results above:

A. There is a metabolic acidosis with a high anion gap
B. There is a metabolic acidosis with a normal anion gap
C. This metabolic acidosis is likely to benefit from intravenous sodium bicarbonate 8.4% infusion given the low HCO_{3-}
D. This metabolic acidosis can be attributed to paracetamol use
E. This patient should be managed with IV dextrose

30. A 63-year-old man underwent a VATS right upper lobectomy for lung cancer. Day 3 post-op, he develops a type 1 respiratory failure and fast AF, for which he is transferred to the ICU. He is loaded with digoxin 500mcg, 250mcg, and another 250mcg, and then finally onto a daily 125mcg dose. Unfortunately, he is unable to clear his secretions and so is intubated and managed as a hospital-acquired pneumonia patient. In addition, his renal biochemistry sufficiently deteriorates, and so he is started on continuous haemodialysis.

Preoperatively he functioned well with activities of daily living, although work-up echo revealed moderate left ventricular dysfunction, and his cardiopulmonary tests are marginal, but not sufficiently poor to not undertake surgical resection of the lung cancer.

Day 10 postoperatively, the situation looks to have improved, and he is extubated. His AF remains controlled, and his biochemistry is such that the renal replacement is stopped.

Day 13, the patient becomes profoundly bradycardic, with heart rate down to 25 beats per minute, and consequent hypotension 80/32mmHg. Blood tests from yesterday reveal:

Na	148	(135–145mmol/l)
K	6.8	(3.5–5.5mmol/l)
Urea	32	(2.5–7mmol/l)
Creatinine	328	(49–90µmol/l)
digoxin	2.2	(0.5–1µg/l)

Select the most appropriate stem for immediate management:

A. Give calcium for its cardioprotective effects in hyperkalaemia
B. Give Digibind (DIGIFab)
C. Give insulin and dextrose to treat the hyperkalaemia
D. Urgently restart continuous haemodialysis
E. Use external pacing to help restore the heart rate

1. C

Eponymous syndromes have somewhat fallen out of favour; however; this clinical case describes Lemierre syndrome.

Lemierre syndrome is thrombophlebitis of the internal jugular vein and bacteraemia following a recent oropharyngeal infection. It is frequently caused by the Gram-negative anaerobe *Fusobacterium necrophorum*, although up to one third of cases are polymicrobial in nature. The primary source of infection is commonly tonsillar, with local invasion of the lateral pharyngeal space and septic thrombophlebitis of the internal jugular. Subsequent complications can include migration of the thrombus inferiorly into the subclavian vein or superiorly into the venous sinuses. Metastatic infections (e.g. to lungs or joints, disseminated intravascular coagulation (DIC), meningitis, and septic shock) can all be associated. Management will include a 2–6 week course of appropriate antibiotics and consideration of anticoagulation for the venous clot.

Bornholm disease = sudden severe pain chest and abdomen on one side, caused by coxsackie B virus

Curtis-Fitz-Hugh = chlamydial perihepatitis in young women

Ludwig angina = rapidly progressive gangrenous bilateral cellulitis of the submandibular space with risk of life-threatening airway compromise

Waterhouse-Friedrichson syndrome = abrupt onset of fever, petechiae, arthralgia, weakness, and myalgias, followed by acute haemorrhagic necrosis of the adrenal glands and severe cardiovascular dysfunction. The syndrome is most often associated with meningococcal septicaemia but may complicate sepsis caused by other organisms, including certain streptococcal species.

Hope R, Longmore M, McManus S, Wood-Allum C. *Oxford handbook of clinical medicine* 4th edition. Oxford: Oxford University Press, 1997.

2. A

Transfusion management has been strongly influenced by the 1999 Transfusion Requirements In Critical Care study which randomly assigned patients to an Hb 'transfusion trigger' of 100g/l (liberal) or 70g/l (restrictive). There was a trend to lower mortality in patients randomized to a restrictive policy, with lower rates of new organ failure and ARDS. A higher transfusion trigger may be beneficial in patients with ischaemic stroke, traumatic brain injury with cerebral ischaemia, acute coronary syndrome, or in the early stages of severe sepsis, but there is no indication to transfuse here with Hb 78g/l. Moderate thrombocytopaenia ($>50 \times 10^9$/l) is common in critical care patients, often associated with sepsis or DIC. 'Prophylactic' platelet transfusion in nonbleeding patients is not indicated. Fresh frozen plasma is not indicated for prophylaxis in nonbleeding patients with abnormal clotting tests. Cryoprecipitate may be used with acute DIC with bleeding and fibrinogen

<1.5g/l. In this clinical scenario, a bolus of balance crystalloid may be given with assessment of fluid responsiveness. Blood tests should be repeated to assess the evolution of DIC.

Joint United Kingdom Blood Transfusion and Tissue Transplantation Services Professional Advisory Committee. *Transfusion in critically ill patients.* https://www.transfusionguidelines.org/transfusion-handbook/7-effective-transfusion-in-surgery-and-critical-care/7-2-transfusion-in-critically-ill-patients [accessed 14 September 2019].

Hébert PC, et al.;Transfusion Requirements in Critical Care Investigators, Canadian Critical Care Trials Group. A multicenter, randomized, controlled clinical trial of transfusion requirements in critical care. *New England Journal of Medicine* 1999;340:409–17.

3. D

Surveillance of influenza and other respiratory viruses in the UK is undertaken throughout the year and collated by the Influenza Surveillance Team at Public Health England's National Infection Service (PHE NIS). Whilst yearly death rates vary considerably, the annual average deaths from 2014–2019 was 17,000 deaths in the UK. Influenza A and B are both RNA viruses. The former has a number of H and N protein surface subtypes, and while both are highly contagious, the latter mutates more slowly and is less likely to cause major epidemics. Prevention through national vaccination programmes is well-established. Management of influenza within critical care is largely supportive, although oseltamivir is recommended for a minimum of 5-days duration. It is a neuraminidase enzyme inhibitor, which facilitates the attachment of virions to infected cell membranes, rather than their release and movement throughout the respiratory tract. As well as atypical cover, clarithromycin also has direct antiviral activity. MRSA is classically associated with post-influenza pneumonia, and for this reason, linezolid should be considered in the presence of superadded bacterial infection. Naproxen has in vitro activity which prevents replication of H1N1 and H3N2 influenza, but the use of naproxen clinically remains uncertain. *VAHS* refers to a state of immune hyperactivation whereby macrophages phagocytose blood cells, including neutrophils and erythrocytes. It is especially associated with the H1N1 and H5N1 subtypes.

Lejal N, et al. Structure-based discovery of the novel antiviral properties of naproxen against the nucleoprotein of influenza A virus. *Antimicrobial Agents and Chemotherapy* 2013;57(5):2231–42.

Beutel G, et al. Virus-associated hemophagocytic syndrome as a major contributor to death in patients with 2009 influenza A (H1N1) infection. *Critical Care* 2011;15(2):R80.

Yamaya M, et al. Clarithromycin inhibits type a seasonal influenza virus infection in human airway epithelial cells. *Journal of Pharmacology and Experimental Therapeutics* 2010;333(1):81–90.

4. D

Deciding on what and how much intravenous fluid a patient should receive is often a complex task, and it requires careful decision-making based on a patient's clinical assessment, history, and investigations. However too much fluid or too little leads to mortality and morbidity. When prescribing intravenous fluid, an individualized approach is required, taking into account resuscitation, routine maintenance, replacement, redistribution and reassessment.

Indicators for resuscitation include systolic <100mmHg, heart rate >90 bpm, capillary refill time >2 seconds, peripherally cool, respiratory rate >20 breaths per minute, and passive leg raise suggests fluid responsiveness, in context of the history. We do not have much history in the question, and there is no mention of additional loss either intra- or postoperatively. However the clinical parameters collectively suggest the patient requires maintenance fluid rather than resuscitation fluid per se. If patients need IV fluid resuscitation, use crystalloids that contain sodium in the range 130–154mmol/l, with a bolus of 500ml over less than 15 minutes. Human albumin 5% may be considered as a resuscitation fluid in severe sepsis. During fluid resuscitation, judicious fluid boluses should be given, with constant reassessment of the patient. If there is no response to fluid, stop and consider alternative therapies in conjunction with the underlying cause of hypotension.

Regarding maintenance fluid, then 25–30ml/kg/day of water and 1mmol/kg/day of potassium, sodium, and chloride are required. Approximately 50–100g/day of glucose is also needed to prevent starvation ketosis. Dextrose 5% will freely spread across all compartments and 9l of free water will approximately provide 1l intravascular expansion transiently. Sodium chloride 0.9% contains the salt equivalent of 20 bags of crisps and leads to hyperchloraemic acidosis. Throughout maintenance fluid prescriptions, allowance should be made for electrolyte losses and abnormal distribution.

National Institute for Health and Care Excellence (NICE). *Clinical guideline 174. Intravenous fluid therapy in adults in hospital.* https://www.nice.org.uk/guidance/cg174/resources/intravenous-fluid-therapy-in-adults-in-hospital-pdf-35109752233669 [accessed 14 September 2019].

5. D

The history provided is suggestive of decompensated cirrhotic liver disease, as per spider naevi, hepatic encephalopathy, and ascites. One of the commonest causes of liver decompensation is cirrhosis associated with alcohol misuse, and the remaining clinical features are in keeping with acute alcohol withdrawal. Collateral history and using a withdrawal scale is helpful, but to prevent further morbidity associated with delirium tremens, a benzodiazepine is required to manage the psychomotor agitation and prevent risk of seizure. Oral chlordiazepoxide is traditionally used as it has a long half-life with active metabolites, and less risk of abuse. However in the context of liver disease and cirrhosis, lorazepam is a preferred alternative because of the shorter half-life and less hepatic metabolism. Alcohol withdrawal is a clinical diagnosis, and consideration of the likelihood of an alternative pathology should be made; however, lumbar puncture without further history and result of blood investigations should not be an immediate strategy. Piperacillin with tazobactam would be an appropriate choice for treatment of spontaneous bacterial peritonitis, and I would advocate an ascitic tap as an early investigation to ensure this is not a contributing factor to the decompensation. It is also important to provide replenishment of B vitamins to prevent Wernicke encephalopathy.

Berry PA, Thomson SJ. The patient presenting with decompensated cirrhosis. *Acute Medicine* 2013;12:232–8.

6. E

In health, pleural fluid volume is small and forms only a very thin film between parietal and visceral pleura. The pH of pleural fluid is 7.6, and under normal circumstances, it contains similar protein levels as interstitial fluid, as well as a small number of cells (mesothelial, macrophages, and lymphocytes) and larger proteins such as lactate dehydrogenase.

Almost 60% of patients with pneumonia may develop a pleural effusion; however, this resolves in the majority with commencing appropriate antibiotics. The progression of empyema develops in stages and includes simple exudate (increased capillary permeability and proinflammatory cytokines). Left untreated, there may be bacterial invasion across the damaged endothelium leading to increases in lactic acid and fall in pH. Leucocyte death leads to rise in LDH, and increased metabolism results in a fall in pleural glucose. This fibrinopurulent stage is associated with pH <7.2, glucose <2.2mmol/l, and LDH >1000iu/l, and is known as a complicated parapneumonic effusion. The presence of pus signifies empyema. Pleural infection may develop in the absence of a pneumonia and is known as primary empyema.

After diagnostic pleural sampling, management includes prompt intercostal chest drain (ICD) for samples that are frankly purulent or turbid. Prompt ICD is also needed for nonpurulent fluid with a positive Gram stain or culture and/or the pleural fluid pH <7.2. Pleural fluid can be measured in a gas analyser; however, measuring frank pus in this way is not advisable or necessary (as ICD is already indicated). Litmus paper cannot be used to assess pleural fluid pH. A small bore ICD is adequate for the majority of pleural infections and can be flushed at regular intervals, using a three-way tap. There is no evidence for a larger ICD being superior, and flushing larger drains is technically more difficult and may introduce further infection. Antibiotics alone can be reserved for pleural fluid that does not meet the aforementioned criteria; however, a low threshold for ICD should be maintained if there is a lack of clinical improvement. Antibiotics should be guided by positive culture, and anaerobic cover should be used unless culture proven pneumococcal infection. Chosen regimes should consider community versus hospital pathogens as well as local policies and antibiotic resistance patterns.

Davies H, Davies R, Davies C. Management of pleural infection in adults: British Thoracic Society pleural disease guideline 2010. *Thorax* 2010;65(Suppl2):ii41–53.

7. **A**

Sodium disorders following brain injury are relatively common and can often be difficult to distinguish. However the correct management is necessary to prevent further morbidity from osmotic shifts and worsening cerebral oedema. Cerebral salt wasting syndrome (CSWS) and syndrome of inappropriate antidiuretic hormone (SIADH) are associated with hyponatraemia and inappropriately high urine sodium and urine osmolality. The distinguishing feature is signs of volume depletion and hypovolaemia is in keeping with CSW, while euvolaemia is in keeping with SIADH. SIADH is often self-limiting, but can be managed with fluid restriction, although this may be difficult to achieve. Other strategies include cautious hypertonic saline use, demeclocycline (inhibition of the renal response to ADH), and conivaptan (ADH-receptor antagonist).

Thorough examination of the patient including clinical parameters such as capillary refill time and JVP, along with a negative balance on ICU charts, daily weights and other blood investigations (increasing urea, increasing haematocrit) can aid the diagnosis of CSWS. Management is replacement of fluid and sodium. Initially 0.9% saline is recommended, but consideration to hypertonic solutions should be made, depending on timing and severity of hyponatraemia. In refractory cases, sodium loss may be prevented with fludrocortisone.

Bradshaw K, Smith M. Disorders of sodium balance after brain injury. *CEACCP* 2008;4:129–33.

8. **E**

This case initially sounds like sepsis, and indeed haemophagocytic lymphohistiocytosis (HLH) has many similar features. HLH is a hyperinflammatory state, characterized by impaired natural killer cytotoxic T cell functions. The excess production of cytokines, inflammatory dysregulation, and end organ damage results in high mortality and due to the considerable overlap with sepsis, is likely an under recognized phenomenon. HLH can be familial, although there is likely interplay between inherited, acquired, and environmental factors. HLH can be triggered by infections such as viruses (EBV is a recognized causative agent as is CMV and HIV), lymphoid malignancy, autoimmune disorders, and some drugs. The main clinical features include high fever, hepatosplenomegaly, two-line cytopaenia, very high ferritin (>10,000μg/l is highly suggestive), high triglycerides, liver transaminitis, and low fibrinogen. While there is no exact definition, there are a number of scoring systems available.

A pragmatic approach should consider HLH in the differential when there is unexplained fever, cytopaenia (especially thrombocytopaenia), and organ dysfunction. A serum ferritin of >500μg/l should prompt repeat measures and beyond >4000μg/l is highly suggestive of HLH. Further diagnostic work-up should continue, as well as institution of supportive organ support, treatment of underlying trigger, and attenuation of cytokine storm. Steroids form the mainstay of immunosuppression, and a 'sepsis dose' of hydrocortisone may need to be converted to a pulsed methylprednisolone course. Lymphomas can be steroid responsive, and therefore attempt to identify these as triggers where possible with the relevant diagnostic pathways. Other potential managements include anakinra (recombinant IL-1 receptor antagonist), intravenous immunoglobulin, and etoposide. Where possible the underlying trigger needs also to be managed (e.g. HAART for HIV associated with HLH).

Bauchmuller K, Manson J, Tattersall R. Haemophagocytic lymphohistiocytosis in adult critical care. *JICS* 2020;21:256–68.

9. D

SARS-CoV-2 virus caused a worldwide pandemic in 2020, resulting in significant mortality and morbidity, and anyone who has worked on an ICU in the UK will undoubtedly have been involved in the care of a patient with significant acute respiratory failure secondary to Covid. Covid, however, marked the evolution of research, technology, and investigation as well as debate. Given the risk of infectivity and often the severity of hypoxaemia, chest CTs failed to be the default investigation of choice, and lung ultrasound established itself as a diagnostic modality. Covid virus particles lodge in the terminal alveoli close to the pleura, and LUS relies on artefacts generated by density changes at air and water or air and tissue interfaces. Such changes result in LUS findings, which include B-lines (originating from pleura and caused by alveolar oedema), subpleural thickening, and consolidation, and C-lines (originate below the pleura from consolidations or defects on the pleural surface and are artefacts caused by viral-induced irregularities of the pleural surface and not caused by alveolar oedema). Pleural effusion, lung consolidation, air bronchograms, and hepatization of the lung may also be visible in advanced disease. Other pathologies can be picked up e.g. pulmonary embolism (echo). Pneumothorax and endobronchial intubation both abolish lung sliding but lung pulse remains with endobronchial intubation. Abnormal lung findings associated with Covid tend to predominate in the posterolateral aspect of the chest. A relatively spared anterior lung field with predominance of postero-lateral atelectasis and consolidation may suggest benefit in prone ventilation. Where there are diffuse anterior bilateral changes with multiple B-lines and pleural abnormalities, the patient may be more likely to respond to increased PEEP. Although there are no hard and fast rules, LUS continues to play a role in this highly variable disease process.

Aziz R, Kaminstein D. Use of lung ultrasound for Covid-19 in the intensive care unit. *BJA Education* 2020;20:400–3.

10. B

There are two issues to address here: one being the acute cause of the dyspnoea and high on the differential would be aspiration pneumonia in a patient with altered airway anatomy and recent increasing frequency of lower respiratory tract infections. The second issue is how best to improve oxygenation in someone anticipated to have a difficult airway. Most cases of pneumonia arise from the aspiration of microorganisms from the oral and nasopharyngeal cavities. A *true aspiration pneumonia* refers to an infection caused by less virulent organisms, such as anaerobes, which are common constituents of normal flora in patients who have compromised defences (e.g. weak cough) or in whom sufficient inoculum stimulates an inflammatory process. In more severe cases, it is prudent to cover for *Staphylococcus aureus*, coliforms, and anaerobes as precaution.

As for respiratory support, I would start with high-flow nasal oxygen (HFNO). It would have the advantage of higher inspired oxygen, humidity, an element of PEEP, and improved patient comfort. Like noninvasive ventilation (NIV), though, caution should be taken with what is potentially an element of airway obstruction and aspiration, and whilst a pragmatic approach may utilize a trial of either HFNO or NIV therapy, there should be readily available equipment and a plan to intubate in this potentially challenging scenario.

Baudoin S, Blumenthal S, Cooper B. Non-invasive ventilation in acute respiratory failure. *Thorax* 2002;57:192–211.

Lorber B, Swenson RM. Bacteriology of aspiration pneumonia: a prospective study of community- and hospital-acquired cases. *Annals of Internal Medicine* 1974;81(3):329.

11. D

Some intravascular devices can be used 'long-term', and the major associated complication is infection, which may be intraluminal blood stream, exit site, or tunnel in origin. Colonization of microorganisms may occur on the external surface (during line insertion or colonization at the exit site) or may be intraluminal, with access of pathogens via a contaminated hub or infusate or as a result of a distant bacteraemia. The commonest pathogens include co Staph (e.g. *Staph epidermidis*, as well as *Staph aureus*) Candida, and some Enterococci. Clinical signs and symptoms of CRBSI can be nonspecific, although fever and rigors after line use, pain along a tunnel site, and signs of exit-site inflammation and pus may be present.

Paired cultures from a peripheral site and through the lumens of the intravascular device should be taken (same volume and same time). Differential time to positivity (DTP) can be used to identify CRBSI. If there is a greater load of pathogens within the lumen, the luminal blood sample will generate an identifiable signal more quickly compared to the peripheral sample, and if the DTP >2 hours in favour of the central sample, then the sensitivity for identifying CRBSI is 72%–94%, and specificity is 91%–95%. Removal of the intravascular device in conjunction with antimicrobials is the most reliable means of eliminating infection. The decision to remove a device depends on the clinical severity of the sepsis or organism-grown or previous infections, the likelihood of CRBSI over other sources, and the choice of alternative vascular access sites. A cannula for fluids could be used in the short term until the bacteraemia had resolved and a new device inserted distinct from the previously inflamed site. Catheter removal alone may be indicated if there is a low-grade pathogen; however, in an immunosuppressed patient, antimicrobial cover is prudent. Intravascular antibiotic line salvage may be indicated where an alternative line is likely to be difficult. However salvage may not be effective when severe sepsis is present or with metastatic infective complications (e.g. osteomyelitis), difficult to eradicate organisms, and persistent bacteraemia despite appropriate antimicrobials.

Pratt RJ, et al. The Epic Project: developing national evidence-based guidelines for preventing healthcare associated infections. Phase I: guidelines for preventing hospital-acquired infections. Department of Health (England). *Journal of Hospital Infection* 2001;47(Suppl):S3–82.

Catton J A, Dobbins BM, Kite P. In situ diagnosis of intravascular catheter-related bloodstream infection: a comparison of quantitative culture, differential time to positivity, and endoluminal brushing. *Critical Care Medicine* 2005;33:787–91.

12. D

At least one in four major airway events reported to the fourth National Audit Project undertaken by the Royal College of Anaesthetists and Difficult Airway Society occurred in the ICU or ED. Often such events resulted from a lack of capnography, displacement of airway with no rescue plan, under-skilled staff, and inadequate equipment. Obese patients were at particular risk. ICU patients will often lack physiological reserve, often requiring some element of respiratory support prior to intubation, which makes prior planning for a difficult airway absolutely essential. Unlike an elective situation, waking the ICU patient up is not often an option, and with saturations in this case low, it is imperative to recognize the 'can't intubate can't oxygenate (CICO)' scenario and prepare for emergency front of neck access (FONA). Ultrasound is increasingly being used to identify the cricothyroid membrane, but it currently does not have a defined role in the difficult airway algorithm as yet. Although where there is a readily available machine and skilled operator not leading to further delay, it could be very helpful in identification of the cricothyroid membrane in this obese patient. It is important to consider the human factors in CICO situations. There is a natural reluctance to accept the CICO scenario and slow progress in a time-critical manner to FONA may add to morbidity and mortality. Priming has been incorporated to try and prevent task fixation (e.g. getting the FONA set to the bedside after one failed intubation attempt, opening the FONA set after a failed rescue attempt, or immediately using the FONA set after declaration of CICO). Avoidance of cognitive overload and having excellent team communication are also essential in promoting best practice. Skill retention is helped with repeated training and simulation. If the cricothyroid membrane is impalpable, then a vertical skin incision followed by 'scalpel-bougie-tube' technique is recommended. Emergency tracheostomy in a CICO scenario takes longer (the tracheal interspaces are deeper, and there is more potential damage to vascular structures and the thyroid gland) and is therefore not recommended as a first-line FONA technique.

Cook TM, Woodall N, Frerk C. Major complications of airway management in the United Kingdom. Report and findings. *Royal College of Anaesthetists, London* 2011;106(5):631–31.

Frerk C, et al. Difficult Airway Society 2015 guidelines for the management of unanticipated difficult intubation in adults. *British Journal of Anaesthesia* 2015;115:827–84.

Price T, McCoy E. Emergency front of neck access in airway management. *BJA Education* 2019;19:246–53.

13. A

There are several causes of this apparent presentation in the patient, and standard CAP and pulmonary TB should be on the differential. However a high index of suspicion should be for infective endocarditis as the patient has a febrile illness, apparent new murmur, and features of heart failure. Ideally three sets of blood cultures should be taken at least 6 hours apart, or the first two sets within an hour if the patient is septic, and ideally before empirical therapy. If there is no sepsis or heart failure, then antimicrobials should be withheld pending blood culture. A microbiological diagnosis enables directed therapy and better treatment success if the pathogen is known. If antimicrobials have been given before blood cultures, then the chance of microbiological diagnosis is reduced. Empirical therapy is warranted with sepsis and heart failure, and a wide range of pathogens with variable susceptibilities cause native infective endocarditis. Intravenous vancomycin and ciprofloxacin are a good starting point, and intravenous flucloxacillin should be reserved for methicillin-sensitive staphylococci. Transthoracic echo is the initial investigation and should be done as soon as possible and certainly within 24 hours of admission. Other valuable investigation may include CT of the head (embolic cerebral abscess, stroke) and abdomen (splenic, renal abscess), and chest (pulmonary embolic abscess). Cardiac surgery may be considered for uncontrolled infection, enlarging vegetation, and worsening heart failure.

Habib G, et al. Guidelines on the prevention, diagnosis, and treatment of infective endocarditis (new version 2009): the Task Force on the Prevention, Diagnosis, and Treatment of Infective Endocarditis of the European Society of Cardiology (ESC). *European Heart Journal* 2009;30(19):2369–413.

14. A

When a patient has a STEMI, coronary reperfusion should be the primary goal, and this can be in the form of fibrinolysis or primary PCI. Reperfusion therapy should be delivered as quickly as possible. Level of consciousness during the acute myocardial event should not be used to determine whether a patient should receive primary PCI or not. Aspirin should be given as a single loading dose, and coronary angiography with follow on primary PCI, as indicated, should be the preferred route if the patient presents within 12 hours of the onset of symptoms, and primary PCI can be delivered within 120 minutes of the time when fibrinolysis could have been given. Coronary angiography with PCI should also be considered in patients who present later than 12 hours and in whom there is evidence of continuing myocardial ischaemia or evolving cardiogenic shock. In patients who are having primary PCI for STEMI, give prasugrel with aspirin as dual antiplatelet therapy (as long as the risk of bleeding is outweighed by the risk of benefit in those >75 years old and the patient is not already on an anticoagulant).

NICE. *Clinical guideline 185. Acute coronary syndromes.* https://www.nice.org.uk/guidance/ng185/resources/acute-coronary-syndromes-pdf-66142023361477 [accessed 24 November 2020].

15. E

Acute aortic syndrome encompasses a spectrum of life-threatening aortic pathologies including aortic dissection, whereby there is disruption of the intimal layer of the aorta and bleeding within the wall. Aneurysms can be true (dilatation of at least more than 50% of the original size and involving all the wall layers) or pseudoaneurysms (a rupture through the layers of the aorta held together by blood and surrounding tissues). Untreated aneurysms of >6cm have an annual risk of dissection and death, and therefore may require some intervention if there is rapid and symptomatic enlargement.

Dissection may result from atherosclerotic ulceration or disruption of the vasa vasorum causing intramural haematoma, or may be *de novo*. Risks include inherited disease such as Marfans, or acquired with aortic wall stress such as hypertension, and structural abnormalities such as bicuspid aortic valve. Patients can present with severe retrosternal chest pain, or interscapular back pain. There may be neurological deficits or other signs of end organ damage and frequently evidence of aortic regurgitation. There are two commonly used classifications: Stanford (type A involving ascending aorta and can extend distally versus type B involving aorta beyond the left subclavian) and DeBakey (type 1 whereby the entire aorta is affected, type 2 confined to the ascending aorta, type 3 whereby the descending aorta distal to the left subclavian is affected). Dissection and rupture can extend up or down, and vessel branch occlusion, aortic regurgitation, and pericardial effusion or tamponade can all occur. Transthoracic echo allows assessment of ventricular and valvular function, but a negative TTE does not exclude a dissection; therefore, transoesophageal echo is superior. A type A dissection is an indication for surgery. Surgery involving the aortic arch requires deep hypothermic arrest during cardiopulmonary bypass as there will be interruption to cerebral blood supply. Once cardiopulmonary bypass is off, reversal with protamine attenuates the effects of residual heparin.

Agawal S, Kendall J, Quarterman C. Perioperative management of thoracic and thoracoabdominal aneurysms. *BJA Education* 2019;4:119–25.

16. D

AF is common postoperatively and it occurs for myriad reasons including electrolyte disturbance and hypovolaemia. Causes are distinct from 'community' AF, although some consideration should be given towards longer term risk of stroke and bleeding if AF persists. Rate control should be the first management strategy in patients unless: the AF has a reversible cause, is the primary cause of heart failure, where AF is new, or whereby atrial flutter may be amenable to an ablation strategy. As the digoxin is within therapeutic levels, it is unlikely further digoxin will help with the fast AF, and it could potentially do more harm. A beta blocker would be a good choice and may well should have been the first-line therapy where the ejection fraction is reduced; however, bisoprolol can only be given orally, which is not feasible post oesophagectomy. Non-dihydropyridine calcium channel blockers such as diltiazem provide reasonable rate control (although should not be used where accessory pathways could be responsible for the AF), and their use is considered where heart failure is associated with preserved ejection fraction. An IV loading dose of 0.25mg/kg is the initial bolus dose. In this circumstance combination therapy with digoxin and IV betablocker such as metoprolol could be useful for rate control. Failing this, substitution and, or addition of amiodarone can be used to manage ongoing suboptimal AF rate. However before starting amiodarone, I would trial a loading dose of magnesium $MgSO_4$, as it has a synergistic effect when given with digoxin in controlling ventricular rate. In a study in which magnesium was administered before amiodarone, many critically ill patients converted with $MgSO_4$ alone, and 90% of patients had converted within 24 hours with both. Magnesium has a low side-effect profile, making it a good choice as an adjunct for cardioversion.

Hindricks G, Potpara T, Dagrres N. ESC Guidelines for the diagnosis and management of atrial fibrillation developed in collaboration with the European Association for Cardio-Thoracic Surgery (EACTS): the task force for the diagnosis and management of atrial fibrillation of the European Society of Cardiology (ESC) developed with the special contribution of the European Heart Rhythm Association (EHRA) of the ESC. *European Heart Journal* Feb 2020;42(5):373–498.

Ho KM, Sheridan DJ, Paterson T. Use of intravenous magnesium to treat acute onset atrial fibrillation: A meta-analysis. *Heart* 2007;93:1433–40.

Sleeswijk ME, et al. Efficacy of magnesium-amiodarone step-up scheme in critically ill patients with new-onset atrial fibrillation: a prospective observational study. *Journal of Intensive Care Medicine* 2008;23:61–6.

17. B

The diagnosis and management of PE can often be straightforward. However, now and again, cases are not as simple as the guidelines suggest. This patient technically has a submassive PE (*massive PE* is defined as haemodynamic compromise of systolic BP <90mmHg for more than 15 minutes, and, or cardiogenic shock and, or circulatory collapse). Submassive PE alone warrants anticoagulation with low molecular heparin; however, the presence of right atrial thrombus is concerning. Right atrial thrombus occurs in 4%–8% of PE and can be type A (long, thin mobile thrombus associated with high mortality), Type B (immobile, nonspecific thrombi which can occur in the absence of PE), or Type C (intermediate in character, being mobile but not worm-like). These have the potential to obstruct the right atrial or ventricular outflow tract. The optimal management remains unclear. Type B is more indolent and may be managed with anticoagulation alone. Type A with the higher associated mortality may benefit from thrombolysis. Surgical embolectomy is recommended for large type C thrombi, which have the risk of dislodging and causing outflow obstruction. Similarly surgical embolectomy has a role for thrombi which may straddle a persistent foramen ovale. As for the meningioma, as this is a stable space occupying lesion, it should not be considered a contraindication to thrombolysis.

Condliffe R, et al. Management dilemmas in acute pulmonary embolism. *Thorax* 2014;69:174–80.

18. C

This patent has abdominal compartment syndrome (ACS), and management should be undertaken in order to reduce his intra-abdominal pressure. This should ideally be done using a stepwise approach as recommended by the World Society of Abdominal Compartment Syndrome. Adding prokinetics is part of the first step in management, whereas the other options listed are all additional measures.

Normal intra-abdominal pressures are between 5–8mmHg. *Intra-abdominal hypertension* (IAH) is defined as a pressure greater than 12mmHg, and ACS is diagnosed when the pressure is greater than 20mmHg with evidence of resulting end organ dysfunction.

Surgical decompression of the abdomen should be considered only when IAH or ACS is refractory to medical management and new end organ dysfunction is present due to the associated morbidity and mortality.

De Laet I, Malbrain M, De Waele J. A clinician's guide to management of intra-abdominal hypertension and abdominal compartment syndrome in critically ill patients. *Critical Care* 2020;24(1):97.

19. A

Oesophageal injury can result from spontaneous perforations (Boerhaave syndrome occurs often after vomiting), trauma, and increasingly iatrogenic injuries as a result of increasing endoscopic procedures. Although there has been an improvement in mortality and morbidity, there needs to be a high index of suspicion and timely management of sepsis, organ failure, and definitive oesophageal perforation. Crucially mortality has been seen to increase substantially if there is a delay of more than 24 hours in initiating treatment.

Confirmation of oesophageal perforation is therefore usually via history, chest radiograph, and CT and, or soluble contrast oesophagraphy. Barium will worsen mediastinal inflammation. Oesophagogastroduodenoscopy (OGD) may be required where there is negative imaging but a high index of suspicion, although there is a risk of extending any perforation. Fluid resuscitation and broad antibiotic cover (anaerobic and aerobic Gram-negative bacillus). Nil by mouth and proton pump inhibitors should be given. TPN is required. Conservative management may be appropriate for small injuries and contained leakage. Endoscopic stent placement may be suitable for patients with contained iatrogenic perforation and no evidence of sepsis. Primary repair is considered gold standard. Surgical technique may involve a hybrid of debridement, drainage, and repair. Primary repair may be difficult in Boerhaave, and so closure may have to occur over a T tube.

King WD, Dickinson MC. Oesophageal injury. *BJA Education* 2015;5:265–70.

20. E

Cytomegalovirus (CMV) pneumonia is a rare opportunistic infection in the setting of HIV, and despite improved laboratory methods for detection, it is important to maintain clinical vigilance for the potential opportunistic infections that can cause pneumonia. The diagnosis of CMV infection by serology involves the detection of CMV-specific IgM antibodies, as well as the observation of at least a fourfold increase in CMV-specific IgG titre in paired specimens obtained 2 to 4 weeks apart. Therefore the necessary time lag is a limitation to this as a diagnostic tool. Quantitative PCR is useful for monitoring disease, as high levels of viral DNA have been found to correlate with clinical symptoms in AIDS patients. CMV is commonly isolated from BAL of HIV patients, and CMV is also commonly isolated along with other pathogens such as *Pneumocystis jiroveci*. The presence of CMV in BAL alone is not an indication for treatment, and so the diagnosis of CMV pneumonia should be made with consistent clinical, radiological, microbiological, and cyto-histopathologic features. Autopsies have been performed to establish the spectrum of disease, as clinically significant CMV infection is difficult to detect. The lung was most frequently affected, followed by the adrenals, retina, and GI tract. Ganciclovir is an antiviral agent that works by competitively inhibiting the binding of dGTP to DNA polymerase, resulting in inhibition of viral DNA synthesis. It is active against CMV and is indicated for treatment of CMV retinitis and prophylaxis in transplant patients.

Wallace JM, Hannah J. Cytomegalovirus pneumonitis in patients with AIDS: findings in an autopsy series. *Chest* 1987:198–203.

Johnstone C, Hall A, Hart I. Common viral illnesses in intensive care: presentation, diagnosis, and management. *BJA Education* 2014;14:213–19.

21. D

The exact definition of haemoptysis is variable throughout the literature; however, expectorated blood loss 200–600ml in a 24 hour period is generally accepted. Massive haemoptysis can be life-threatening due to airway obstruction and respiratory arrest or profound hypovolaemia. The commonest causes of haemoptysis include TB, bronchiectasis, mycetomas, necrotizing pneumonia, and bronchogenic carcinomas. Management should focus on optimizing ventilation, protecting the airways, and ensuring haemodynamic stability. Given the described low oxygen saturation and high respiratory rate, urgent intubation is the first step. If the site of bleeding is known, place the patient in the lateral decubitus position bleeding side down. Similarly if the bleeding is suspected to be from the right, one could consider putting an uncut single lumen tube down the left to ventilate selectively the nonbleeding site to protect airways from further contamination. Bronchial blockers or double lumen tubes could also be used; however, in the ED, it is unlikely this equipment is readily to hand even if the site of bleeding is known. Resuscitation should be instituted, and this may also include reversal of warfarin and bleeding risk with either vitamin K or more rapidly acting pro thrombin complex. Tranexamic acid may also be useful. During the acute management of massive haemoptysis both a CT scan and bronchoscopy may localize the site of haemorrhage. Flexible bronchoscopy can be done at the bedside and could have the advantage of being able to instil vasoactive drug into the bleeding bronchus (epinephrine diluted at 1:20,000). Rigid bronchoscopy may allow better suctioning and visualization of proximal pathologies, but again will take time to organize so should not precede the safety of immediate intubation. CT angiogram is likely to be helpful once the patient is stabilized, and bronchial angiography may be needed as approximately 90% of all episodes of massive haemoptysis arise from the bronchial artery circulation, and it will allow embolization.

Radchenko C, Alraiyes A, Shojaee S. A systematic approach to the management of massive hemoptysis. *Journal of Thoracic Disease* 2017;9:S1069–S1086.

22. B

LVAD are increasingly becoming common as life-prolonging therapy in patients with advanced heart failure. Current devices are now used as definitive treatment in some patients given the improved durability of continuous flow pumps. LVADS function as a separate circuit pumping blood from the left ventricle to the aorta. The pump is connected via a driveline externally through the skin to a controller which houses the electronics and monitors pump function. This is often connected to two battery packs holstered on the patient's shoulders. Current generation LVADs use a propeller-type mechanism (technically called an impellar) creating constant nonpulsatile blood flow through the circuit. As such, these patients often lack palpable pulses, and heart sounds are usually absent.

However there are well-recognized complications to LVADS including gastrointestinal bleeding. This is a result of arteriovenous malformations, thought to arise as a result of a decrease in pulsatile blood flow, local hypoxia within gastrointestinal mucosa, and vessel dysplasia. Octreotide can be used for recurrent GI bleeding but probably has a limited role in the acute setting. In addition, patients are on aspirin and anticoagulated and the impellar may cause thrombocytopaenia and shearing of von Willebrand factor, all leading to bleeding diathesis.

Obtaining an ECG is important, but the radial arterial line can be obtained via ultrasound guidance. Similarly fluid resuscitation should be first-line therapy, and crystalloid, and blood as necessary to ensure adequate preload. In the absence of sufficient preload or dysrhythmias, the negative pressure generated by the LVAD that pulls blood from the LV to the aorta can cause collapse of the LV wall. This causes decreased flow through the LVAD and decreased cardiac output. The LVAD controller can often detect these events and will attempt to decrease the pump speed to account for this. An absent hum on auscultation suggests pump failure, and like patients with mechanical valves, LVADs are at risk of thrombosis. The presentation varies quite widely, from increased pump power consumption and pump overheating to pump failure, cardiogenic shock, and death. Thrombosis can also present as distal embolization causing stroke or limb or intestinal ischaemia. Regarding reversal of anticoagulation, it is a balance of risks. In short, patients with an LVAD who present with immediate life-threatening bleeding, not responding to other measures, can have their anticoagulation reversed, but LVAD thrombosis can have devastating complications, so this decision should be made in consultation with a cardiologist specializing in LVAD. In this instance, assessment of the response to resuscitation should be made before reversal.

Patel S, Vukelic S, Jorde U. Bleeding in continuous flow left ventricular assist device recipients: an acquired vasculopathy? *Journal of Thoracic Disease* 2016;8:E1321–E1327.

Vedachalam S, Haas G. Treatment of gastrointestinal bleeding in left ventricular assist devices: A comprehensive review. *World Journal of Gastroenterology* 2020;28:2550–8.

23. E

Hypernatraemia is defined as a sodium >145mmol/l and is relatively common on the ICU, despite being suggested as a hallmark of poor care. It occurs as a consequence of either net sodium gain, net free water loss, or a combination of both. Hypernatraemia rarely resolves without active management, and therefore prompt correction is necessary. Goals of fluid mobilization in critically ill patients should be focused on increasing urine output to achieve overall net negative fluid status (without haemodynamic compromise), promoting a urine composition that is similar to plasma, and avoiding the deleterious effects of diuretics such as dehydration, hypernatraemia, and alkalosis. The traditional approach to fluid removal on the ICU is with furosemide, a loop diuretic. While furosemide is familiar and largely devoid of adverse effects, it promotes diuresis and not natriuresis, and as a consequence, a greater amount of free water is lost compared to sodium, leading to dehydration. In addition, various drugs and feeds are formulated in sodium containing fluids, and hence hypernatraemia commonly ensues. A management strategy could include continuing the furosemide and replacing free water with NG water or 5% dextrose. The latter may lead to high patient glucose levels, and large quantities of enteral free water may be necessary, mitigating the overall net negative fluid balance. To enhance natriuresis, a combination of a loop diuretic, which prevents sodium absorption in the loop of Henle, and a thiazide diuretic, which promotes sodium loss in the distal nephron, can work really well. Dual diuretic therapy may result in hypokalaemia, and other strategies promoting natriuresis include loop diuretic with aminophylline, acetazolamide, and spironolactone.

Lindner G, Funk G. Hypernatraemia in critically ill patients. *Journal of Critical Care* 2013;28:216.e-11–20.

Morris C, Plumb J. Mobilising oedema in the oedematous critically ill patient with ARDS: do we seek natriuresis not diuresis? *JICS* 2011;12:92–7.

24. E

Incidence of aortic stenosis increases with increasing age secondary to calcification but also as a result of abnormal aortic valve structure (e.g. bicuspid valve). There are haemodynamic changes as the aortic valve area approached 1cm^2 (normal values are 2.6–3.5cm^2). The left ventricle hypertrophies, and there is an increasing pressure gradient across the valve. However progressive hypertrophy leads to reduced left ventricle compliance and diastolic dysfunction. There is increased reliance therefore on atrial filling during diastole. Hypovolaemia and AF are therefore poorly tolerated. Therefore adequate preload is necessary in this scenario, and furosemide is not indicated.

As a pure alpha-1 agonist, phenylephrine increases diastolic blood pressure and thus improves coronary perfusion. Phenylephrine also may result in a reflex bradycardia, which is a favourable pharmacodynamic property in this situation. Phenylephrine also can be run peripherally without the use of invasive lines. Whilst there may be a reversible element to the managing the sepsis, conversations with the patient, family, and oncology team should be considered regarding levels of critical care input and possible ceilings of care in the context of severe aortic stenosis and active cancer. Beta blockade may lead to further hypotension and coronary ischaemia. Further discussions with microbiology may help direct the most appropriate antimicrobial management in light of any blood cultures and samples sent.

Brown J, Morgan-Hughes N. Aortic stenosis and non-cardiac surgery. *CEACCP* 2005;5:1–4.

25. D

Ethylene glycol exerts a similar effect on the central nervous system as alcohol. However as it undergoes metabolism, it produces glycolic acid (severe anion gap metabolic acidosis, and nephrotoxicity) and calcium oxalate (deposits in brain, myocardium, muscles, and renal tubules leading to acute kidney injury). It is these compounds that exert the dangerous effects of ethylene glycol, a substance commonly found in garages, radiator fluid, and antifreeze. This particular patient was renown amongst his colleagues for taking their drinks, and to 'get him back as a joke', they laced his drink with antifreeze. A high anion gap acidosis, with high lactate, hypocalcaemia, and rising creatinine is highly suggestive of ethylene glycol intoxication. Ethylene glycol levels should be taken, but as it is not a routine laboratory test; suspicion and management should be started before the results are back. Ethanol levels can be helpful as overdoses can be mixed, and before the availability of fomepizole, alcohol was used as a substrate for alcohol dehydrogenase (the enzyme responsible for producing the toxic metabolites in ethylene glycol breakdown). Urinalysis is useful, as the presence of oxalate crystals confirms the diagnosis of ethylene toxicity. Calculation of osmolar gap is useful, as it is high early on with the presence of ethylene glycol. As metabolism occurs, anion gap is high due to glycolic acid and high lactate. Management is supportive and is fomepizole infusion. In the absence of fomepizole, alcohol infusion can be used. Haemodialysis may be indicated if severe acidosis or acute kidney injury. Serum beta-hydroxybutyrate is useful in alcoholic ketosis.

Mégarbane B, Borron SW, Baud FJ. Current recommendations for treatment of severe toxic alcohol poisonings. *Intensive Care Medicine* Feb 2005;31(2):189–95.

Caravati EM, et al. Ethylene glycol exposure: an evidence based consensus guideline for out-of-hospital management. *Clinical Toxicology* 2005;43:327–345.

26. A

The combination of a prodromal flu-like syndrome and subsequent psychotic stage, followed by seizures, raises the suspicion of anti-NMDA receptor encephalitis. While it is not a common occurrence on the ICU, it is important to consider it in the differential of all meningitis or encephalitis presentations, as approximately 60% of patients with anti-NMDA receptor encephalitis have an associated malignancy (teratoma being common). Definitive diagnosis is achieved with positive NR1 and NR2 antibodies in CSF combined with a characteristic clinical picture. Auto antibodies can be found in serum, but this is less sensitive than CSF samples. Other close differentials include paraneoplastic encephalitis (autoantibodies against Hu, Ma2, CV2, and amphiphysin) and voltage gated potassium channel antibody associated limbic encephalitis. Immunotherapy (steroids, IV immunoglobulin, and plasma exchange) and tumour removal are the management strategies for anti-NMDA receptor encephalitis, and up to 50% of patients will make a full recovery.

Barry H, et al. Anti-*N*-methyl-d-aspartate receptor encephalitis: review of clinical presentation, diagnosis and treatment. *BJPsych Bulletin* 2015;39(1):19–23.

Dalmau J, et al. Anti-NMDA-receptor encephalitis: case series and analysis of the effects of antibodies. *Lancet Neurology* 2008;7:1091–8.

Wandinger KP, Saschenbrecker S, Stoecker W, Dalmau J. Anti-NMDA-receptor encephalitis: a severe, multistage, treatable disorder presenting with psychosis. *Journal of Neuroimmunology* 2011;231:86–91.

27. C

The CURB 65 score is used to guide diagnostics and treatment, and 1 point is scored for:

Confusion (new Abbreviated Mental Test score 8 or less)

Urea (>7mmol/l)

Respiratory rate (≥30)

Blood pressure (systolic <90mmHg or diastolic ≤60mmHg)

Age ≥65 years

Legionnaire disease is an atypical pneumonia mostly caused by *Legionella pneumophilia*. The bacterium is naturally found in fresh water, and classically Legionnaire disease is associated with outbreaks in hotels (air conditioning units), hot tubs, and cooling towers and is spread by breathing in mist or aspirating the water directly. Therefore it typically does not spread directly from person to person. It is diagnosed by urinary antigen, which should be sent in all severe episodes of CAP. Recommended treatment is with levofloxacin, and if the CURB 65 score is high, this should be intravenously. Alternative antibiotic regimes include macrolides or ciprofloxacin with rifampicin.

British Thoracic Society Standards of Care Committee. BTS guidelines for the management of community acquired pneumonia in adults: update 2009. *Thorax* 2009;64:iii1–iii55.

28. A

Multiple sclerosis (MS) is a common immune-mediated demyelinating disease of the central nervous system. It has a variably progressive course and widespread symptoms including motor weakness, paraparesis, spasticity, heat sensitivity, ocular involvement, depression, cognitive impairment, and brainstem lesions such as pseudobulbar palsies (upper motor lesions of cranial nerves, which result in increased gag, spastic tongue and absent fasciculations and palatal movement) are found in advanced disease. I would escalate the antibiotics to include anaerobic cover. Further collateral history is required from the family and next of kin to establish quality of life, progression of disease, and their wishes, bearing in mind the refusal of previous medical advice regarding PEG, before moving to the ICU for full critical care escalation or conversely putting ceilings of care into place.

Lublin FD, Reingold SC, Cohen JA. Defining the clinical course of multiple sclerosis: the 2013 revisions. *Neurology* 2014;83:278.

Mandell LA, Niederman MS. Aspiration pneumonia. *NEJM* 2019;380:651.

29. C

Anion gap = sodium − (chloride + bicarbonate) and is typically between 4 and 12mmol/l. Therefore there is a raised anion gap (think lactate, toxins, ketones, and renal failure). Ketones were subsequently measured and were high, and the history is suggestive of starvation ketosis. This is managed with replacement of carbohydrate (IV dextrose 5%) +/− insulin as required and with the addition of thiamine and vitamin B to prevent refeeding syndrome.

The bicarbonate has decreased by more than the anion gap has increased, and therefore there is a coexistent normal anion gap metabolic acidosis (think chloride excess or GIT or renal loss of bicarbonate). This reflects the hyperchloraemic metabolic acidosis generated by giving too much normal saline (while she was fasted for her surgery for fractured femur). Potentially paracetamol can cause a high anion gap acidosis but also depletion of glutathione levels and accumulation in pyroglutamic acid. This woman is thin, and 1 g paracetamol qds could lead to toxicity. Sodium bicarbonate is useful in hyperkalaemia, sodium channel blocker overdose, urinary alkalization, and normal anion gap acidaemia due to bicarbonate loss. However it can lead to hypernatraemia, 'overshoot' alkalosis, worsened intracellular acidosis, increased phosphofructokinase activity, and increased lactate. Therefore it is generally better to treat the underlying cause of acidosis rather than just give bicarbonate.

Forsythe SM, Schmidt GA. Sodium bicarbonate for the treatment of lactic acidosis. *Chest* Jan 2000;117(1):260–7.

Yeow, C, Wilson, F, Walter, E. Perioperative diagnosis of euglycaemic ketoacidosis. *Journal of the Intensive Care Society* 2016;17:79–81.

Dempsey GA, Lyall HJ, Corke CF, Scheinkestel CD. Pyroglutamic acidemia: a cause of high anion gap metabolic acidosis. *Critical Care Medicine* 2000;28(6):1803–7.

30. C

Digoxin is a cardiac glycoside that directly inhibits the cardiac Na/K/ATPase and has indirect effects slowing AV node conduction by increasing acetylcholine. Digoxin has a narrow therapeutic window and relies primarily on renal excretion. This particular patient accumulated digoxin when the renal replacement was stopped, but renal function had not completely recovered. Acute digoxin toxicity can manifest as enhanced automaticity (atrial tachycardia with AV block or ventricular tachyarrhythmia) or bradyarrhythmia. Hyperkalaemia is an early sign of significant toxicity, and patients may also complain of gastrointestinal upset. Resuscitation should address any life-threatening dysrhythmias and address the hyperkalaemia. Administration of intravenous calcium has traditionally been considered a contraindication for the treatment of hyperkalaemia in the presence of digoxin toxicity. This is based on the 'Stone Heart' theory, whereby calcium may lead to an irreversible noncontractile state, due to impaired diastolic relaxation from calcium-troponin C binding, and calcium excess may also predispose to dysrhythmia by causing delayed after-depolarizations. This seems to be theoretical, and calcium may be necessary in extreme hyperkalaemia. Digibind/DIGIFab is the specific antidote and consists of digoxin-specific antibody Fab fragments. It is expensive and often difficult to immediately access; hence, the first-line approach should be managing the hyperkalaemia whilst waiting for the vials. Dosing can be calculated using the digoxin level and weight. Digoxin levels cannot be accurately measured for up to 3 weeks after administration of Digibind, as assays measure free and bound digoxin giving falsely high levels.

Levine M, Nikkanen H, Pallin DJ. The effects of intravenous calcium in patients with digoxin toxicity. *Journal of Emergency Medicine* 2011;40(1):41–6.

Antman EM, Wenger TL, Butler VP Jr, Haber E, Smith TW. Treatment of 150 cases of life-threatening digitalis intoxication with digoxin-specific Fab antibody fragments. Final report of a multicenter study. *Circulation* 1990;81(6):1744–52.

INDEX

Page numbers: **bold** denotes questions; *italic* denotes answers.